HEALING BODIES, SAVING SOULS

MEDICAL MISSIONS IN ASIA AND AFRICA

THE WELLCOME SERIES IN THE HISTORY OF MEDICINE

Forthcoming:

British Military and Naval Medicine, 1600-1830

Edited by Geoff Hudson

The Wellcome Series in the History of Medicine series editors are V. Nutton, M. Neve and R. Cooter.
Please send all queries regarding the series to Michael Laycock, The Wellcome Trust Centre for the History of Medicine at UCL, 210 Euston Road, London NW1 2BE, UK.

HEALING BODIES, SAVING SOULS

MEDICAL MISSIONS IN ASIA AND AFRICA

Edited by David Hardiman

Rodopi

Amsterdam – New York, NY 2006

First published in 2006
by Editions Rodopi B.V., Amsterdam – New York, NY 2006.

Design and Typesetting by Michael Laycock,
The Wellcome Trust Centre for the History of Medicine at UCL.
Printed and bound in The Netherlands by Editions Rodopi B.V.,
Amsterdam – New York, NY 2006.

Index by Indexing Specialists (UK) Ltd.

British Library Cataloguing in Publication Data
A catalogue record for this book is available from the British Library
ISBN 10: 90-420-2106-3
ISBN 13: 978-90-420-2106-8

'Healing Bodies, Saving Souls
Medical Missions in Asia and Africa –
Amsterdam – New York, NY:
Rodopi. – ill.
(Clio Medica 80 / ISSN 0045-7183;
The Wellcome Series in the History of Medicine)

Front cover:

A medical missionary attending to a sick African.
Oil painting by Harold Copping, 1930. Courtesy: Wellcome Library, London.

Printed in The Netherlands

All titles in the Clio Medica series (from 1999 onwards) are available to download from the IngentaConnect website: http://www.ingentaconnect.com

Contents

List of Illustrations

Acknowledgements

This volume has grown from a conference on 'Medical Missions in Asia and Africa' that was held at the University of Warwick in May–June 2002. As the organiser of this conference, I would like to thank the Centre for the History of Medicine and the Department of History at Warwick, the Wellcome Trust in London, and the Wellcome Unit for the History of Medicine in Oxford for help in funding. Besides the contributors to this volume, I would like to thank the following who attended and helped to make of it a most stimulating occasion (in alphabetical order): Bridie Andrews, David Arnold, Rosemary Fitzgerald, Deborah Gaitskell, Sue Gronewald, Mark Harrison, Sarah Hodges, Shruti Kapila, Maneesha Lal, Murray Last, Vicky Long, Sloane Mahone, Shula Marks, Hilary Marland, Richard Newman, Daniel O'Connor, Jo Robertson, Sheryl Root, Lyn Schumacher, Samiksha Sehrawat, Helen Tilly, Megan Vaughan, Gregory Wells, and Michael Worboys. In addition, I would like to thank Rosemary Fitzgerald, Mark Harrison, and Brian Stanley for their very helpful comments on the manuscript.

1

Introduction

David Hardiman

During the colonial era, mission doctors exercised a powerful hold over the Western imagination. They worked with sick people in remote parts of the globe, treating maladies that were seen to be as much social as physical. They laboured not only to restore health to the bodies of 'natives', but also to save their souls. Writing of southern Africa, Jean and John Comaroff argue that missionary rhetoric was one in which: 'images of healing and social amelioration infused each other, in which the blighted body served as a graphic symptom of moral disorder. Physical affliction suggested a "sin-sick soul".' Just as it had been Europe's responsibility to heal the wound caused by slavery, so it had become its duty to cure physical illness and moral sloth.[1] These heroic figures were seen to carry on their difficult and dangerous work through a moral courage that was derived from strong religious faith. They provided a combination of Christian conviction, imperial mission, and science, a compelling amalgam for an age in which each such value was held in high regard. For many Christians, the medical missionary appeared to be straddling the ever-growing chasm between religious belief and secular science. In providing what seemed to be a Christian resolution to the challenge of modernity, they appeared – for a time – to be the new Man or Woman for the Age.

In the past two decades there has been a lot of excellent research and writing on the history of biomedicine in European colonial territories during the nineteenth and twentieth centuries. The chief focus has been on the ways in which colonial states sought to promote biomedical forms of treatment. Following Foucault, this has often been analysed in terms of the exercise of a disciplinary control. This was seen most strongly in the initiatives taken to combat epidemic diseases that threatened white functionaries of the colonial state. It is clear that few colonial powers were prepared to engage in major spending on medical facilities for the masses and it is generally recognised that the main purveyors of such medicine at the local level were missionaries.

Yet, as Megan Vaughan has argued in a book that provided a groundbreaking analysis of colonial medicine in Africa, much of this literature 'is strangely silent on the activities of mission doctors and nurses.'[2]

Vaughan – who has a lot to say about medical missionaries – brings out how during colonial times the Europeans were fascinated by the image of the white doctor working in tropical climes. In the nineteenth century, this encounter was often:

> [F]ramed in a jungle-like setting, as in many pictorial depictions of David Livingstone. The white doctor stands confronting both the 'nature' and the 'culture' of the dark continent, the boundaries between which are disturbingly ill-defined. Armed only with his faith and his medicine, he is stalked both by the animals of the bush and by men in animal skins.[3]

In the early-twentieth century, the scene tended to move to the hospital ward. The outside tropical world – with all its menace – was glanced through the hospital window, while inside the skilled mission doctor fought the insidious diseases of that environment, providing a ray of hope in the surrounding darkness. The mission rhetoric stressed the drama of the situation, with images 'of death, disease, degeneration, inscribed through a set of recurring and simple dualisms – black and white, good and evil, light and dark.'[4] The mission 'jungle doctor' was depicted as fighting witchcraft, superstition, ignorance and degeneracy, with disease being both a natural and a socio–cultural force.[5] Encounters with animals always loomed large, the prototype being Livingstone's own near-fatal attack by a lion.[6] Mission doctors were also scientists, collecting specimens, observing their surroundings and exploring new territory. In this way, the light of Christian reason was seen to be gradually dispelling the surrounding darkness.

Vaughan maintains that mission doctors above all sought to bring about a mental change within their patients, creating new subjectivities. Each sick person was a potential convert, each had an individual soul to be won. 'Healing, for medical missionaries, was part of a programme of social and moral engineering through which "Africa" would be saved.'[7] Yet, even today, few in the West believe that Africa – and indeed the non-Western world in general – has been 'cured' of its 'sickness'. The image of the social and cultural malignancy of the 'Other' that was propagated and popularised by the missionaries continues to resonate in the West to this day.

Vaughan argues that there were some important qualitative differences between secular and mission medicine in the colonies. Whereas secular colonial medics tended to concentrate on society in general, with sweeping and often coercive campaigns to eliminate the causes of certain diseases,[8] mission doctors focused on healing individuals and inculcating a belief amongst their patients that ill health was caused as much as anything through their own moral failings. She has also argued in a review of the literature on the social history of medicine in Africa that mission medicine, unlike colonial state medicine, competed with indigenous healers on their own terrain. She states that the missionaries saw their activities in a holistic way, as being part of a wider process of healing the body politic by providing faith along with health. Curing the sick was connected with social reform and the saving of souls. Local people as a result saw mission doctors as being of a completely different species to official colonial doctors.[9] Vaughan accepts, however, that the two shared some characteristics. Secular colonial medicine was, she argues, influenced by Christian perceptions about healing, and both had a tendency to understand sickness in social terms. Also, colonial governments often supported and even funded medical missionaries, and individual doctors and nurses sometimes moved between the two sectors, so the distinction could at times become blurred.[10]

Vaughan delineates what she sees as a distinct medical missionary discourse on issues of maternity and child health and other women-related medical problems. For Christian missionaries, African women were often seen as the repository of all that was dark and evil about Africa, being centrally-involved – it was argued – in initiation ceremonies, fertility cults and crude and unhygienic midwifery. The missionaries sought to liberate them from their 'backwardness' in these respects. Medical missionaries made maternity and child health their particular concern, while governments neglected these areas. It was only quite late in the day – Vaughan contends – that a secularised version of this discourse began to appear in government documents.[11]

Vaughan's work – with her insightful and revealing critical analysis of mission texts – has been important in pioneering a new postcolonial approach towards the study of colonial and missionary medicine, and her work provides a point of reference for much of the scholarly discussion and debate on the topic today. She was not, however, the first scholar in recent times to cast a critical gaze over the activities of medical missionaries, for Terence Ranger had already made an important intervention in two articles on mission medicine in Tanzania and Zimbabwe. He argued that the missionaries' expectations that medical work would transform popular beliefs and facilitate the spread of alternative Christian values were not generally realised in practice, due to the enduring hold of alternative notions about disease causation and cure. In part this was because the missionaries were unable to cure many diseases found in Africa. As important was the fact that for certain categories of illness, local people demanded exorcism, witch-finding and faith healing, and the missionaries were not generally willing to give them what they wanted in these respects.[12]

Writing in 1997, Jean and John Comaroff were rather more sympathetic about mission medicine in a long chapter of their major study of religion in the making of modern South Africa. Noting the great popularity of mission doctors, they argued that such medical work brought about a level of contact between whites and blacks that was lacking in almost all other areas of life in that highly segregated society. In this sphere:

> [T]he hybridizing effects of colonial evangelism were perhaps most fully realised... healing remained, in large measure, a tactile process, one in which the physical separations of the civilizing mission were most often ruptured – and where feelings of recognition, even compassion, flowed across the cleavages of a racially divided society.[13]

In an important study of a medical mission in the Belgium Congo published in 1999, Nancy Rose Hunt has, by contrast, argued that medical missionaries were quite prepared to implement a coercive approach in their work. In the Congo, medical missionaries served as active agents of the state in the implementation of a policy of highly intrusive medical vetting of the population for cases of sleeping sickness. She provides evidence that medical missionaries were not averse to using the whip against evaders. In return, their work received state subsidies. They also accepted financial support from colonial rubber companies in return for running dispensaries on their plantations. She states:

> Missionary medicine has often been portrayed as an anomaly within colonial medicine, as a benevolent, persuasive, sentimental form, an interpretation that has served to underscore the coercive aspect of colonial medicine as practiced by company and state doctors. It has also been in the benevolent, missionary domain that medical work with women and children has been most often situated. State medicine was frequently not gender sensitive, the story goes, and African women were patients in much smaller numbers than men. The correctives of feminist scholars have tended to elaborate what began as an opposition ripe with gendered meanings (soft/hard, gentle/forced), accepting the underlying supposition that missionary healing was the soft side of colonial medicine. The dichotomy does not work here. Colonial evangelism was not soft, and 'the' colonial state was not (always) strong.[14]

To what extent this harsh side to the medical mission was a product of the particular colonial history of the Congo – a notoriously brutal one – remains, nonetheless, to be determined.

These studies were all of medical mission work in Africa. Historians largely ignored other areas of work, even though the majority of medical missionaries were found in Asia, particularly in India and China. The scholar who more than anyone has opened up this area of research for India has been Rosemary Fitzgerald. In a series of articles from 1996 that have focussed on medical work among Indian women in Delhi, she has brought out how missionaries in India neglected medical work in general until the late-nineteenth century. She shows how attitudes gradually changed and demonstrates the ways in which a more professional attitude came to prevail in mission circles. Like Ranger, she doubts whether such work brought many converts in the long run.[15]

It is clear from the writings of these pioneering historians that the mission archives contain a vast amount of material on medical work that has been greatly under-utilised by scholars. They provide a particularly important resource for a history of the colonial clinic – whether of the dispensary, the hospital, or the maternity home. Also, they contain voluminous information on the many ways in which colonised peoples reacted to and received western biomedicine. Given their under-utilisation up until now, it is apparent that a lot more can be said on the subject. Almost all of the major writings until now have been on Protestant medical missionaries from a British background, even though large numbers came from the USA. Also, although the move towards medical missions was largely initiated by American and British Protestants, European Protestants and Roman Catholics became involved in such work over time. The medical mission archives of the latter two groups have as yet been hardly explored at all.[16]

The present collection of essays provides a number of case studies of medical missions in China, India, and Africa south of the Sahara. They were presented first at a conference held in May–June 2002 at the University of Warwick on 'Medical Missions in Asia and Africa'. A wide range of historians, sociologists, and anthropologists working on medical missionaries came together to explore the topic in more detail. A number of major themes emerged, and in this introduction, I shall explore these in the light of both previous writings and the contributions to this volume. In contrast to the practice of many editors of such volumes, I do not intend to summarise the individual chapters in this introduction, but rather refer to them as and when they have a bearing on these major themes, showing how they augment or challenge existing understandings of the subject.

I shall start with an overview of the history of medical missions, which seeks to show out how this project changed profoundly over time. I shall then focus on the major themes. I shall look at the attitude of different Christian denominations towards medical mission work, then go on to examine the theory and practice of Christian medicine, saying something on the attitude of mission theologians towards supernatural cures. Many medical missionaries were women, and this feature will be studied in the next section. Another theme concerns leprosy, a disease that missionaries considered their special sphere. We shall then go on to adopt a more patient-centred approach, by examining in the next section how local people perceived disease, healing, the medical missionaries, and the ways in which such work often drew the missionaries into contentious local politics. The place of mission medicine within the overall history of medicine is the next theme, followed by that of the ways in which local converts began gradually to replace white medical workers in the mission establishments. I shall end with a few words about the ethos of service that was found in medical mission work at its best.

A history of medical missions

From an early stage, missionaries who travelled to Asia and Africa sought to heal those they intended to convert. The Jesuits at Macao, for example, had taken their medical knowledge to Beijing in the late-sixteenth century, and they did the same in Goa. It was however by no means apparent that their skills were superior to those of Chinese or Indian medical practitioners. Many Europeans acknowledged this, and sought to learn from those doctors. In India, for example, Europeans had been impressed by the practices of Ayurvedic physicians, and they propagated their knowledge in Europe.[17]

Within the evangelical movement that gave rise to the great Protestant missionary movement of the early years of the nineteenth century, very little emphasis was placed on medical work. In 1842, for example, the Anglican Church Missionary Society (CMS) informed a surgeon that they would employ him on the understanding that medicine 'was only to be an occasional occupation'.[18] The Secretary of this association told an applicant in 1861 who was considering medical training not to waste his time, as 'it very seldom answers any good purpose'.[19] In 1852, missionary societies throughout Europe employed only thirteen medical missionaries. Between 1851 and 1870, the CMS recruited seven doctors out of a total of 307 new missionaries. These ratios continued into the 1870s.[20]

There were several reasons for this. One was that at the time the Protestant missionary movement began to develop on a large scale – that is, the late-eighteenth and start of the nineteenth centuries – physicians were not much respected in evangelical circles. They depended on elite patrons – tending to pander to their whims – and were associated with the establishment as a result. In the eighteenth century, many dissenters and puritans had avoided such physicians on principle, seeing them both as dubious healers and in thrall to the rich. Following the old Calvinistic belief, they saw cleanliness as 'a prophylactic against sin and sloth, the mark of the elect,'[21] and insisted that true health rested on piety and 'plain living'.[22] In contrast to the old aristocracy – which was obsessed with heredity and 'blood' – the assertive new middling orders were concerned above all with their health and fitness, both physical and moral.[23] Following in this vein, John Wesley preached that moral salvation lay in bodily hygiene, a clean house, a temperate life and an ordered and industrious daily routine. As he once stated: 'Every one that would preserve health should be as clean and sweet as possible in their houses, clothes and furniture.'[24] Wesley believed that doctors tended to obfuscate an understanding of the true principles of health, and held a generally low opinion of them.[25] He believed that his own healing arts were generally superior, and he was in the habit of prescribing for his sick followers a range of folk remedies – such as powdered toads, cowdung plasters and live puppies on the belly – along with the power of prayer.[26] Doctors, in return, were similarly disdainful of Wesley's methods.

Evangelicals often depicted paganism as a sickness of both mind and body, requiring an all-round therapy administered by an evangelist. The 'native' of the European colonies was seen as a source of moral and physical contamination and infection. Such being the case, illness hardly required the attention of a qualified medical man; any Godly person who understood the rudimentary principles of hygiene and sanitation was in a position to bring health to the 'native' by cleansing their bodies with soap and their minds with the Gospel.

Another cause for mission antipathy at that time towards any strongly-focussed medical work was that European medicine – as then practised by physicians, surgeons and apothecaries – was not at all efficacious in the colonies. Indeed, the treatment resorted to by such practitioners was frequently more iatrogenic than curative. Purgatives and emetics were prescribed frequently and lancing was used to extract blood or drain pustules to cleanse the body of what were seen to be accumulations of noxious substances or to correct its 'nervous tone'. When treating malaria, for example, David Livingstone administered strong purgatives that were designed to cleanse the body of the 'noxious miasmas' that had been supposedly ingested.[27] European doctors also dressed wounds and carried out some basic surgery, such as amputations, excisions and teeth pulling. With uncertain hygiene, such procedures could provide an entry for dangerous infections. The secretary of the CMS had good reason to wonder in 1851 'whether a missionary does not lose rather than gain influence with the natives by the exercise of medical knowledge.'[28]

Although missionaries were frequently incapacitated by illness and often died, the missionary organisations were generally unwilling to employ doctors to look after them. In part this was to save money, in part because it was known that the medicine of the day was inadequate to the task. The chief remedy prescribed by the missionary societies was extra moral vigilance. As a London Missionary Society booklet called *The Means of Preserving Health in Hot Climates* stated in 1819:

> There are *moral* as well as *medical* means of preserving health: and the former are hardly less important than the latter...especially in climates which render the duration of health even more dependent on habits and associations, than it is in colder countries.[29]

The book gave careful instructions on how to maintain 'evenness of feeling' so as to counteract the 'nervous state of body' and 'torpid state of the bowels' caused by tropical climates. Following the humoral theory of the day, the associations advised their missionaries to locate their stations in healthy places, such as on elevated ground away from the swamps that were believed to emanate malaria – causing miasmas. Unfortunately, even these 'healthier' sites often proved malarial as well. The overriding attitude was that missionaries had to go seeking for converts, and that health considerations could only be secondary.[30] In general, the wives of missionaries, if they were with them, were expected to nurse them in illness. As result, mortality rates continued high well into the second half of the nineteenth century.[31]

It was an American missionary working in Canton in the 1830s called E.C. Bridgman who first appreciated the strategic importance of missionaries who could carry out certain treatments in which Western doctors were proving superior to the Chinese – in particular in eye surgery for cataract removal. He saw that British East India Company physicians had managed to gain a unique access to Chinese society through medical work in a situation in which most contacts between Chinese and foreigners were forbidden by the Chinese authorities. In response to Bridgman's appeal, the American Board of Commissioners for Foreign Missions – an interdenominational body formed in 1810 – sent Dr Peter Parker to start such work in 1834, and he became the first Protestant medical missionary. Parker had been trained in both theology and medicine at Yale. He opened a hospital in Canton that specialised in eye disorders, and particularly the treatment of cataracts. As Michael Lazich shows in his chapter in this volume, Parker was soon attracting large numbers of patients, and calls were sent to America for more medical missionaries.[32] This led to the formation in 1838 of the Medical Missionary Society in China. Parker visited Britain in 1841 to put the case for Christian doctors to work with the missionaries in China. He was heard with particular interest in Edinburgh by leading physicians of the city, who established the Edinburgh Medical Missionary Society, the first medical mission society in Europe.[33]

This early initiative did not however set trends. The Edinburgh Society found it extremely hard to persuade qualified doctors to serve as missionaries. In America, the members of the American Board soon began to have their doubts about medical work by its missionaries, as they felt that it led to a neglect of evangelism, and they began to pressurise the missionaries to curtail their non-religious work. Eventually, in 1847, Parker severed his connection with the Board on the issue.[34] This tension – between evangelical and medical mission work – was one that was to continue in missionary circles for many years.

One of the first and most important medical missionaries was David Livingstone (1813–73). Working at Robert Moffat's long-established mission station at Kuruman in South Africa from 1841, he soon gained a reputation for his healing abilities. Moffat reported in 1842 that Livingstone 'was quite besieged by blind & halt and lame.' Some patients were even walking over a hundred miles for treatment by him.[35] Livingstone did not, however, regard his medical practice as a priority. His very popularity as a healer made him fearful of where this work was leading him. In a letter written home at that time, he said that a sort of 'mania' had seized him when he had first studied medicine in Scotland, and feared that his medical success in Africa might engage his fascination with medicine again, so that he would be led astray from his evangelical work and become 'a useless drone of a missionary'.[36] He found day-to-day medical practice tedious, and soon doubted whether by itself it would bring conversions. After a relatively short period in Kuruman, he set out on his travels to the interior, devoting his life to exploration and the fight against the slave trade. His much-publicised work in these respects inspired the imagination of a generation of idealistic young Christians, encouraging an ever-growing number to devote their lives to missionary careers, including medical missionary work. In this, young doctors followed Livingstone's advice to take advantage of 'the opportunity which the bed of sickness presents' for evangelism, and in the process 'imitate as far as you can the conduct of the Great Physician, whose followers we profess to be.'[37]

Throughout the world, colonial rule itself was frequently responsible for creating a new need for medical work during the nineteenth century. Agriculture was increasingly commodified, local ecosystems were fractured, and rural society became more stratified, with disparities growing between rich and poor. Many colonial subjects sought work in the towns, mines, and plantations, where living conditions were extremely poor. By the end of the nineteenth century, diseases which were virtually unknown in many interior regions in the early years of that century – such as venereal disease and tuberculosis – had become major problems. All of this provided an opening for greater biomedical intervention and medical mission work.

This came at a time when Western medicine was gaining a new status and sense of moral direction. In Britain, the Medical Act of 1858 allowed for greater regulation of the profession, by creating a register of doctors that allowed incompetent practitioners to be struck off.[38] Policies of public hygiene and the implementation of preventive health measures were bringing observable benefits, and breakthroughs were being made in surgery. As the Comaroffs have noted, medicine began to replace the Church as the guardian of public and private health.[39] Missionary organisations responded to this development by trying to keep a foot in both camps – the spiritual and the medical. In the process, mission medicine developed a new arrogance – no longer was it prepared to accept the validity of 'native' treatments, or seek to learn from local healers, who were now described as 'quacks' or 'witch doctors'. The missionaries were in accord here with the climate of the age of high imperialism, with its Social Darwinism and belief in the racial and cultural superiority of the white man, all of which provided a closure against the culture and practices of those who were not white. The new mission clinic was not, however, to be the exclusive preserve of the secular medic; it was to be a hybrid in which the priest and the doctor worked side-by-side, one preaching while the other healed.

From the 1870s onwards the demand for medical missionaries became more vociferous. Increasingly, medicine was viewed as a powerful aid to conversion. It was argued that in the heathen mind, religion and healing went hand-in-hand. As John Lowe stated in 1886:

> In India, China, Africa, Madagascar and in almost every heathen land, crude systems of medicine are intimately associated with the religions of the people, and the treatment of disease, such as it is, is monopolised by the priests, or by others under their control.[40]

In the words of another missionary, writing in 1901: 'among all rude races, magic and medicine are wedded, the priest and the doctor are one.'[41] Twelve years later R. Fletcher Moorshead argued that western medical treatment undermined the superstitions on which 'false religious systems' depended:

> It follows, therefore, that no more fatal blow can be dealt at this awful evil, cursing alike body and soul, than by proving by living demonstration the fallacy, fatuity, and powerlessness of the superstitious methods of treatment employed by the medicine man. Destroy the faith of the non-Christian man in his 'doctor' and you have very frequently taken the surest and simplest course towards the destruction of his faith in the superstition of his religion.[42]

Miss M. Andrews wrote five years later that: 'Every attendance at the dispensary is a defiance of evil spirits.'[43] Heathenism, in other words, had to be attacked on the medical front as well as through belief-systems, and

Christianity had to provide 'an all-encompassing cosmology that addressed the needs of body, mind and soul.'[44]

In an important book on American women missionaries, Dana Robert has argued that the assertion of women within the missionary movement from the 1860s onwards led to a new focus on medical work amongst missionaries in general. Some influential women missionaries held that 'heathen' beliefs and culture could only be attacked effectively within the home, and that female missionaries were required to work with native women, winning their sympathy, and through them influencing their children. This strategy became known as 'Woman's Work for Woman'.[45] Medical work was a key element within this. Robert notes that in many cultures, women were expected to heal, and this allowed women mission doctors to find an opening. This was in contrast to educators, who generally encountered strong opposition when they tried to teach women. This came at a time when women were gaining new freedoms and responsibilities in American society. The Woman's Foreign Missionary Society (WFMS) of the Methodist Episcopal Church was the foremost woman's mission organisation. Founded in 1869, it was not auxiliary to any male-dominated mission board. It appointed and paid for its own missionaries, and it sent the first female physicians to India, China and Korea. It opened the first women's hospitals in India, China, and Korea also.[46] Robert maintains: 'The embracing of medical missions by American Protestant women in the late-nineteenth century was one of the most important missiological advances of "Woman's Work for Woman".'[47]

Until the 1870s, no hard and fast distinction was made between the evangelical and the medical missionary. Many medically unqualified missionaries turned their hand to medical work, believing that for Jesus and the Apostles healing and ministry had gone hand in hand. Indeed, in Britain before the Medical Act of 1858, just about anyone could call themselves a doctor if they so wished.[48] Thereafter, there was a growing regulation of the profession. This process led to the emergence of a clear demarcation between careers in medicine and the church, and a clear distinction began accordingly to be made between the evangelical and the medical missionary. Although many medically unqualified missionaries continued to provide rudimentary medical care as a part of their work, such people were no longer considered to be 'medical missionaries'. This title was now reserved in missionary parlance for those who had full medical training and qualifications. In this way, medically qualified missionaries distanced themselves from untrained missionary practitioners. They were, nonetheless, expected to have some theological training, to know their Bible and engage in evangelism to some extent.[49] This all created a demand for medically qualified missionaries.

For these ends, the Medical Missionary Association was established in London in 1878. This provided grants for potential medical missionaries to study medicine, and it opened a hostel for their residence in the city while they studied.[50] The New York Medical Missionary Society (later the International Medical Missionary Society) was founded in 1881, with a dispensary being opened in 1882. It also provided funding to students undergoing training, and the first of them graduated in 1884. Dr Martyn Scudder, who had been a medical missionary in India, founded the American Medical Missionary Society in Chicago in 1885. In Germany, The Medical Missionary Society of Stuttgart was founded in 1898 as an auxiliary of the Basel Missionary Society.[51]

Closer relationships were also being fostered between churches and the medical profession. The Christian Medical Association had been founded in 1853 to encourage an active faith amongst doctors in Britain. This and its successor-organisation from 1874, the Medical Prayer Union, worked actively with medical students, encouraging them to study the Bible and pray regularly. Up to a quarter of all students attended its meetings in some medical colleges.[52] The Student Christian Movement had a similarly strong medical following – of its members in 1893, thirty-eight percent were medical students.[53] Young Christian doctors were often moved strongly by a sense of benevolent compassion and a desire to do good in the world, and they saw their medical work as providing a means to this end. At the same time that the medical profession was expanding vigorously in size and prestige, a career in the Church was fast falling from favour.[54] Despite this, recruitment for missionary work remained buoyant in the last three decades of the nineteenth century, and this was due in no small part to the new emphasis on engaging qualified doctors. Many such doctors might not have found such fulfilling employment in Britain, especially as the medical profession was becoming overstocked at that time.

The numbers of medical missionaries grew rapidly. In 1858 there had been only 7 such missionaries in India and China, this rose to 28 in 1882, 140 in 1895, and 280 in 1905. By the 1890s there were 680 medically qualified Protestant missionaries working worldwide, of whom 338 were American, 288 British, 27 Canadian, 7 Australian, and 20 from continental Europe. By 1916 the Protestant medical mission force worldwide had grown to 1,052 doctors and 537 nurses. Of these, 420 (40%) of the doctors were serving in China and 281 (27%) in India; while 127 (24%) of missionary nurses were in China and 108 (20%) in India. By 1916, missionaries in India were running 183 hospitals and 376 dispensaries that treated over one-and-a-quarter million patients each year.[55]

Until the later years of the nineteenth century, most medical missionaries practised from their own houses or in rented buildings that had not been

Figure 1.1

'Preaching to Native Patients at the Kashmir Medical Mission.'
The Church Missionary Gleaner, December 1884, p.139.

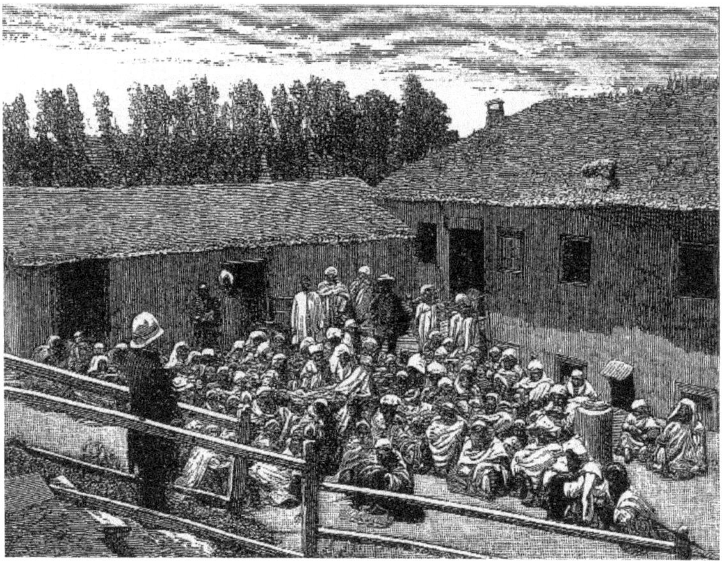

The Church Missionary Society medical mission in Kashmir had been up-and-running for just less than twenty years at the time that this print was published. It shows that the hospital buildings were still rudimentary, with patients having to wait patiently for their treatment outside in the sun, providing an opportunity for preaching.

built with this purpose in mind and which were often poorly suited to the task. Patients were preached to as they waited to be treated by the mission doctors. Indigenous evangelists often performed this task as they had a better command of the local language. They read stories from the Bible, said prayers and distributed tracts and Bible texts. In this way, what was called in 1901 a 'good dose of the Gospel' was administered along with treatment. As biomedical work grew in sophistication, the emphasis gradually shifted towards the construction of purpose-built hospitals – which required much planning, organisation and extensive fund-raising. The great advantage of hospitals – from the missionary point of view – was that patients were confined and thus amenable to preaching and other 'Christian' influences.[56] Indeed, in China many were reluctant to undergo surgery in mission hospitals because they associated the prolonged stay required with conversion.[57] It was also understood by the missionaries that as inpatients tended to be more seriously ill, they would be in a frame of mind that was more amenable to the message of the Gospel. There were frequent bedside prayers, with services in the wards on Sundays. Often, non-believers were deliberately placed next to Christians so that they could witness the Holy Communion. Scenes from the Bible decorated the walls. The hospital wards themselves were meant to demonstrate Christian order and cleanliness, with their beds in neat rows with clean white sheets. It was hoped that the patient would learn to be punctual, self-disciplined and sober – virtues that were seen as preconditions for 'Christian' rationality and civilisation.[58] Some people were even kept in hospital after being cured to win their souls.[59] Vaughan comments:

> A lengthy stay in hospital as a patient thus provided a medical and spiritual training for the job. It was a kind of rite of passage not unlike that experienced by many African healers whose status as former clients was central to their reputation.[60]

The downside to this new hospital-oriented strategy was that running such an institution placed great burdens on mission doctors. The place had to be equipped and staffed with at least two doctors – allowing the work to continue when one was indisposed or on leave – nurses and trained local assistants. The doctors had, as a rule, to turn their hands to many areas of specialisation, often combining general practice with surgery, eye, ear and dental work. In addition, they had to administer the hospital and raise funds. Often, driving themselves too hard, they broke down under the strain.[61] In other cases – unable to develop their institutions in the manner they felt necessary for efficient and effective medical work – they gave up the struggle. John Stanley, in this volume, has described how one such doctor in China abandoned the mission to which he had devoted many years of his professional life due to his frustration with the dismal conditions in which he was forced to work and after his attempts to raise funds for improvements to the hospital failed due to lack of support from his mission organisation.[62]

Until the 1920s, it was expected that medical missionaries would devote a substantial part of their time to evangelical work. The emphasis began to shift towards a more exclusive focus on medical work after the First World War, for a number of reasons. There was a growing demand by medical missionaries that they be allowed to devote their full energies to the work in which they had been trained. In the nineteenth century, the missionary was expected to be a jack-of-all-trades, with medicine as one among many tasks. Everyone, regardless of qualification, was expected to devote generous time

Figure 1.2 and 1.3

'Dr A.R. Cook writing prescriptions, Mengo Hospital.'
The Church Missionary Gleaner, July 1912, p.99.

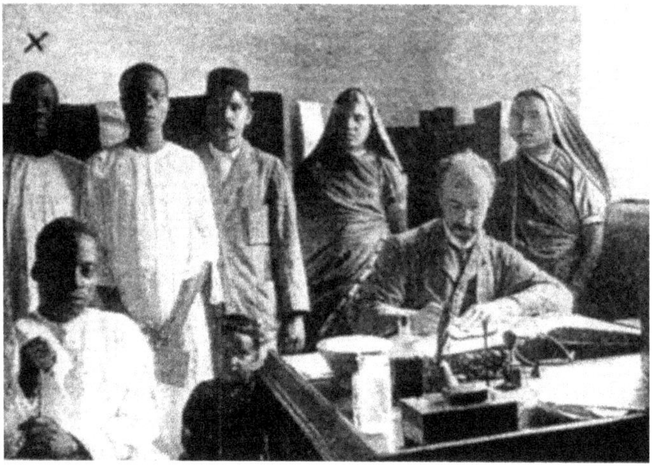

'An operation in Mengo Hospital.'
The Church Missionary Gleaner, July 1912, p.99.

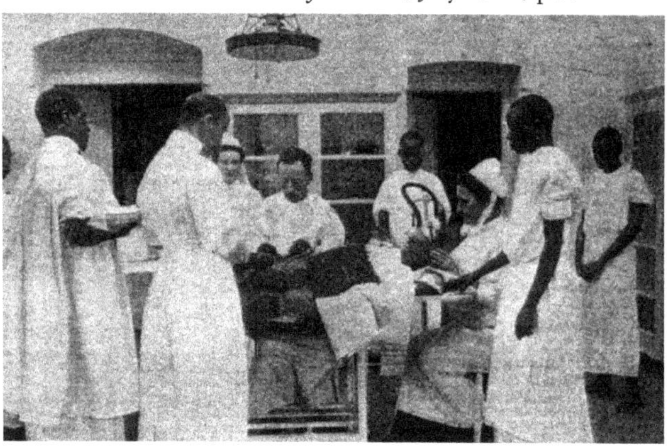

Mengo, opened by Dr Albert and Mrs Cook in Uganda in 1897, was the flagship hospital of the Church Missionary Society in East Africa. The first photo shows Albert Cook with outpatients, three of whom are from the Indian community in Uganda. The missionaries believed that the Indians, who had often broken caste rules by leaving their country to work in East Africa, were open to conversion. The second photo shows Dr E.N. Cook, Albert's brother, operating, assisted as anaesthetist by Mrs Albert Cook. 'Trained native boys' are shown assisting them.

to evangelising. By the early-twentieth century, missionaries with full medical qualifications were no longer prepared to work in such a way. The old corner cutting and making do was becoming increasingly outmoded in a world of more exacting and sophisticated medical therapy. No longer was the 'native' likely to be dazzled by second-best treatment. In addition, local Christians were increasingly carrying out evangelistic activity, while foreign missionaries focused on supervisory, organisational or professional work.[63]

This was happening at the same time that the challenge of nationalist movements in European colonial territories and a growing respect amongst many Christians for other religions saw the development of a belief that missionaries should try to work with indigenous people rather than merely convert them to Christianity. Gandhi, and his strand of Hinduism and strong spirituality, was particularly admired. There was a growing emphasis on the shared project of many religious people. The old certainties were thus being replaced with an attitude of greater circumspection and humility. It was felt increasingly that missionaries should seek to exemplify a Christian way of life in their own persons through their compassion and good work. Medical work for its own sake provided an exemplary means towards this end. As a result, missionaries in the field became more and more involved in social work, and they often saw this as their authentic life mission. In the process, preaching became secondary.[64]

The status of medical missions within the missionary movement in general was enhanced in the post-First World War period as new sources of funding for medical work opened up. The mission societies were funded from voluntary contributions and always operated on tight budgets. Often, it was hard for them to find the resources to finance the building and running of large and sophisticated modern hospitals. John Stanley has shown in his chapter in this volume how medical missions in China were transformed by the new availability of funding from a secular charity, the Rockefeller Foundation. This body had established a China Medical Board in 1914 that made large grants available for medical work by mission organisations. Henceforth, medical missionaries could carry on their work for its own sake rather than have to justify it in terms of its evangelical potential. To gain and maintain such funding, missions had to demonstrate a high standard in their medical work. This, Stanley shows, could have a knock-on effect, with missions being encouraged to improve their medical services, even in cases in which no such funding was obtained.[65]

After the Second World War, colonial medical departments became more interventionist, and more began to be spent on medicine. In the process, they began to intrude on what had been regarded before as mission territory. For the missionaries, the growing involvement of the state in 'their' sphere presented something of a crisis – what was their role to be in future?

This was happening at the same time as a gradual secularisation of medical discourse and practice amongst the mission doctors themselves. Mission hospitals were growing in size, and their treatment was becoming more impersonal and technical, while faith and belief were less emphasised. After 1945, the only area that was still, on the whole, considered the realm of the missionary was leprosy treatment, and even in that realm a purely secular cure became available in the 1950s.[66]

With the waning of European colonial power and influence in the period after the second world war, medical missions had to face an increasingly hostile political climate. Pressures grew for mission hospitals to be either closed down or taken over and run as government institutions. In China, the new communist rulers were hostile to mission work of any sort, and medical missionaries were soon forced to leave. Dr Chris Maddox, for instance, had worked in the mission hospital at Paoning in Sichuan Province since 1938, and had remained there right through the war with Japan, communicating with the outside world through Vietnam. He and his wife found the communists to be far more concerned with the welfare of the local people than the former nationalist regime, and they donned Maoist outfits and participated enthusiastically in the 'barefoot doctor' scheme. The Korean War, however, saw all westerners in China being stigmatised, and in 1952 the couple left to practice in Thailand.[67]

Many mission hospitals had to close in India too, though the process was spread over a longer period than in China. During the 1950s and 1960s, the Indian government became increasingly hostile towards foreign missionaries, whom they saw as agents of western neo-colonialism. More and more, it refused to issue visas to missionaries. Controls were placed on foreign funding, and mission-run institutions found it increasingly hard to obtain clearance for donations. The government also began to develop its own network of Primary Health Centres, which were often located near to mission hospitals and in direct competition with them. Mission hospitals had a choice of either closing down or deciding to become entirely indigenous organisations, staffed and financed by Indians.[68] In many cases, the new Indian-led churches decided that they no longer were prepared to support such a transition on grounds of cost. In Gujarat, for example, six of the eleven Protestant mission hospitals were closed for this reason in the period between 1956 and 1965.[69]

By the 1960s, it was clear that Christian missionary organisations had to review their strategy towards medical missions. The topic was debated in Tübingen in Germany at a special meeting on medical missions convened in 1964 by the World Council of Churches. Lesslie Newbigin, a former bishop of the Church of South India, argued that in many respects the work begun by medical missions had been fulfilled as the state took responsibility for such work in Asia and Africa. 'The whole business of secularisation and the Welfare State is obviously something which could never have arisen out of the ancient pagan religions of Asia. It is a by-product of Christianity.'[70] Now that missionaries had achieved this objective, he wondered whether the distinctive elements to Christian medical mission work were sufficient to justify a continuation of the work. It was perhaps best to encourage Christian doctors and nurses to act as good Christians within a secular medical system. Erling Kayser, a Norwegian who had served as a medical missionary in Indonesia, pointed out that medicine had lost some of its lustre in recent years, with scandals such as the thalidomide affair, 'which was in a sense, an epidemic of a very handicapping disease, brought about by a modern drug, the result of the physician's work.' There was a widespread feeling that something was seriously wrong with modern medicine. Much disease was hardly understood, and it was increasingly realised that many maladies were psychosomatic. This being the case: 'Can the medical profession...continue to ignore or look askance at pre-scientific forms of healing?' Citing Freud, he argued that disease was likely to develop if strong emotions were repressed or were in conflict. 'The point is that there is no dichotomy between soul and body.' The real dichotomies were those of creation and destruction, the urge to life and the urge to death, God and the devil, and crucifixion and resurrection.[71] The implication here was that Christianity might be better served if it focused on spiritual rather than biomedical healing.

Denominational differences

In what ways did the various Christian denominations differ in their approach to medical work? C. Peter Williams has argued that Scottish Presbyterians were the first group in Britain to become enthusiastic supporters of medical mission work – from the 1840s onwards – due to their firm belief that the civilisational superiority of Christianity should be revealed through good works. Scots had played a pioneering role in the development of medical science, and they were likewise in the vanguard of a new emphasis on a Christian medicine that emphasised the spiritual dimension to healing.[72] This is a suggestive idea, though Williams hardly develops it adequately in his essay. As it was, the first important initiative in medical mission work came from American missionaries of a variety of denominations working in China. Peter Parker, who was the leading figure in this, was an American Presbyterian, but E.C. Bridgman, also of great importance, was a Congregationalist.[73] Also, not all Scottish Presbyterians were enthusiastic about medical mission work. When Dr Colin Valentine applied to the United Presbyterian Church of Scotland Mission in 1860 to serve as a medical missionary, there was considerable opposition within the mission board, and his appointment went through with great difficulty.[74] Clearly, Scottish Presbyterianism cannot explain all.

What seems to have underlain this new development in Britain was a more general emergence of a new theory, practice, and class base to medicine that was associated with Edinburgh University and the dissenting medical academies that emerged after the Napoleonic Wars. Doctors trained in these new institutions were often patronised by dissenting and nonconformist businessmen. Such doctors generally held a low opinion of the established physicians who had studied at Oxford or Cambridge and who were associated with the Tory-Anglican gentry classes. The dissenting doctors established their own local and national medical journals from the 1820s onwards, all of which helped to develop medicine as a profession with national standards. Doctors of this sort were frequently evangelical Christians who were eager to improve the health and the morals of the poor, both of which had, they believed, been callously neglected by the older establishment medics. They sponsored Town Missions to investigate the conditions of the working classes and educate them in healthy living. Dispensaries were established where the poor could obtain treatment at a moderate cost. This work had been pioneered in Edinburgh, where the first charitable dispensaries had been opened for the sick poor in 1776, followed by others in later years. All of this created a climate in which medical missionary work abroad became a logical extension of such work, and in this, Edinburgh had been in the lead in Britain from the start.[75] The Americans who were also to the fore in such work seem to have been driven by broadly similar considerations, being from a class that had rejected the British establishment during their war of independence, and which also had strong dissenting, evangelical and philanthropic concerns.

The Anglican Church, by contrast, was slow to adopt medical work. In India, it was largely as a result of pressure put on the Church by the Government in 1864 that this Church agreed to open a medical mission in Kashmir in 1865.[76] The missionary appointed for this work was not however an Anglican, but Dr William Elmslie of the Free Church of Scotland.[77] Even this did not provide a breakthrough – twelve years later Bishop McDougall was complaining that Anglicans continued to lag behind in this important new area – one that other denominations were now adopting with enthusiasm.[78] It was only after 1885, under a threat that a separate medical society would be formed, that this church became centrally involved in such work.[79] Opposition continued amongst Anglican missionaries even after this date. For example, the Universities' Mission to Central Africa always retrenched on medical work first of all when there were any financial cutbacks, on the grounds that it was 'woman's work'. Its bishop stated in 1918 about this branch of their activity: 'I feel myself bound to say that till the stations are *manned*, the women's work must wait… We must have more men.'[80]

The Roman Catholic Church took even longer to become involved. Both in Europe and the United States, Catholic orders for women were involved strongly in health care in the nineteenth century, but this work had not been extended in any formal way to colonial territories at that time. As it was, the Church believed that the chastity of priests and nuns was endangered in medical work, and members of religious orders were banned by canon law from studying medicine, engaging in obstetrics, or coming into intimate contact with the human body. The nuns who provided nursing care were not therefore trained, and as nursing became more professionalised in the late-nineteenth century, this put them at a grave disadvantage against their Protestant rivals.[81] Individual male Catholic missionary priests appear to have provided basic treatment as a means of gaining converts from the late-nineteenth century onwards, as Uoldelul Chelati Dirar reveals in his chapter on Capuchin missionary work in Eritrea in this volume. Many Catholics believed that they were losing out badly to Protestant missions through a lack of systematic work in this sphere, and demands for a change in policy began to be voiced more vociferously in the early years of the twentieth century. The breakthrough came with the accession to the papacy of Pius XI in 1922, a keen promoter of missionary evangelism who approved of medical work for this purpose. A Missionary Vatican Exhibition was held in Rome in 1925 that devoted a whole section to medical issues. In 1926 Pius published an encyclical that gave a firm place to medical work in mission activities in the European colonies. This led to the formation of a number of Catholic medical missions over the next decade.[82] The Society of Catholic Medical Missionaries was established in the USA in 1925. In 1936, members of female orders were finally permitted to study medicine, though male priests were still not allowed to attend medical schools.

The Catholic Church rapidly became a leading player in this sphere. It was able to both train and deploy large cadres of priests and nuns, and it had the funds to make a major impact. In particular, it was able to staff its new hospitals and maternity homes with nuns, and rarely suffered the personnel problems that constantly hampered the Protestant denominations in their medical work. John Manton's chapter in this volume provides a case study that shows how Irish Catholic missions came to dominate medical mission work amongst leprosy sufferers in Ogoja Province of Nigeria from the 1930s onwards. He also argues that by the 1960s, the growing prevalence of contraceptive-oriented population control policies in such areas led the local Catholic missionaries to depict their medical work as a bastion against 'Protestant' forms of family planning. Catholic doctors and hospitals were needed urgently to save 'Christian Homes'.[83] As yet, there are few studies of

Figure 1.4

'Out of darkness:
Dr Iliff removes the bandages from a cataract patient, Bannu.'
CMS Outlook, October 1951.

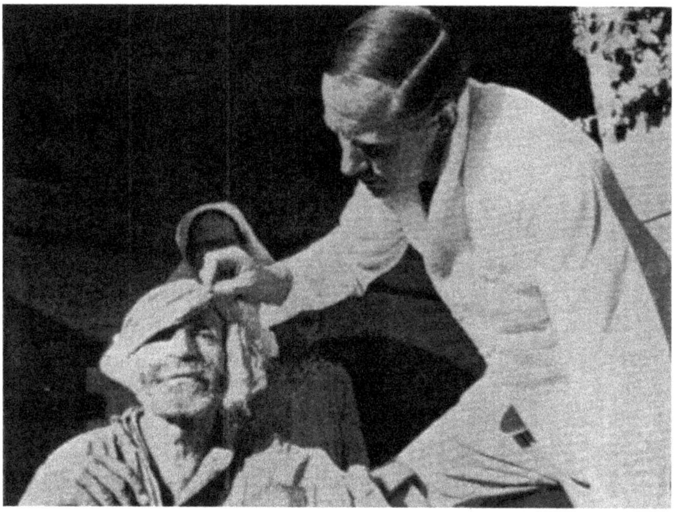

Bannu was in the North West Frontier Province, which after 1947 was in Pakistan.

Roman Catholic medical mission work, and it is an area deserving far more research.

The theory and practice of Christian medicine

The standard view of medical missionary work within missionary circles in the late-nineteenth century was that it was not done for a purely medical purpose, but used as a beneficent means to spread Christianity. Work was carried out where most converts could be won, not necessarily where the need was greatest. Treatment was seen to put people in a receptive frame of mind to the message of the Gospel.[84] The mission dispensary and hospital were designed to act like a 'magnet', drawing patients from near and far to the missionaries. The work also demonstrated that Christians practiced what they preached, in a way that emphasised the superiority of their religion.[85]

The medical missionary was seen to be walking in the path of Christ. In a prize essay written for the Edinburgh Medical Missionary Society in 1854, W. Burns Thomson emphasised that Jesus had urged his followers to 'Heal and Preach'. Healing provided an entry into the hearts and minds of 'simple people' who, like children, were often taught best by objective demonstration. In this way the rationality and science of the time could contribute towards the spread of Christianity.[86] Numerous quotations from the four Gospels could be cited to make the point that Jesus himself had sanctioned such work. It was claimed that Jesus was 'the ideal medical missionary'. 'He is the Founder and Patron of medical missions; and He has given us an example that we should follow in His steps.' It was argued that all the diseases and disabilities mentioned in the New Testament abounded in the 'heathen lands' of the day. Everywhere the crippled and diseased could be seen – the lepers, the maimed, the paralysed, the blind, those scourged by plague – providing a harrowing sight that the inhabitants of the 'civilised' nations were spared. In such an environment, the mission doctors could, through their skill, carry out what seemed to be 'marvels of healing'. They could give sight to blind, make the deaf hear, the lame and paralysed walk, and make fever flee at their approach. As the 'battle front of the Church was in the heathen lands', the best doctors and surgeons were needed for this great work, and medical colleges were needed to train Christian doctors.[87]

Medical missionaries were not, however, expected to heal in a miraculous way by casting out evil spirits or practising supernatural healing, as the Gospels had shown Jesus doing. Protestant theologians largely followed the doctrine of dispensationalism, which held that God gave a dispensation for miracles for only a limited time and purpose. Both Luther and Calvin had propounded this theory. Luther, for example, held that the day of miracles had passed, and that now that the Gospel stood revealed, all that was necessary was to preach it. As he stated: 'now that the apostles have preached the Word and have given their writings, and nothing more than what they have written remains to be revealed, no new and special revelation or miracle is necessary.'[88] Calvin stated similarly that:

> The gift of healing disappeared with the other miraculous powers which the Lord was pleased to give for a time, that it might render the new preaching of the gospel for ever wonderful. Therefore, even were we to grant that anointing was a sacrament of those powers which were then administered by the hands of the apostles, it pertains not to us, to whom no such powers have been committed.[89]

This doctrine informed the medical mission upsurge of the later nineteenth century. Sir Robert Anderson argued at that time in *The Silence of God* that the display of divine power through miracles had been appropriate for its time, but in modern times God required a higher form of belief, that of faith by those 'who have not seen and yet have believed'.[90] Modern Christians would accordingly be in error if they sought to emulate the healing practices of the Jesus of the Gospels. The medical mission theologians argued that such miraculous cures were not central to Jesus' ministry. He performed them out of a sense of compassion, not to impress or win converts.[91] In contemporary times, it was argued, miracle-workers were generally charlatans, and their supposed cures fraudulent.[92] They accepted, however, that it was wholly legitimate to pray for the recovery of a patient. As it was, in missionary reports from the field there was often considerable ambiguity over whether or not a cure came through medical intervention or prayer.

The prevailing Protestant missionary hostility towards supernatural healing was above all the product of a class history, for there had always been a tension in practice between the stern theologies of Luther, Calvin, and their successor and a popular Christianity based on a belief in supernatural intervention in everyday life. In Britain, for example, dissenting groups had emerged during the seventeenth-century revolution that believed in supernatural healing. George Fox, founder of the Quakers, is recorded as having carried out frequent cures of this kind from the late-1640s onwards.[93] The Anglican hierarchy had sought to dampen such enthusiasm after the restoration of 1660 as they feared that such practices might give rise to a dangerous populism that would not only undermine church discipline, but could cause wider social disruption if allowed to flourish.[94] Even William Booth, the founder of a denomination – the Salvation Army – that was known for its evangelical enthusiasm, and who was himself sceptical of modern medicine, refused to countenance any supernatural healing, on the grounds that it tended to be associated with 'one or another form of fanaticism'. Stuart Mews has argued that he, in common with the leaders of other churches, feared that such charismatic practices by lower-level clerics or members of the laity would undermine their ecclesiastical authority.[95]

The Roman Catholic Church was more open to the idea of supernatural intervention in everyday life, with its cults of saints, Marian healing shrines, sacraments, and healing rituals. Writing on this in the context of Sri Lanka, R.L. Stirrat has argued that the French Roman Catholic missionaries were often ambivalent towards miracle cures. On the one hand, they were prepared to allow such practices so that their shrines could attract pilgrims, and they made no attempt to prevent the sale there of pamphlets that were full of miracle stories connected with that place. Yet, aware that their Protestant competitors despised them for this, they tended to feel somewhat defensive on the matter. Their education in France had imbued them with post-Enlightenment values, so that they themselves must have been somewhat sceptical – as indeed was often the case in nineteenth-century France, where an educated clergy tolerated what they now saw as popular superstitions. On the whole, they believed in the superiority of biomedical treatment.[96] Amongst Protestants, Anglo-Catholics shared this ambivalence. They often performed the ceremony of unction – anointing with oil – for the sick, a practice that was eventually given full sanction by the Church in the 1920s as a counter to the growing popularity of charismatic Christian faith-healers who were less easily controlled than High Church clerics.[97] In the colonies, however, missionaries of this persuasion tended to be highly suspicious of these supposed 'Roman' practices. As Father Puller of the UMCA – a High Church body – stated in 1897: 'To my mind, it is most deplorable that the cultus of images and the invocations of saints should be instilled into the minds and affections of the infant church… I consider that practices of that sort are dangerous among European Christians, but they are tenfold more dangerous among newly converted African natives.'[98] The Anglo-Catholic missionaries were eager to rebut charges from other Protestants that they were encouraging Africans to develop a 'magical' view of Christianity. Converts were believers, they insisted, through freely willed choice. They tended as a result to oppose anything other than 'scientific' healing.[99]

Christian spiritual healing was, in consequence, mainly the preserve of either independent African churches or American Pentecostalist-style missions. This process began early on. In South Africa 'charismatic bricoleurs' – in the phrase of the Comaroffs – began to emerge from new Christian communities from as early as the 1830s. They were often women – in contrast to the tradition healers. 'They applied the power of Christian rites to ends shaped by vernacular ideas of healing; among them, divination, rainmaking, and the husbandry of wealth and well-being.'[100] This tendency was reinforced with the arrival of American Pentecostalist missions in South Africa in the early-twentieth century, which proved popular initially with white Afrikaaners, and then blacks. There were enthusiastic meetings, with shouting and hand clapping. People who saw the light were baptised on the spot. Preachers – both black and white – laid hands on people and healed them. The movement spread north into central Africa in the second decade of the century. Despite the involvement of whites in some areas, the colonial authorities saw this as a threat to social order, and many chiefs backed them in this. In the Belgium Congo, such sects were persecuted and their prophetic leaders arrested and jailed.[101] In Rhodesia, the British authorities saw the religious enthusiasm as a sign of madness, just as their Anglican forebears had done in the eighteenth century. Attempts were made to exclude such preachers from African areas, but the idea had taken root, leading to the emergence of new hybrid sects.[102]

These sects catered for the poor and lowly, being sources of great creativity and energy. They were concerned above all with the idea of the power of the Holy Spirit to address sickness, poverty, and social and family problems. Unlike in mission medicine, healing came from within the local community rather than from outside. Made thus redundant, missionaries tended to be highly critical of such sects. They tried to depict the new charismatic sects as a reversion to a 'primitive' irrationality. This ignored the fact that Pentecostalism and other such apostolic movements had emerged amongst the nineteenth-century urban poor in Europe and America, and that in Africa these sects established themselves initially in the cities before they attracted a rural following.[103]

In general, therefore, missionaries were reluctant to alter their practice in ways that would have been in tune with local beliefs about disease causation and treatment. In particular, they were hampered by their refusal to utilise exorcism, religious charms and the laying on of hands by members of the church hierarchy – practices that had been historically an important element within the Christian tradition. Instead, they insisted that those who took advantage of their medical facilities, whether Christian or non-Christian, had to disavow such treatments. This was ironic, seeing that the process of conversion from paganism to Christianity in Europe had depended markedly on miracle cures. The seventh-century saint of Northumbria, Cuthbert, is, for example, depicted by Bede as healing the sick through prayer and the laying-on of hands, all of which cemented the faith of the people in their new religion.[104] There was during medieval times no clear dividing line between healing and Christian ministry, with the shrines of saints being major therapeutic centres.[105] This whole historical experience was being ignored by the missionaries of the colonial era.

Woman medical missionaries

Dana Robert has shown in her history of American women missionaries that until the mid-nineteenth century, women were to a large extent accepted in the mission field only if they went as the wives of missionaries. In this role, they were expected to establish Christian homes in mission outposts, demonstrating to indigenous people the domestic arrangements and gender relations of a Christian family. In fact, from the start, women had gone beyond the domestic boundary, helping with basic educational and medical work amongst local women and children. This was carried out either on the veranda of the mission house or in the homes of the local people, and it was seen as an extension of domestic work.[106] Attempts by single women to gain support from the missionary societies to be sent as missionaries were in almost all cases blocked.[107]

This changed in the second half of the nineteenth century as women began to found their own missionary societies that were committed to sending single women to the mission field. They claimed that women had a particular and unique role to play as educators, healers, and workers among

Figure 1.5

'Attending female out-patients in an Indian hospital.'
The Church Missionary Gleaner, July 1892, p.101.

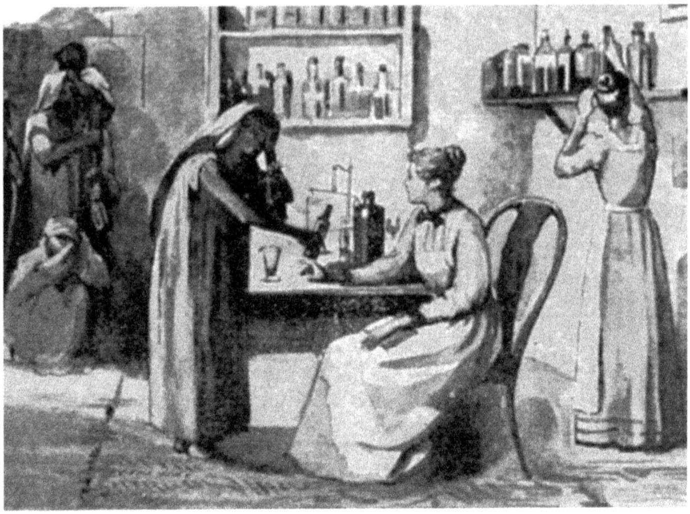

'heathen women'. From this developed the theory of 'Woman's Work for Woman'. This, according to Robert, 'was based on a materialistic, albeit idealistic, belief that non-Christian religions trapped and degraded women, yet all women in the world were sisters and should support each other.'[108] They were moved by pity – as they saw it – to provide the blessings of Christian civilisation to such women – religious, educational, and medical. A central focus was on converting mothers so that they would influence their children. They would purify their homes, and provide a shining example of Christian values. 'The emphasis on the conversion of mothers, and through them their children, and through children, the society, continued as a justification for the movement into the twentieth century.'[109]

The first fully trained woman medical doctor to become a foreign missionary was Clara Swain. She was sent to India by the pioneering women's society – the Woman's Foreign Missionary Society, founded in 1869 in Boston – in that same year.[110] Swain's success silenced the objections of male missionaries, allowing medicine to become the most universally acclaimed aspect of women's missionary work in the late-nineteenth century. By 1909, the woman's missionary movement had sent out 147 physicians and ninety-one trained nurses, representing ten percent of the woman's mission force, and it was supporting eighty-two dispensaries and eighty hospitals around the world. Robert argues that the effect of this work was far greater than the numbers alone suggest, as the work gave an opening for missionaries in otherwise hostile places, and because missionary doctors made the training of indigenous women a top priority, and in the process 'revolutionised the medical treatment of women in India and China.'[111]

America took the lead in this, as women's medical education had been pioneered there, while Britain lagged behind. The first British medical school for women – the London School of Medicine for Women – was founded only in 1874, and three more such single-sex institutions followed in 1886, 1888 and 1890. The women who received such training did not find it easy to obtain employment equal to their skills due to continuing discrimination by males in the profession, and it soon became clear that missionary work provided one of the most fulfilling openings available to them.[112] Fanny Butler, who was in the initial batch of students at the London School of Medicine for Women, was sent to India by the CMS after qualifying in 1880. She was the first British woman doctor to practice in India.[113] By 1890 there were twelve women missionaries with British qualifications, ten of whom were serving in India. In 1900 there were 258 women on the British Medical Register – of these seventy-two were serving as medical missionaries, forty-five of them in India.[114] In 1910, Protestant missions – American, British and European – employed 341 women physicians throughout the world. Of these, half were serving in India and one-third in China.[115]

In India, the initial focus of women's medical work was the secluded quarter for women – the *zenana*. A special hospital for *zenana* women was founded in Delhi in 1885. In the early years, it proved hard to attract suitably qualified women doctors and nurses to work there, and only after an adequate number become available in the 1890s did it prove a success.[116] Such work was consolidated with the opening of the North India School of Medicine for Christian Women at Ludhiana in 1894. Its prime object was to train Indian Christian women for *zenana* medical work. In the early twentieth century it began to admit non-Christian students, and changed its name to the Women's Christian Medical College. A course there lasted four years, and students gained a diploma from Lahore University.[117]

In Africa, where women were not kept in seclusion as in many parts of Asia, there was no comparable woman's work. However, as Michael Jennings shows in his chapter in this volume, a strong emphasis developed in medical mission circles in Africa from the 1920s onwards on maternity and childcare work. Babies born in mission maternity wards became known as 'mission babies'. They were then, ideally, brought to the child welfare clinics run by the missions. Such babies won regular prizes in baby shows organised by the colonial rulers. Child welfare clinics were said to rear contented but disciplined babies, their effect being as much moral as physical. It was asserted that until child-rearing practices changed in Africa, Africans would not develop a 'well-balanced' personality and good character. The missionaries criticised mothers who brought their babies to the clinics with 'heathen charms' around their necks; they praised those who dressed their babies 'in simple coloured frocks, sent out by friends in England...'[118] Many African women responded positively to the provision of maternity care, as European midwifery was safer and it provided an alternative context in which to give birth. Giving birth in a mission maternity home sent out a clear message, and for some it provided an escape from kinship groups. In time, such a delivery became a status symbol, a signifier of superior class. Men appreciated it for this reason, and encouraged wives to attend.[119]

Colonial governments in Africa encouraged this missionary work, as child mortality rates had risen generally under colonial rule. Grants-in-aid were provided to missions for this task, though in British territories these were meagre before the late 1940s.[120] In the Congo, where the population decline had been most dramatic as a result of the slaughter carried out by the early Belgian colonisers, the colonial state tried to redeem the situation by developing the most extensive system of clinicalised childbirth of any sub-Saharan African territory, most of which was operated by missionaries.[121] In 1935 it was estimated that only about one per cent of Congolese deliveries were medically supervised, by 1952 this figure had risen to twenty-eight per cent, and in 1958, forty-three per cent. By 1958, every administrative territory in the Congo had a medical centre with a surgical section, a maternity ward, and prenatal and infant facilities. Births attracted bonuses, inscription books, and rations for pregnant women. Fathers of more than four children received relief from taxation in some areas.[122] Jennings argues that the colonial authorities provided funding to mission organisations for this work after 1945 largely because they had proved far superior in this sphere. The missionaries had the patience to educate local communities in the need for better maternity and childcare, and they developed their service in more culturally sensitive ways.[123]

In the nineteenth century, many mission women without any formal training acted as nurses. By the closing years of the century, there was a growing demand from missions for properly qualified nurses. They were needed to staff hospitals for women and children, and to educate local women to become nurses.[124] By getting in first in developing nursing in new areas, missionaries saw an opportunity to exert a Christian influence over women's medical and nursing education. This would, it was hoped, imbue their future professional practice with an ethos of selfless service and devotion to duty rather than with a spirit of commercialism.[125] In India, the missions were in the vanguard in this respect; by the second world war, some ninety per cent of Indian nurses were Christians, and eighty per cent of all Indian nurses had been trained in mission hospitals. This 'proved to be one of the most enduring legacies of the female medical missions of the colonial era,'[126] and it laid the basis for the profession of nursing in India since that time. During the first four decades of the twentieth century, many women medical missionaries began to go beyond the 'Woman's Work for Woman' model, becoming involved in running general hospitals and in administration. They were, however, rarely accorded equality with the male missionaries. It proved, for example, hard for women to be accepted as equal colleagues and teachers in mission hospitals. Many male doctors still felt that women should focus on woman's work and the training of female nurses. At home, the mission-supporting public, and particularly the women's societies that funded special work for women, had difficulty in moving away from the old image of benighted Eastern women dependent on their Western 'sisters' for leadership and protection from abuses. 'Missions certainly remained gendered spaces in the interwar era....'[127]

Leprosy

Missionaries saw leprosy in strongly Biblical terms, as a malady of the cursed, with its disfigured and crippled sufferers living in squalor and rags, crying out for Christ's healing touch.[128] They considered the disease to be unique and different from all others.[129] Those who were infected were designated with a label that subsumed any other identity they might have: that of 'leper'. Missionaries went out of their way to help such people, encouraging them to come for treatment and live in 'leper' colonies. In part, this was because stigmatised people were seen as good material for proselytism, in part because such work was seen as particularly Godly, requiring faith, grace, and courage in the face of a gruesome and contagious affliction. Leprosy work was perhaps the ultimate test of a missionary's commitment to his vocation. Furthermore, colonies of sufferers became locations for Christian social engineering, with the creation of new Godly communities. The sick 'were encouraged to think of themselves as having been quite literally erased by the disease, and then encouraged to adopt a new, salvatory and collective identity as "the lepers".'[130] The missionaries claimed that they were saving a socially cast-off people. In practice, leprosy patients were not always so excluded in their own societies.[131]

In the early years of the nineteenth century, missionaries ran leprosy asylums more as sanctuaries than as medical institutions. They often took in poor people who were infected by other diseases that caused disfigurement, such as leucaderma or syphilis. as well as leprosy. No medical treatment was provided as a rule. Indeed, many experts at the time believed that leprosy was an hereditary complaint and thus not curable. In 1873, Armauer Hanson discovered that the illness was caused by a bacterium, and was thus infectious. The discovery led to calls for sufferers to be segregated, as they were seen to threaten white people in the colonies. In India, the colonial authorities held that voluntary organisations – and particularly missionaries – should take the initiative in this respect, with some financial support from the state. The Mission to Lepers in India was founded in 1874; by 1893 it was running ten leper asylums.

Leprosy received a lot of publicity in 1889 when Father Damien de Veuster, a Belgium missionary who worked with leprosy sufferers in Hawaii, died from the disease. There were calls in Europe for compulsory confinement of patients. In India, the colonial rulers were particularly disturbed by the high visibility of sufferers who exhibited their sores and disfigurements in public as they begged. In 1898 the authorities consequently passed the Lepers Act, which allowed for the forcible segregation of all such 'pauper lepers' in special colonies. This policy had little medical justification, for it was known that leprosy was not highly contagious. However, it suited the non-medical agendas of both colonial governments and missionaries alike.[132] Missionaries largely ran the asylums that were established as a result. In 1911 there were seventy-three of them in India, with about 5,000 inmates in all. The numbers rose in subsequent years. All of this helped to legitimise the work of medical missions in this sphere.[133] Similar measures were taken in other colonies, such as the Lepers Proclamation of 1911 in Northern Nigeria which ordered that all leprosy sufferers should be detained for enquiry, and which threatened with punishment anyone who withheld information about those with the disease from the authorities.[134] As in India, the leprosy colonies were predominantly mission-run organisations, being funded by local governments or the British Empire Leprosy Relief Association (BELRA). As it was, no other single disease attracted such attention and funding in the colonial territories. Tuberculosis was equally prevalent, and a growing problem that received greater government attention in the colonies from the First World War onwards, yet few tuberculosis patients were put in special sanatoria, as was the practice in Europe and America at that time.[135]

In leprosy settlements, patients were 'rescued' from the influences of traditional society, and in the process a new identity was created for them. The inmates were represented in mission magazines as the subjects of the mission organisation; a missionary would write of 'my lepers'.[136] They were depicted as wretched people in a desolate condition, but special in the eyes of Christ and thus redeemable in death through faith in Him. Missionaries tended to depict the diseases as a consequence of sin, redeemable through conversion and conformity to mission morality.[137] In these institutions, religion was to the fore, with medicine in the background. The missionaries felt that they were justified in enforcing a 'Christian' way of life on inmates, for their own good. This could be seen in the common policy of sexual segregation in asylums, for which there was no medical justification. Sexes had been segregated in medieval leper asylums, and donors to such projects expected this practice to be continued. Violations of this rule could lead to the excommunication of patients by the missionaries.[138] As a rule, Christian worship was mandatory for the patients, and they were forbidden to practice any other religion. Although the missionaries denied that they carried out forced conversions, the atmosphere in these institutions was such that it was hard to resist becoming a Christian.[139]

The asylums were generally grim-looking places, resembling prisons.[140] Inmates were often distressed at being cut off from their families and relatives. The sexes, were as a rule, segregated in the asylums, even thought there was no medical evidence that the disease was transmitted sexually.[141] Mothers who suffered from the disease might even be segregated from their children. In her chapter in this volume, Shobana Shankar argues that many women in northern Nigeria avoided missionaries, as they feared that they might be forced into leprosaria and so segregated.[142] Inmates were usually made to labour for their livelihood by missionaries who saw this as a necessary part of their redemption. They ran the places in a paternalistic and autocratic manner. The patients sometimes broke the rules and disobeyed the missionaries, complaining of being overworked or poorly provided for.[143]

Before the mid-twentieth century, the most effective medical intervention available for leprosy sufferers was careful nursing and sanitation, as this helped prevent further damage to their limbs and allowed ulcers to heal. Surgery, particularly for the eyes, could also help, though this was not much developed before the important pioneering work of the Baptist medical missionary, Paul Brand, at the Christian Medical College in Vellore, in south India, from the late-1940s onwards.[144] In practice, such attention was the exception rather than the rule. Instead, the resident doctors practiced dubious 'cures' that were often more harmful than therapeutic, such as daily injections of chaulmoogra oil. These treatments were often continued even after they had been discredited.[145] The sulphone drugs that were developed in the 1950s provided the first effective cure for the disease. They made the settlements redundant as the malady could now be treated successfully within the home.[146] More rigorous investigation of patterns of disease also showed that leprosy was far more widespread in many parts of Asia and Africa than hitherto realised – those who bore the obvious marks of the disease were just the tip of the iceberg. Whereas the missionaries had based their appeals for support for such work on the idea that the 'leper' was a person apart, it now became clear that he or she was not.

The local politics of mission medicine

While much of the writing on medical missions has focused on the white missionaries and their work, there has been an increasing interest in recent years in discovering how the objects of the missionaries' attentions – the local people – understood and reacted to their medical work. The pioneering study in this respect was by John Jantzen, who studied the 'quest for therapy' pursued by patients who sought treatment at some stage in the progress of their illness at a mission hospital in the Congo. He found that there was much mutual incomprehension between the mission medics and their patients as to the nature of disease and its cure. The local people made a distinction between a 'natural'-cum-'divine' and a 'human' cause of illness. If a disease responded readily to therapy, or was predictable – as when very old people fall sick and die – it was normally seen as 'natural'-cum-'divine'. If a disease was intractable, it was frequently believed that it was caused by human malevolence. Patients and their kin had to decide within which category to place an illness before consulting a specialist. Western medicine was generally considered efficacious in the treatment of 'natural'-cum-'divine' illnesses, as were some herbalists. But, if a disease took an unusual or slow course, or if there was conflict within the social group of the sufferer, human causes were suspected. Attempts were then made to resolve conflicts, cast counter spells, and perform rituals of purification.[147]

Scholars working on other parts of Africa south of the Sahara have found similar beliefs operating in their areas of study, with disease and illness likewise being viewed in terms that did not accord with European categories of thought. Ranger has pointed out in the context of Zimbabwe: 'Paradoxically, then, diseases of God were the sphere of herbal and other secular remedies; diseases of Man were the sphere of *spiritual* treatment of diseases, since the afflictions themselves were caused by actions of the spirits.'[148] The healers of maladies caused by 'human' agency sought to reverse harmful processes that had affected socially-connected people. It was thus believed that the rivalries of relatives and neighbours or the anger of the dead could cause people to suffer misfortune or fall ill. Sickness, rainfall, plant growth, and other natural phenomena were considered to be interconnected, requiring similar remedies applied by shamanistic healers. Tswana healers in South Africa, for example, used oracles to discover the source of such a malady, and they fought the evil with spells. 'They cooled bodies inflamed by conflict, warmed ones chilled by bereavement, steadied relations disrupted by human carelessness and greed.'[149]

The Tswana initially understood the missionaries in terms of their own beliefs about disease, well-being and healing. Hearing them promise dramatic relief from death, disease, and affliction, they believed that the missionaries were claiming to possess strong supernatural powers of healing.[150] The Tswana were always on the lookout for powerful healers of any sort, and had a tradition of importing them from elsewhere if necessary. The missionaries appear to have been regarded in such a light – as a valuable therapeutic resource.[151] The Tswana did not distinguish between the roles of priest and doctor. They misread the equipment and apparatus that the missionaries carried – their Bibles, sacred communion, medicine chests and guns – as fetishes that were animated by a mysterious 'medicine of God's Word'.[152] John Moffat was once asked to his surprise whether his books were '*bola*' (prognosticating dice).[153] Missionaries were often asked to make rain – one of the major tasks of royal ritual practitioners. But it was soon seen that they lacked any aptitude in this sphere. Gradually, it became apparent that the chief skill of the missionary lay in the sphere of 'natural'-cum-'divine' disease. In this way, Western medicine could be incorporated into African popular belief without undermining its rationale. In cases in which western medicine proved effective in treating previously intractable – or 'human' – diseases, then that disease and its range of symptoms might be moved into the category of 'natural'-cum-'divine' diseases. The 'human' disease category continued to be applied in those many cases in which Western medicine proved ineffective.[154]

This led to a situation in southern Africa in which many medically unqualified missionaries felt that they had to provide medical services if they were to maintain their credibility. John Moffat, for example, had no medical training, but found that he obtained a more ready audience for his preaching through healing the sick.[155] David Livingstone – one of the few qualified mission doctors – was seen as having particularly compelling powers. Unlike other missionaries, he had the competence to perform surgery and treat more difficult cases. Rumours as to his skill – even in matters in which he claimed no ability, such as being able to cure sterility – led rapidly to him being almost overwhelmed by would-be patients, many of whom came from great distances to consult him and purchase his remedies.[156]

As the boundaries between the different forms of healing were always in flux and always disputed, the missionaries with their medicine tended to be constantly drawn into struggles for power at the local level. Drawing on the work of Steven Feierman,[157] Megan Vaughan has noted how the common belief in a connection between illness and sorcery led to a contest between the sorcerer and the bewitched, each backed by their own relatives and political allies, and with the victory tending to go to the more powerful. The power of the chief depended on his ability to mobilise such discourses in his favour.[158] When the missionary was relatively powerless against local chiefs – a situation that was the norm until the closing years of the nineteenth century – it could lead to a struggle between chiefs to appropriate the power

Figure 1.6

'Dr Drewe gives an injection to a witchdoctor. Holy Cross, Pondoland.'
Conquest by Healing, December 1942, p.54.

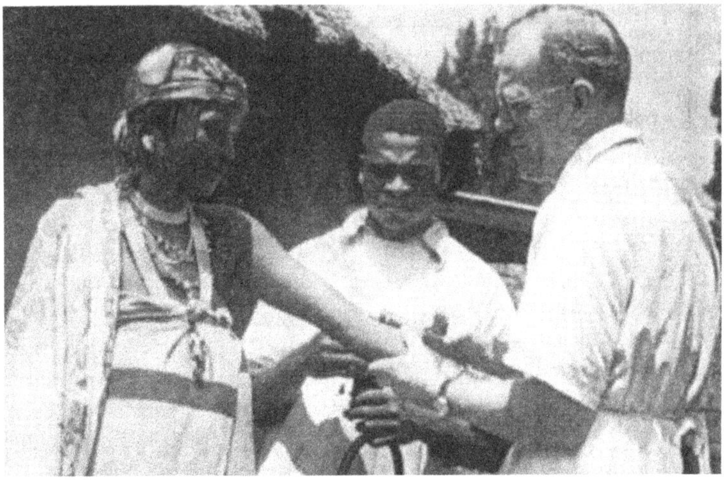

The Holy Cross Hospital, Pondoland, was in South Africa. The photo accompanies an article describing the baneful effects of the medicine provided by 'witchdoctors'. The unstated implication of the photo is that even 'witchdoctors' are now prepared to receive treatment from the medical missionaries, signalling an anticipated 'conquest by healing' of what was viewed as a particularly obstinate foe.

of the European, as represented by the missionary. Here, the quest was for that elusive power that underlay European technology, literacy, and healing.[159] For example, in the interior of southern Africa in the early- to mid-nineteenth century, all missionaries, including medical missionaries, were working in a situation in which local chiefs still retained effective power. They had to deal with this situation through tact and a certain amount of tolerance. In turn, the chiefs tended to treat the missionaries as useful resources, able to provide new technology and skill, including the power to heal.

Once, however, these chiefs had been defeated and subjugated by the colonial state, many missions became like an alternative local state, being centres for education, medical treatment, relief provision during periods of dearth, agricultural activity – which might include the provision of cooperative credit for farmers – and local craft production. They were

Figure 1.7

'Dispensary Tent of the Cashmere Medical Mission.'
The Church Missionary Gleaner, November 1874, p.122.

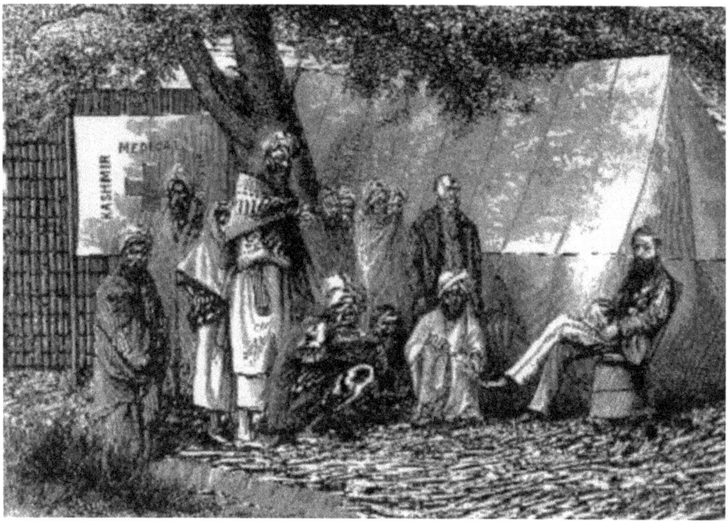

Missionaries were unable to gain an entry into Kashmir, which was a Muslim majority region ruled by a Hindu prince, before 1865, when Dr Elmslie of the CMS founded a medical mission at Srinagar. Elmslie died in 1872, and the print shows his successor, Dr Theodore Maxwell sitting before the tent used on itinerating medical tours in the valley of Kashmir.

backed in this work by the colonial authorities.[160] In this situation of enhanced power, many medical missionaries began to oppose the practice of indigenous healers more actively, and they often tried to stop local converts from taking treatment from them. This might lead to conflicts over medical treatment that had a strong political content. Such battles were often depicted in mission literature as ones between the mission doctor and the 'witchdoctor' or 'wizard'. When called to treat a patient in their hut, the missionary was frequently shown as being drawn into an encounter with such practitioners of the 'dark' arts. The struggle became one between the Light of Christian Reason and the Forces of Evil. In some cases the missionary triumphed, in others he or she was forced to withdraw, for the time being at least. Unlike the 'rational' patient of Europe, the native was depicted as being frequently too 'primitive', stubborn and ignorant to heed the doctor's wisdom. This was shown to be deeply frustrating, requiring a staunch Christian forbearance on the part of the missionary.[161]

In India, we can observe a difference between the response to medical missionaries in regions ruled by Indian princes and the areas ruled directly by the British. The former ruled about one-third of the landmass of British India. When the United Presbyterian Church of Scotland, for example, initiated missionary work in India, it decided to focus on Rajasthan, as other mission bodies had neglected this area. Indian princes ruled most of this region, and to work in their states, the missionaries had to cultivate their goodwill. Dr Colin Valentine managed to gain a base for his medical mission work in Jaipur State after he had successfully treated a member of the Maharaja's household. The ruler pressed him to remain as his personal physician, and paid him a salary. Valentine thus combined medical missionary work in the city with employment as a servant of the state.[162] In part, the princely rulers of Rajasthan appreciated the medical missionaries as they wanted trained western doctors without having to provide any great outlay, and mission doctors came at a bargain price. The Hindu princes were not much concerned about their being Christians, for they had a longstanding tradition of patronising a whole range of religious bodies and sects, and they saw the missionaries as just one more such group worthy of support. Their subordinate feudatories – who were rulers of localities consisting of often just a few villages – extended such support to missionaries for similar reasons. The local village elites tended, however, to be less tolerant, as was seen in some areas ruled by such feudatories in southern Rajasthan and northeastern Gujarat. As I have argued in my chapter in this volume, many leaders of the Bhil peasantry of this region resented the challenge that the medical missionaries posed to their ritual power and did their best to undermine their work.

Similar tendencies appear to have operated in areas in Africa under a comparable system of colonial indirect rule. Shobana Shankar argues in her chapter in this volume that the emirs of Northern Nigeria allowed missionaries to establish colonies for sufferers from leprosy under strict controls designed to restrict proselytisation to a minimum. The missionaries accepted these onerous terms as hitherto they had not been permitted to operate at all in the region. This led to a situation in which Islam and Christianity were considered to have separate medical spheres, with leprosy treatment being labelled as 'Christian'. Individuals crossed from one sphere to the other, but had to justify it by saying – if they went to the mission doctors – that they were suffering from leprosy, or that they were merely using 'Christian' medicine as an outpatient. Mission medicine was thus kept at arm's length from Muslim society as a whole.[163] Whether or not the same was true for other societies over which the European colonial powers had

Figure 1.8
Advertisement insert in *Medical Missions at Home and Abroad*, October 1895, p.32.

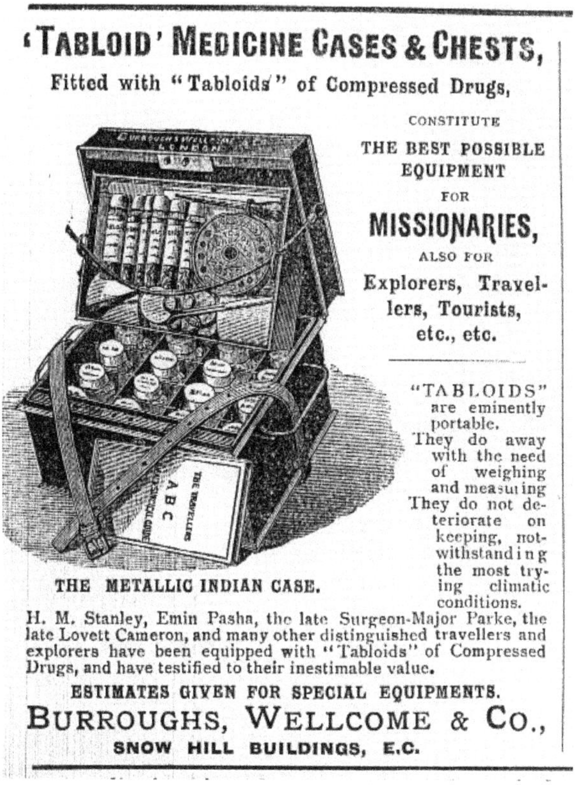

This quarterly was the journal of the London-based Medical Missionaries Association, and it catered for a wide range of Protestant denominations.

only a limited, or perhaps no power – areas such as inland China, Thailand, Afghanistan or Ethiopia – can only be determined by further study.

Mission medicine in the history of medicine

The practice of mission medicine had a noted impact on western medical knowledge and theory in general. Western biomedicine evolved during the European colonial era, and it was inevitably affected by that experience. Empires provided vast fields for research, allowing for the production of a new globalised system of scientific knowledge.[164] 'Tropical medicine' became a particularly popular and prestigious field of specialisation, and it attracted large numbers of European medical graduates from the later years of the nineteenth century.[165] Becoming a medical missionary provided one entry into this field of work and research; a practice on a remote mission station was a path to possible medical fame, especially as the work of medical missionaries was read as 'a saga of heroic science' in the home countries.[166] There were, moreover, no profound intellectual barriers between missionary and medical work, and many doctors were strong Christians. Rhodri Hayward has noted how the language of biomedicine is suffused with religious imagery:

> Although there have been persistent attempts to revise and mathematise the language of medicine, the modern discipline still reveals rich traces of its religious inheritance. Neurology is still permeated by Christian notions of order and hierarchy whilst modern pathological concepts of viruses and germs remain rooted in the magical language of agency.[167]

This all facilitated a continuing dialogue between Christian religious workers and biomedical practitioners – occupations that in the case of medical missionaries were in any case combined.

The pioneer figure in this respect was David Livingstone. Although he had little enthusiasm for day-to-day healing, he was keen to contribute to knowledge about Africa through medical observation, and he continued to be willing to treat cases that he felt had scientific importance. He wrote up and published his findings in this and other respects, and propounded them on his lecture tours, in the process reaching a wide and highly receptive medical audience. In common with most other Victorian missionaries, Livingstone believed that there were physiological differences between Europeans and Africans that could be attributed to the 'excess' sexuality of the black. He was, for example, struck by the low incidence of malaria among African women, and he put this down to their 'excessive' menstrual discharges that, he argued, purged their bodies of the disease. He was also impressed by the ease with which Tswana women gave birth, as compared to women in Britain, and he continued to practice obstetric medicine so that he could discover the reasons for this. Whether he intended it or not, this all fed into popular European racist notions about Africans.[168] There was a common medical belief that blacks were sexually different to whites, to the extent that one African woman whose physiognomy happened to match the stereotype was exhibited naked in the West to make the point.[169] When Livingstone's findings ran counter to popular medical prejudice, they were often ignored. Thus, it was commonly asserted by medical men that venereal diseases had originated amongst African women, who had then infected

Europeans. Livingstone himself had in fact reported that he had found a remarkable absence of syphilis amongst Africans in the interior, and the evidence suggests that white people, particularly colonial soldiers, later brought the disease to the interior.[170] Mission doctors might therefore be listened to when their findings were acceptable, but ignored when they were not.

Medical research that required the inspection of bodies, the taking of blood samples, and autopsies could cause considerable suspicion, leading often to a deliberate avoidance of medical missions. In the Congo, for example, it was commonly believed that autopsies were a form of butchery by whites, who then canned and ate the bodies. Such rumours were fuelled by the fact that some doctors removed body parts furtively for later study, returning an incomplete corpse to relatives. Hunt describes one such incident from the 1940s, in which the doctor, a syphilis specialist, secretly removed the foetus from a syphilitic woman who had died in her eighth month of pregnancy, keeping it for his research. While he was doing this, the woman's suspicious relatives stood outside the autopsy room, wailing. Hunt comments that 'a key incentive for colonial medical research in gynaecology, obstetrics, and paediatrics was implicitly the ready availability of a dead and dissectible subject population.'[171]

In his chapter in this volume, James Mills provides a case study of the missionary contribution to medical knowledge in the case of opinions about cannabis in the late-nineteenth century. Little was known about this drug in nineteenth-century Britain, but in India the colonial regime derived considerable sums of revenue from the excise on its sale. This was an anathema to temperance reformers in Britain, and they obtained the information that they needed about the allegedly harmful effects of cannabis from missionaries there. Mills argues that the missionary antipathy towards the drug came from a mix of temperance commitments, a belief that it stimulated a wild sexuality, and knowledge that it was used by Indian mendicants – their religious rivals – to open themselves and their followers to heightened spiritual experiences. They thus had a vested interest in condemning the drug as a pernicious and immoral substance. Although the temperance reformers failed to obtain a ban on the drug in the late-nineteenth century, Mills argues that the missionary input into the debate helped to form a generally negative view of cannabis that was to inform metropolitan discourses on the drug in important respects during the twentieth century.

Vaughan has argued that missionary prejudices also fed into early-twentieth century eugenics, with its multiple fears of rampant sexuality, miscegenation, and 'racial degeneration'.[172] Missionaries were generally obsessed with the 'primitive', 'uncontrolled' and 'excess' sexuality of the native, and frequently sought in this a cause of illness. Morality and illness were seen to be inextricably intertwined. This was considered to be the case particularly with Africans, and the views of the missionaries in this respect informed wider European perceptions of 'the Negro'.[173] Such views underpinned medical debates, even in cases where there were divergent views between secular and mission doctors in other respects. For example, when there was a supposed epidemic of venereally-transmitted syphilis in Buganda in the first decade of the twentieth century, colonial doctors argued that African women – who 'were, in effect, merely female animals with strong passions'[174] – had in the past been kept in check by strong patriarchs, but social changes brought by Christianity had loosened male controls, leading to the women giving vent to their lust. The argument was informed by a view of 'primitive morality' that accorded with that of the missionaries, but the conclusion – that Christianity was to blame for their getting out of hand – was not of course acceptable to the latter. In their ripostes, mission doctors blamed the colonial state for destroying the old feudal system of Buganda, arguing that it was only Christianity that could provide a new moral base that would allow syphilis to be brought eventually under control. As it was, the mission doctors had largely misdiagnosed the disease, for it was later found that what they called 'native syphilis' was in many cases yaws, or a form of syphilis that was not transmitted sexually. Their moralistic views had established the terms for a seemingly erudite medical debate about an 'epidemic' of a sexually-transmitted disease that later research revealed as a figment of their imagination.[175]

Transitions to indigenous practice

Medical mission work was taken over by local converts earliest of all in China, as Timothy Wong reveals in his chapter in this volume. In India, Dr Colin Valentine established the Agra Medical Missionary Training Institution in 1881. Christian converts were provided with grants to stay in Agra, and housed in a special Christian hostel while they trained at the Government Medical College in the city. Many indigenous Christian doctors were trained there, and without their work many of the medical missions in India would have been unable to function.[176] In much of Africa, by contrast, there was minimal indigenisation at this level during the colonial period.

Although it took time for indigenous Christians to train as doctors and take over the medical work of the missions, medical missions depended on indigenous medical assistants from the start. In the early years, these were normally trained on the job, and they lacked any formal qualification. Missions began to establish special training centres for such people from the late nineteenth century onwards. In India, for example, the London

Figure 1.9

'Raw material' and 'A Nurse at Holy Cross – finished product!'
Conquest by Healing, December 1942, p.55.

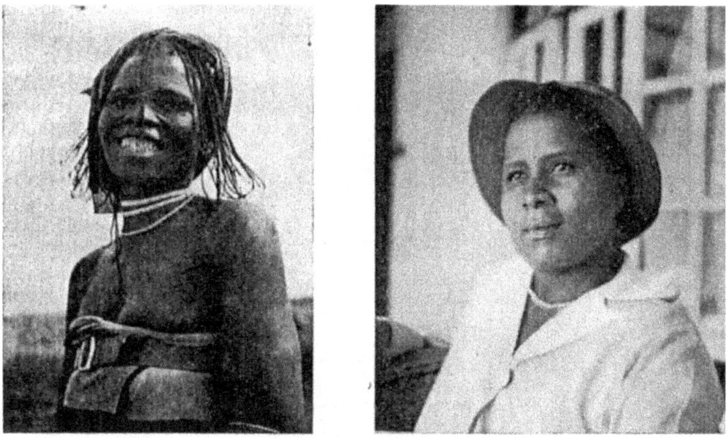

The accompanying article states that: 'It is hard to believe that, within fifteen years of opening the hospital, girls taken from a background of such primitive superstition could be trained to take, in English, the full examination of the South African Medical Council.' It was also reported that the nurses were in extremely high demand in South Africa, which was hardly surprising in view of the fact that there had been almost no training available before the 1930s. The Holy Cross nurses were at that time an exception in Africa; most nurses were still male.

Missionary Society and the American Presbyterians founded medical-cum-theological schools to train Indian Christians. Students received a diploma after four years which enabled them to become 'Medical Evangelists'. Such people generally worked as assistants to Western-trained medical missionaries in mission hospitals, or ran branch dispensaries in outlying stations.[177]

Such positions were, ideally, reserved for Christian converts, as the aim was to have a thoroughly Christian staff. It was not always easy, however, to ensure this, and non-Christians were not infrequently employed on pragmatic grounds. In some cases, Christians were appointed who were not suitable for the task.[178] In Africa, the missions found it hard during the early years to recruit local people in such a role, as the work was regarded as lowly and demeaning. The majority at that time were former patients who had become converts and who had stayed around the mission compound after they were healed.[179] Later, most came to be recruited from those who had

Figure 1.10

'An anxious mother brings her baby to St Luke's Hospital, Hiranpur. Here Dr Bryan Thompson and nurse Mary Draper try to find out what's wrong. More doctors – men and women – are needed throughout Africa and Asia.'
CMS Outlook, January 1966, p.6.

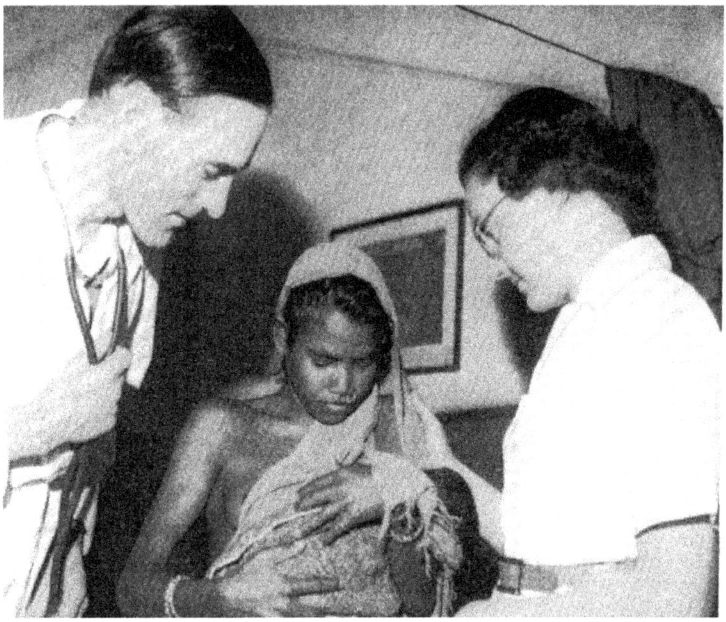

Hiranpur was located in a particularly poor tribal area in southern Bihar, India. The photo is used for an appeal for more medical missionaries. The 1960s were designated by the United Nations as the 'Decade of Development,' and many optimistically believed that with skilled western help and guidance the ex-colonial countries could be modernised rapidly. While putting over an image of benevolent Christianity in action, the photo also inadvertently highlights the huge inequalities of power that existed between western missionaries and the underprivileged patients in their care.

studied at the mission schools. They were almost always male, and were known as *dawa* (medicine) or dispensary 'boys'. To a large extent this was because few African women had the necessary education for such a task. There was also a long-standing prejudice against the use of African women. As one colonial official in Northern Rhodesia wrote in 1926: 'The native female of this territory is at present inherently unsuited to such work, and I hold the opinion that she should be at present altogether disregarded in this connection'.[180] Even in the late-1940s, some medical missionaries were still resisting the employment of female nurses.[181] The use of males, however, brought its own anxieties, for the missionaries were concerned about the appropriate roles for men and women and were worried lest there be sexual improprieties in the treatment of women patients.[182]

As the mission stations were always short of European personnel, such assistants were critical for the running of their hospitals and medical work. The assistants communicated with the patients in their own language, explaining unfamiliar hospital regulations. They often played an important role in popularising western medicine more generally in their society.[183] Despite this, mission doctors were constantly displeased with their assistants, whom they tended to regard as hard to train, lazy in their work, and often guilty of misdemeanours. They felt that such work was not 'natural' to natives. Those who were considered to have made a success of the job were a cause for rejoicing.[184]

Kumwenda describes such tensions between the white medical personnel and their assistants in her chapter in this volume on Northern Rhodesia. The alleged misdemeanours of the assistants included insubordination, shoddy medical work, drunkenness, sexual improprieties with patients and other local women, and the appropriation of medical stores for private gain. They in turn were often upset with the harsh disciplinarian bent and racist behaviour of many of the white medical staff, and also the low pay they received in mission stations compared to what they could have commanded in government institutions or working for mining organisations. Several who had been trained under the auspices of the missions later quit them for such better positions.

In Africa, most of the nurses in government and mission hospitals were male until almost the end of the colonial period. In some areas, missions rather than the colonial governments took the lead in trying to attract women into nursing. In Northern Rhodesia, for example, a new Anglican bishop, who was appointed in 1941, championed this measure for the first time.[185] Mission girls' schools provided the best recruiting ground for trainee nurses. It was not easy, however, to find qualified nurses to train the recruits, and the girls often ended up only half trained and holding an inferior certificate. Even this was of value, as there was a continuing high demand for nurses with any sort of training from both missions and secular medical institutions.

The paucity of African medical personnel was even more apparent at more senior levels. There were almost no African doctors working for the medical missions before the 1960s. Terence Ranger has argued in the context of Tanzania that educated African Christians tended to shun the medical profession until after the second world war as they resented the intolerant way in which the mission doctors tried to impose their cultural values in the sphere of healing. Instead, they preferred to become teachers or priests.[186] This situation was to cause some embarrassment to the missions as independence loomed in the different colonies, leading to some hasty measures to train Africans to work at this level alongside the missionaries.

Conclusion

There is no doubt about the great popularity of medical work by missionaries. All over the world, people came in large numbers for treatment at their local mission dispensaries and hospitals. But did this bring many converts? Shobana Shankar addresses this question in a persuasive way in her chapter in this book. In her research in Islamic Northern Nigeria, she interviewed former patients of mission leprosaria – both converts and non-converts – and found that those who had become Christians placed very little emphasis on their experience of medical treatment by mission medical staff. What seems to have determined conversion in many cases was the course of life that they decided upon after they were cured. There were openings for ex-patients as teachers or workers in the Christian leprosaria, and those who took these options would convert, whereas those who decided to return to their villages were likely to remain Muslim. She also found that particularly pious people – often students previously of a Qur'anic school – might find an affinity with the missionaries and become Christian. She mentions one such patient whom the missionaries singled out for attention because of his obvious piety. He felt fulfilled by their attentions at a time when he was experiencing the pain of separation from his family and community, and converted as a result. Treatment in a mission hospital or medical establishment was thus one element within an extended narrative of conversion, and it was not necessarily a determining cause.

A more lasting legacy of medical missions most probably lay not so much in the number of converts they won, but in their popularisation of biomedicine, or at least certain aspects of biomedicine, in many parts of the world. There was, moreover, an informing medical ethos in such institutions that was of immense value – namely that medical people from rich countries had a moral duty to provide good medical care for those who would otherwise have had no access to it. C. Peter Williams has pointed out that many Victorian missionaries were moved not only by a desire to win converts, but also to provide an example to the world of Christian benevolence and compassion, and that medical work was seen by many to provide an excellent expression of this moral imperative. The Reverend James Lewes thus argued in 1860, echoing Livingstone, that if European civilisation was 'an embodied Christianity', then it was important for the missionary to represent that civilisation in a full sense.[187] According to Williams: 'This underlining of the place of benevolence in missionary strategy is probably the most important factor in explaining the growth of medical missions.'[188] Many outside missionary circles who were critical of evangelical activities were often far more sympathetic to medical missionary work. Christianity was losing its intellectual credibility for many, but there was still a strong belief in social duty, social reform, and sympathy for the weak and powerless.

In Johannesburg, for example, the work at the Bridgman Memorial Hospital, founded by Clara Bridgman in 1928, had such a quality. It taught black women child-care and hygiene, seeking to make them into exemplary mothers. It became extremely popular, and was always crowded with patients. Although run on racial lines, with whites doing the caring and teaching, there was an ethos of providing compassionate care to black women that lifted it above most white-dominated institutions. Eventually, due to its success in this respect, it was in 1965 forcibly closed by the apartheid regime. The greatest impact in such work was probably in the training given to Africans as nurses and midwives. They spread a new medical knowledge and practise informed by an ethos of care within the context of a community suffering from terrible problems of poverty and squalid living conditions. Such women became role models for girls in the black community. They were inspired by their religion, which was reinforced by the religious atmosphere of the mission maternity hospital. They were used to working in an atmosphere of prayer and religious imagery. They devoted their lives to good work in their communities.[189]

Through work imbued with such qualities, mission medicine was often able to transcend its many limits and shortcomings. Today, such a spirit lives on in the work of dedicated non-governmental workers – Christian and non-Christian alike – throughout the world. In the long term, this may prove to be the most lasting and positive contribution that mission medicine – at its best – has provided for medical practice and the art of healing in general.

Notes

1. J. and J. Comaroff, *Of Revelation and Revolution: The Dialectics of Modernity on a South African Frontier*, Vol. 2 (Chicago: Chicago University Press, 1997), 324. The quote of 'sin-sick soul' is from J. Lowe, *Medical Missions: Their Place and Power* (New York and Chicago: Fleming H. Revell Company, 1887), 218.
2. M. Vaughan, *Curing their Ills: Colonial Power and African Illness* (Cambridge: Polity Press, 1991), 55.
3. *Ibid.*, 1.

4. *Ibid.*, 2.
5. *Ibid.*, 158.
6. See for example J.I. Macnair, 'The Lion and Livingstone' in *Livingstone the Liberator: A Study of a Dynamic Personality* (London and Glasgow: Collins, 1940), 82–5.
7. Vaughan, *op. cit.* (note 2), 74.
8. On this, see Vaughan, *ibid.*, 39–52.
9. M. Vaughan, 'Healing and Curing: Issues in the Social History and Anthropology of Medicine in Africa', *Social History of Medicine*, 7 (1994), 295.
10. Vaughan, *op. cit.* (note 2), 57.
11. *Ibid.*, 23.
12. T. Ranger, 'Godly Medicine: The Ambiguities of Medical Mission in Southeast Tanzania, 1900–1945', *Social Science and Medicine*, 15B (1981), 261–77, and T. Ranger, 'Medical Science and Pentecost: The Dilemma of Anglicanism in Africa', in W.J. Shiels (ed.), *The Church and Healing* (Oxford: Basil Blackwell, 1982), 333–65.
13. The chapter is titled 'The Medicine of God's Word.' Comaroff, *op. cit.* (note 1), 323–64, quote on 323–4.
14. N.R. Hunt, *A Colonial Lexicon: Of Birth Ritual, Medicalization and Mobility in the Congo* (Durham: Duke University Press, 1999), 161.
15. R. Fitzgerald, '"A Peculiar and Exceptional Measure": The Call for Women Medical Missionaries for India in the Later Nineteenth Century', in R.A. Bickers and R. Seton (eds), *Missionary Encounters: Sources and Issues* (Richmond: Curzon Press, 1996), 174–96; R. Fitzgerald, 'Rescue and Redemption – The Rise of Female Medical Missions in Colonial India during the Late Nineteenth and Early Twentieth Centuries', in A.M. Rafferty, J. Robinson and R. Elkan (eds), *Nursing History and the Politics of Welfare* (London: Routledge, 1997, 64–79); R. Fitzgerald, '"Clinical Christianity": The Emergence of Medical Work as a Missionary Strategy in Colonial India, 1800-1914', in B. Pati and M. Harrison (eds), *Health, Medicine and Empire: Perspectives on Colonial India* (New Delhi: Orient Longman, 2001)88–136.
16. This lacuna is addressed in U.C. Dirar, 'Curing Bodies to Rescue Souls: Health in Capuchin's Missionary Strategy in Eritrea, 1894–1935', in this volume, 251–80, and J. Manton, 'Administering Leprosy Control in Ogoja Province, Nigeria, 1945–67: A Case Study in Government–Mission Relations', in this volume, 307–331, on Roman Catholic work in Eritrea and Nigeria respectively. For French West Africa, Bertrand Taithe has informed me that French Catholic missionaries were carrying out medical work there in the late-nineteenth and early-twentieth centuries in a fairly widespread way. As yet, however, there are no proper studies of their work. Personal

discussion with Bertrand Taithe. For German East Africa, Walter Bruchhausen has collected evidence that suggests that German Protestant missionaries had a very different approach to healing than their British and American counterparts. For example, they had a particular interest in herbal remedies and were keen to collect local herbal-based medicines to use in their work. Extract from an unpublished conference paper sent to me by Walter Bruchhausen.

17. On this, see R. Grove, *Green Imperialism: Colonial Expansion, Tropical Island Edens and the Origins of Environmentalism 1600–1860* (Cambridge: Cambridge University Press, 1995), 80–90. Mark Harrison is at present carrying out research on missionaries who carried out medical work and collected botanical knowledge in eighteenth-century India. Among others, Moravian and Lutheran missionaries were engaged in such work.
18. C.P. Williams, 'Healing and Evangelism: The Place of Medicine in Later Victorian Protestant Missionary Thinking', in Sheils, *op. cit.* (note 12), 271.
19. *Ibid.*, 271.
20. *Ibid.*, 271–2.
21. R. Porter, 'The Patient's View: Doing Medical History from Below', *Theory and Society*, 14: 2 (1985), 186.
22. J.V. Pickstone, 'Establishment and Dissent in Nineteenth-Century Medicine: An Exploration of Some Correspondence and Connections between Religious and Medical Belief-Systems in Early Industrial England', in Sheils, *op. cit.* (note 12), 169–70.
23. M. Foucault, *The History of Sexuality: An Introduction* (Harmondsworth: Penguin, 1984), 124–5.
24. Quoted in Comaroff, *op. cit.* (note 1), 336.
25. Pickstone, *op. cit.* (note 22), 171.
26. H.D. Rack, 'Doctors, Demons and Early Methodist Healing', in Sheils, *op. cit.* (note 12), 139 and 143–4.
27. Comaroff, *op. cit.* (note 1), 357 and ft. 55, 497–8.
28. Williams, *op. cit.* (note 18), 272.
29. Quoted in Comaroff, *op. cit.* (note 1), 327.
30. For a study of this problem in an African context, see M. Jennings, '"This Mysterious and Intangible Enemy": Health and Disease amongst the Early UMCA Missionaries, 1860–1918', *Social History of Medicine*, Vol 15, (2002), 65–87.
31. *Ibid.*, 66.
32. See Lazich, 'Seeking Souls Through the Eyes of the Blind: The Birth of the Medical Mission Society in Nineteenth-Century Chine' in this volume. 59–86.
33. J. Wilkinson, *The Coogate Doctors: The History of the Edinburgh Medical Missionary Society 1841 to 1991* (Edinburgh: The Edinburgh Medical

Missionary Society, 1991), 1–3 and 6–7.
34. See Lazich in this volume, 78–9.
35. Comaroff, *op. cit.* (note 1), 338.
36. Macnair, *op. cit.* (note 6), 77.
37. Vaughan, *op. cit.* (note 2), 58.
38. Williams, *op. cit.* (note 18), 273.
39. Comaroff, *op. cit.* (note 1), 325.
40. Lowe, *op. cit.* (note 1), 148; quoted in R. Fitzgerald, 'Clinical Christianity', *op. cit.* (note 15), 115.
41. J. Wells, 'The Sixth Gospel', *Medical Missions in India*, 27 (October 1901), 73, quoted in Fitzgerald, 'Clinical Christianity', *op. cit.* (note 15), 115.
42. R. Fletcher Moorshead, *The Appeal of Medical Missions* (Edinburgh: Oliphant, Anderson and Ferrier, 1913), 76.
43. M. Andrews, 'Speech to the Anniversary', *Central Africa*, 36 (1918), 149, quoted in Ranger, 'Godly Medicine', *op. cit.* (note 12), 262.
44. Fitzgerald, 'Clinical Christianity', *op. cit.* (note 15), 115.
45. D.L. Robert, *American Women in Mission: A Social History of their Thought and Practice*, (Macon: Mercer University Press, 1996), 130.
46. *Ibid.*, 137.
47. *Ibid.*, 166.
48. Comaroff, *op. cit.* (note 1), 326.
49. A. Neve, 'The Calling of a Medical Missionary', *Mercy and Truth*, 15: 180 (December 1911), 400–1; C.F.H. [*sic*], 'Principles and Practices of Medical Missions, Chapter II, A Definition', *Mercy and Truth*, 16: 182 (February 1912) 48–9.
50. Wilkinson, *op. cit.* (note 33), 22–3.
51. *Ibid.*, 23
52. 'Introduction' and 'The Christian Medical Association the Predecessor of the Medical Prayer Union', *Medical Missions at Home and Abroad*, 1 (July 1878), 3–4. The London School of Medicine for Women had a flourishing Bible and Prayer Union at this time. See Antoinette Burton, 'Contesting the Zenana: The Mission to make "Lady Doctors for India",' *Journal of British Studies*, 35: 3 (1996), 379.
53. Williams, *op. cit.* (note 18), 278.
54. *Ibid.*, 273.
55. Fitzgerald, 'Clinical Christianity', *op. cit.* (note 15), ft. 10, 77 and 67.
56. See the statement by Lowe, *op. cit.* (note 1), 48; quoted in Fitzgerald, 'Peculiar and Exceptional Measure', *op. cit.* (note 15), 192.
57. A.F. Walls, '"The Heavy Artillery of the Missionary Army": The Domestic Importance of the Nineteenth-Century Medical Missionary', in Sheils, *op. cit.* (note 12), 293–4.
58. Ranger, 'Godly Medicine', *op. cit.* (note 12), 262.

59. For an example, see *Mercy and Truth*, 65 (1902), 6, quoted in Vaughan, *op. cit.* (note 2), 62.
60. Vaughan, *op. cit.* (note 2), 61–2.
61. Walls, *op. cit.* (note 57), 291–2.
62. J. Stanley, 'Professionalising the Rural Medical Mission in Weixian, 1890–1925', in this volume, 115–36: 122–27.
63. R.C. Brouwer, *Modern Women Modernizing Men: The Changing Missions of Three Professional Women in Asia and Africa, 1902–69* (Vancouver: UBC Press, 2002), 10–13.
64. J. Stanley in this volume, 119–21; Brouwer, *op. cit.* (note 63), 3–4 and 7–10.
65. Stanley in this volume, 125–31.
66. Vaughan, *op. cit.* (note 2), 70–71, 74–5.
67. R. Porter, 'Chris Maddox: Obituary', *The Guardian*, 31 January 2004.
68. R.K.M. Sanders, 'Metamorphosis of Medical Missions in India: The Emmanuel Hospital Association', *Saving Health* (June 1972), 33.
69. R. Boyd, *A Church History of Gujarat* (Madras: The Christian Literature Society, 1981), 190.
70. L. Newbigin, 'The Healing Ministry in the Mission of the Church', in F. Davey (ed.), *The Healing Church: The Tübingen Consultation 1964* (Geneva: World Council of Churches, 1965), 10.
71. E. Kayser, 'Medicine and Modern Philosophy: An Introduction', in Davey, *ibid.*, 18 and 20–1.
72. Williams, *op. cit.* (note 18), 277 and 281.
73. Personal communication from Michael Lazich, 16 March 2003.
74. Fitzgerald, 'Clinical Christianity', *op. cit.* (note 15), 117.
75. This paragraph is based on Pickstone, *op. cit.* (note 22), 170–4, and Wilkinson, *op. cit.* (note 33), 22.
76. Williams, *op. cit.* (note 18), 280; 'The Medical Mission in Cashmere', *The Church Missionary Gleaner*, 1 (1874), 122–3.
77. Walls, *op. cit.* (note 57), 290.
78. W.G. [*sic*], 'The C.M.S. and Medical Missions', *The Church Missionary Intelligencer and Record*, 9 (new series) (May 1884), 315–6.
79. Williams, *op. cit.* (note 18), 280.
80. L.B. Kumwenda, 'African Medical Personnel of the Universities' Mission to Central Africa in Northern Rhodesia', in this volume, 193–226: 196. My italics.
81. Robert, *op. cit.* (note 45), 271.
82. See Dirar and Manton in this volume, 251–80 and 307–331 respectively.
83. *Ibid.*
84. 'Report by Drs A. Lankester and A.H. Browne on the Suitability of the Peshawar Valley for Medical Mission Work', *Mercy and Truth*, 1: 10 (October

1897), 219–21.

85. A. Lankester, 'Medical Mission in Theory', *Mercy and Truth*, 4: 38 (February 1900), 39–41.
86. Thomson's article summarised in Comaroff, *op. cit.* (note 1), 332.
87. All the quotations after footnote 86 are from C.F. Strange, 'The Raison D'Être of Medical Missions', *Mercy and Truth*, 25: 278 (February 1921), 33–4.
88. M. Luther, *Sermons on the Gospel of St John*, Ch. 14–16, in *Luther's Works*, American Edition, 55 vols. (St Louis: Concordia Publishing House 1955-86), Vol. 24, 367, quoted in M. Kelsey, *Healing and Christianity* (Minneapolis: Augsburg, 1995), 17.
89. J. Calvin, *Institutes of the Christian Religion* (Grand Rapids, MI: Wm. B. Eerdmans, 1953), VI.18, 2: 636, quoted in Kelsey, *ibid.*, 17.
90. R. Anderson, *The Silence of God* (Grand Rapids: Kregal Publications, 1953), 153–4, quoted in Kelsey, *ibid.*, 19.
91. W.F. Buroughs, 'Our Title', *Mercy and Truth*, 1: 1 (January 1897), 2.
92. C.F.H. [*sic*], 'Principles and Practices of Medical Mission', *Mercy and Truth*, 16: 181 (January 1912), 24–5.
93. H.J. Cadbury, *George Fox's Book of Miracles* (Cambridge: University of Cambridge, 1949); D. Hodges, *George Fox and the Healing Ministry* (Guildford: Friends Fellowship of Healing, 1995).
94. M. Macdonald, 'Religion, Social Change and Psychological Healing in England 1600–1800', in Shiels, *op. cit.* (note 12), 101–26.
95. S. Mews, 'The Revival of Spiritual Healing in the Church of England 1920–26', in Sheils, *ibid.*, 300–01.
96. R.L. Stirrat, 'Shrines, Pilgrimage and Miraculous Powers in Roman Catholic Sri Lanka', in Sheils, *ibid.*, 397.
97. Mews, *op. cit.* (note 95), 324–5.
98. Quoted in Ranger, 'Medical Science and Pentecost', *op. cit.* (note 12), 344–5.
99. *Ibid.*, 334 and 344–5.
100. Comaroff, *op. cit.* (note 1), 359.
101. J. Janzen, *The Quest for Therapy in Lower Zaire* (Berkeley: University of California Press, 1978), 52.
102. Ranger, 'Medical Science and Pentecost', *op. cit.* (note 12), 360–1.
103. T. Ranger, 'Introduction', in Sheils, *op. cit.* (note 12), xi–xii.
104. Venerable Bede, 'The Life of Cuthbert', in D.H. Farmer (ed.), *The Age of Bede* (Harmondsworth: Penguin, 1988), 39–102.
105. For the healing cult of St Winifred of Holywell see J.F. Champ, 'Bishop Milner, Holywell, and the Cure Tradition', in Sheils, *op. cit.* (note 12), 153–8.
106. Robert, 'The Missionary Wife', in *op. cit.* (note 45), 1–38.

107. *Ibid.*, 127–28.
108. *Ibid.*, 133.
109. *Ibid.*, 135.
110. Swain's career in India is described in *ibid.*, 164–5.
111. *Ibid.*, 162.
112. A. Burton, *op. cit.* (note 52), 394. Burton argues that medically-trained women faced redundancy if they limited their employment horizons to the United Kingdom. Anne Crowther, who has carried out research on the careers of male and female doctors trained in late-nineteenth-century Scotland, argues, against this, that adequate employment was available for women in Britain. Personal communication from Anne Crowther. Nonetheless, missionary propandists who were trying to recruit British women doctors held out to them the attraction of being able to practice a particularly wide range of skills in mission hospitals. See the 1896 appeal by the Delhi-based missionary Charlotte Hull in J. Cox, *Imperial Fault Lines: Christianity and Colonial Power in India, 1818–1940* (Stanford: Stanford University Press, 2002), 175.
113. Burton, *ibid.*, 378.
114. Fitzgerald, 'Peculiar and Exceptional Measure', *op. cit.* (note 15), 195.
115. Fitzgerald, 'Rescue and Redemption', *op. cit.* (note 15), 69.
116. Fitzgerald, 'Peculiar and Exceptional Measure', *op. cit.* (note 15), 190–2.
117. Fletcher Moorshead, *op. cit.* (note 42), 153.
118. *Central Africa*, 576 (1930), 260, quoted in Vaughan, *op. cit.* (note 2), 69.
119. Vaughan, *op. cit.* (note 2), 69–70.
120. See M. Jennings, '"A Matter of Vital Importance": The Place of Medical Mission in Maternal and Child Healthcare in Tanganyika, 1919–39', in this volume, 227–50.
121. Hunt, *op. cit.* (note 14), 3.
122. *Ibid.*, 3–4.
123. See Jennings in this volume, 227–50.
124. Fitzgerald, 'Rescue and Redemption', *op. cit.* (note 15), 74–5.
125. E.K. Paget, *The Claim of Suffering: A Plea for Medical Missions* (London: 1913), 87–90, quoted in Fitzgerald, 'Rescue and Redemption', *op. cit.* (note 15), 75–6.
126. Fitzgerald, *ibid.*, 76–7.
127. Brouwer, *op. cit.* (note 63), 3–17, 21–5 and ft. 3, 131.
128. Vaughan, *op. cit.* (note 2), 79.
129. See Manton in this volume, 309.
130. Vaughan, *op. cit.* (note 2), 14.
131. See S. Shankar, 'The Social Dimensions of Christian Leprosy Work among Muslims: American Missionaries and Young Patients in Colonial Northern Nigeria, 1920–40' in this volume, 281–305: 297, and Manton on southern

Nigeria, also in this volume, 311–2; also Vaughan, *op. cit.* (note 2), 80–1.
132. S. Kakar, 'Medical Developments and Patient Unrest in the Leprosy Asylum, 1860 to 1940', in B. Pati and M. Harrison (eds), *Medicine and Empire: Perspectives on Colonial India* (New Delhi: Orient Longman, 2001), 195.
133. S. Kakar, 'Leprosy in British India, 1860–1940: Colonial Politics and Missionary Medicine', *Medical History*, 40 (1996), 217–22.
134. 'Proclamation No. 8', *The Nothern Nigeria Gazette* (1911), 39–40.
135. Vaughan, *op. cit.* (note 2), 95–6.
136. *Ibid.*, 83.
137. S. Kakar, 'Leprosy in British India: The Intervention of Oral History', *Oral History*, 23 (1995), 43.
138. *Ibid.*, 225.
139. *Ibid.*, 224.
140. Kakar, *op. cit.* (note 132), 198.
141. Kakar, *op. cit.* (note 133), 224.
142. See Shankar in this volume, 292.
143. Kakar describes some of such protests in India – in 1934, 1938–40 and 1946 – in *op. cit.* (note 132), 209–11.
144. J. Young, *Paul Brand* (London: SCM Press, 1980), 12–21; obituary of Paul Brand, *The Guardian*, 27 August 2003.
145. See Shankar in this volume, 283–4.
146. Kakar, *op. cit.* (note 133), 226.
147. Janzen, *op. cit.* (note 101), 8–9.
148. Ranger, 'Medical Science and Pentecost', *op. cit.* (note 12), 339.
149. Comaroff, *op. cit.* (note 1), 344.
150. *Ibid.*, 333.
151. *Ibid.*, 338.
152. *Ibid.*, 346.
153. *Ibid.*, 345.
154. Ranger, 'Medical Science and Pentecost', *op. cit.* (note 12), 340.
155. Comaroff, *op. cit.* (note 1), 325.
156. *Ibid.*, 338.
157. S. Feierman, *Peasant Intellectuals: Anthropology and History in Tanzania* (Madison: The University of Wisconsin, 1990).
158. Vaughan, *op. cit.* (note 9), 285–6.
159. Comaroffs, *op. cit.* (note 1), 347.
160. I am grateful to David Arnold for this point.
161. Vaughan, *op. cit.* (note 2), 162–6.
162. George Carstairs, *Shepherd of Udaipur and the Land he Loved* (London: Hodder and Stroughton, 1926), 117–18.
163. See Shankar in this volume, 281–305.
164. R. Macleod, 'Introduction', in R. Macleod and M. Lewis (eds), *Disease,*

Medicine and Empire: Perspectives on Western Medicine and the Experience of European Expansion (Routledge, London 1988), 1–18.

165. M. Worboys, 'Manson, Ross and Colonial Medical Policy: Tropical Medicine in London and Liverpool, 1899-1914', in Macleod and Lewis, *ibid.*, 21–37.
166. The quotation is from Comaroff, *op. cit.* (note 1), 357.
167. R. Hayward, 'Demonology, Neurology and Medicine in Edwardian Britain', *Bulletin of the History of Medicine*, 78: 1 (2004), 58.
168. Comaroff, *op. cit.* (note 1), 354–6.
169. Vaughan, *op. cit.* (note 2), 20–1.
170. Comaroff, *op. cit.* (note 1), 249–50 and ft. 56, 498.
171. Hunt, *op. cit.* (note 14), 190–1.
172. Vaughan, *op. cit.* (note 2), 132.
173. *Ibid.*, 129–30.
174. Colonel Lambkin, of the Royal Army Medical Corps, 'An Outbreak of Syphilis on Virgin Soil', in D.A. Power and K. Murphy (eds), *A System of Syphilis*, Vol. 2 (London: 1908), quoted in Vaughan, *op. cit.* (note 2), 133.
175. Vaughan, *op. cit.* (note 2), 132–38.
176. Wilkinson, *op. cit.* (note 33), 30–1.
177. Fletcher Moorshead, *op. cit.* (note 42), 98–9.
178. See A. Neve, 'The Place of Medical Missions in the Evangelisation of the World', *Mercy and Truth*, 9: 108 (December 1905), 370.
179. Vaughan, *op. cit.* (note 2), 61.
180. Quoted in Kumwenda in this volume, 210–1.
181. *Ibid.*, 211.
182. *Ibid.*, 210.
183. D. Arnold, 'Disease, Medicine and Empire' in D. Arnold (ed), *Imperial Medicine and Indigenous Societies* (Manchester: Manchester University Press, 1988), 2.
184. Vaughan, *op. cit.* (note 2), 64–6. See also Kumwenda in this volume, 193–226.
185. Kumwenda in this volume, 211.
186. Ranger, 'Godly Medicine', *op. cit.* (note 12), 270–2.
187. Williams, *op. cit.* (note 18), 276–7.
188. *Ibid.*, 279–80.
189. Gaitskell, 'The Zulu have no Zenanas: Comparing Female Medical Missions in Africa and Asia', paper delivered at a conference on Medical Missions in Asia and Africa, Warwick University, May-June 2002, 11–14.

2

Seeking Souls through the Eyes of the Blind: The Birth of the Medical Missionary Society in Nineteenth-Century China

Michael C. Lazich

The establishment of small hospitals and dispensaries was among the most effective strategies employed by the earliest Protestant missionaries to China. Encouraged by the initial success of such enterprises, yet aware of the need for an administrative apparatus to facilitate their operation, a group of merchants and missionaries established the Medical Missionary Society in 1838 to promote and oversee the work of missionary physicians. This chapter examines the birth and early achievements of the Medical Missionary Society in the context of the period immediately prior to the Opium War, when most Western trade and contact with the Chinese was confined to the southern port city of Canton.

The Protestant missionary movement that emerged from the high tide of European and American evangelicalism in the late-eighteenth and early-nineteenth centuries played a key role in the development of modern Sino-Western relations. Unlike the merchants and traders who preceded them, the earliest Protestant missionaries to China were determined to penetrate the cultural and political barriers that isolated Chinese society from the Western world. Among the most effective strategies employed by these missionaries was the establishment of small hospitals and dispensaries. In bringing the benefits of Western medical science to the Chinese, missionaries were provided with a means of social intercourse with the common people – an opportunity that was otherwise denied them by the various restrictions of the Chinese government. Encouraged by the initial success of such enterprises, a group of merchants and missionaries established the Medical Missionary Society in 1838 to promote and oversee the work of missionary physicians in China. This essay will examine the birth and early achievements of the Medical Missionary Society in the context of the period immediately prior to the Opium War, when most Western trade and contact with the Chinese was confined to the southern port city of Canton.

The 'Canton system' and the Protestant missionary enterprise in China

Although Western merchants had carried on trade with China since the mid-sixteenth century, the Chinese Imperial Government had strictly limited the range of their commercial activities. The presence of foreigners in China had historically represented a threat to the ruling dynasty to which the Chinese authorities normally responded by restricting contact between such outsiders and the general population. Since 1760, for example, the ruling Qing dynasty had confined its trade with most Westerners to the southern port city of Canton located a short distance up the West River in Guangdong Province. The only major exception to this arrangement was the Portuguese centre of trade at Macao, located not far from Canton on the western edge of the river estuary.

Foreigners doing business in Canton were restricted to a block of Western-style buildings along the river outside the southwest corner of the city walls. These 'factories', as they were called, served as the offices and residences of Western traders while they carried out their transactions with the various Hong merchants (*hang* or *hong* means business firm) that comprised the Cohong, a merchant guild supervised by a Court-appointed chief official called the Hoppo. A list of 'Eight Regulations,' dating from 1760 and subsequently reconfirmed by an edict of the Jiaqing Emperor in 1819, restricted the foreigners to a narrowly prescribed range of activity with the intention of limiting the impact of their presence on the population of the city. Among other things, these regulations prohibited the foreigners from entering the city of Canton, or from otherwise wandering from the confines of the factories.[1]

Although Catholic missionaries had established a limited presence in China since their arrival with Portuguese traders in the late-sixteenth century, Protestant missionaries did not appear until 1807, when Robert Morrison of the London Missionary Society discreetly established a mission in Canton by connecting himself with the British East India Company. Laboring virtually alone for over twenty years, Morrison was finally joined in 1830 by Elijah Coleman Bridgman of the American Board of Commissioners for Foreign Missions. These two men quickly developed a warm camaraderie as they attempted to expand their understanding of Chinese culture and acquire the language skills necessary for establishing a secure foundation for an expanded China mission. Morrison, naturally, had a significant head start in this process and served as a mentor to his devout and energetic younger colleague from America.

In his original instructions from the American Board, Bridgman had been directed to acquire, among other things, a thorough knowledge of the Chinese language and to 'make as full communications respecting the character, condition, manners, and rites of the people, especially so far as these things are affected by their religion, as your labors and other circumstances will permit.'[2] Above all, Bridgman was told to keep in mind that his primary objective was to introduce the Christian Gospel among the Chinese, a work for which 'the providence of God may soon open a wide and effectual door'.[3] Bridgman accepted the challenge of these instructions very enthusiastically, and within a few years had assisted in the publication of a variety of religious tracts in Chinese that were cautiously distributed to the Chinese residents of the region around Canton. Although such activities were prohibited by the regulations of the Qing government, the Chinese authorities generally ignored them as long as they did not prove threatening or disruptive.

In 1832, Bridgman also began the publication of the *Chinese Repository*, an English-language journal of sinology that would become a major venue for scholarly investigations of Chinese civilisation and an important instrument for the promotion of missionary work. As the chief editor of the *Chinese Repository*, Bridgman would remain one of the most influential figures in the missionary community as it slowly expanded its presence in the years prior to the Opium War (1839–42). Indeed, it was through articles selected for publication in the *Chinese Repository* that many Europeans and Americans first began to learn about life in China and the activities of foreigners in the factories of Canton. Among these activities was some pioneering medical work undertaken by Western physicians in China in the early years of the nineteenth century. Bridgman was particularly interested in these activities for their exemplary display of Christian philanthropy and because of their great potential as instruments of religious proselytisation.

Pioneers of Western medical practice in China

Providing various medical treatments to the Chinese was not an entirely new activity for Westerners in China in the early-nineteenth century. Physicians associated with the Portuguese outpost at Macao had occasionally offered their services to the Chinese, and the Jesuits had brought their medical knowledge along with them to Beijing as early as the late-sixteenth century. But prior to modern times, the medical practices of Westerners offered little that could improve significantly upon the traditional skills of Chinese practitioners, who over their long history had developed some very effective and sophisticated treatments of their own. This relative parity in medical knowledge and practice would change dramatically, however, as medical science in the West began to advance significantly in the early-nineteenth century. One of the most noteworthy examples of the impact of these advances on China was the introduction of vaccination procedures to stem the raging smallpox epidemics that frequently afflicted the coastal population.

The effective vaccination procedures pioneered by Edward Jenner were first introduced to China by a Portuguese subject who brought the vaccine from Manila to Macao in the spring of 1805.[4] The practice was further propagated among the Chinese by Dr Alexander Pearson, the senior surgeon in Macao for the British East India Company.[5] The East India Company enthusiastically promoted the practice both to protect its agents from the epidemics and to win the favour of the Chinese authorities by stemming the spread of the disease among the civilian population. In time, Chinese Cohong officials had even established a fund for the inoculation of the poor, which offered monetary incentives for families to bring their children forward for this purpose. The work of Pearson was later supplemented by Dr John Livingstone, who took up residence in Macao in 1808 as physician for the East India Company. From Macao, the practice of vaccination was spread with great effect to the neighbouring provinces of Jiangsu and Fujian by Chinese practitioners who had been trained in the procedure by Pearson and Livingstone.[6]

In 1820, Dr Livingstone teamed up with Robert Morrison to open a joint Sino–Western dispensary with a respected Chinese practitioner named Dr Lee. Pearson also contributed a portion of his time to this enterprise. The purpose of this clinic was to provide some basic treatment and effective medicines to Chinese patients and to acquire some understanding of traditional Chinese therapies. During the height of its operation, the dispensary stocked a variety of both Western and Chinese medicines and accumulated an extensive library of Chinese medical treatises.[7] The clinic apparently ceased operating in 1823, when Morrison took a temporary leave of absence from his post in China. The effort nevertheless served as the inspiration for another pioneering clinic opened by Dr T.R. Colledge in 1827.

Like Pearson and Livingstone, Dr Colledge had formerly served as a ship's surgeon for the British East India Company before settling in Macao as a Company physician in 1826. While in Macao, Colledge devoted a significant portion of his time treating the various maladies of the local Chinese. He focused particularly on those afflicted with 'diseases of the eyes', which according to Colledge were 'very prevalent, and from which the utter incapacity of native practitioners denies to them all other hope of relief.'[8] The most common surgical procedure employed by Colledge was a technique called 'couching' for the treatment of cataracts. Europeans had used this procedure since the early-eighteenth century. It involved inserting a small needle into the defective lens and impaling it within the eye to the side of the visual axis where it would hopefully remain without causing additional problems. Because the procedure required only a small puncture wound, the recovery time was short and the rate of success relatively high. Such invasive surgical procedures were rarely used in Chinese medical practice for they conflicted with the more holistic conceptions of healing and physical well being embodied in the Daoist and Confucian traditions.

Colledge's dedicated efforts treating Chinese patients in Macao soon attracted the attention of his Company colleagues and employers, who began contributing funds for the upkeep of a small hospital capable of housing about forty patients. In time, Colledge also received contributions from some of the wealthier Chinese residents of the city, as they too grew increasingly impressed with the beneficial results of his labours. Indeed, by 1832 Colledge's small ophthalmic hospital had treated about 4,000 patients who, according to Colledge, 'have been relieved of impending blindness, resumed their usual occupations, and have supported, in lieu of remaining a burden on, their families.'[9] Unfortunately, Colledge was forced to close his hospital when his medical duties for the Company increased following the departure of Dr Pearson in the winter of 1832/3.

The success of Colledge's hospital in Macao was heartily praised by Bridgman and his missionary colleagues in Canton, who, in October 1833 published a laudatory account of the doctor's achievements in the *Chinese Repository.* This account included translations of two effusively grateful testimonials in Chinese sent to Colledge by former patients whose eyesight he had restored. In a brief introduction to the article, the editors of the *Chinese Repository* expressed their hope that 'the publication of such facts will do good by inciting others to go and do likewise.'[10] They also asked their readers to consider 'whether the modern teachers of Christianity, who have gone forth to the desolate places of the earth, have not overlooked too much the bodily infirmities of those whom they would benefit.'[11] After all, as the editors pointed out, 'the conduct, as well as the precept of our divine Lord is very full on this point; he not only *taught* from place to place, but "he went about *doing* good"; he not only healed the sick and cured the lame, but "unto many that were blind he gave sight."'[12]

Inspired by the example of Dr Colledge, physicians in Canton, led by Dr James H. Bradford, opened a public dispensary in 1828 in order to distribute medicines to the Chinese residents of that city.[13] In an article praising the success of the clinic in the *Chinese Repository*, the writer described the typical scene one might behold there:

> At an early hour in the morning, one may daily witness the sick, the blind, and the lame – of all ages and both sexes – crowding around the doors of the

> Dispensary. We have seen helpless children brought there in the arms of their nurses – or more commonly lashed, according to the custom of the country, upon the back of a young servant. We have seen old, blind, decrepit men, 'with staff in hand', led thither by their little grandchildren; while others, who were in better circumstances, were brought in their sedans.[14]

The article then described in captivating detail some of the typical cases successfully treated at the clinic, such as the young man who had swallowed a deadly dose of raw opium because his father had forbidden him the charms of a prostitute with whom he had become enamoured. But particular emphasis was directed to those who came to the dispensary with diseased eyes, the treatment of which 'they could never have obtained from native practitioners'.[15]

Applauding the achievements of these earlier enterprises as shining examples of Christian philanthropy and marvelling at the splendid opportunity they provided to teach Christianity to the Chinese, the editor declared that their successes 'both warrant and encourage a continuation and extension of these benevolent exertions, and at the same time excite others to follow examples so worthy of imitation.'[16] It is not surprising therefore, that Bridgman began around this time to plead emphatically with the American Board to send out an individual adequately trained as a physician in order to establish a small missionary-run hospital in Canton. Indeed, when Ira Tracy, one of the American Board's recently arrived representatives in Canton, decided in December of 1833 to transfer to Singapore, Bridgman insisted that his replacement be a missionary trained in the medical profession. Referring to the articles he had published several months earlier in the *Chinese Repository*, Bridgman wrote:

> I desire that his place here may be reoccupied immediately by an able physician. By referring to the Oct. No. of the Repos. [*Chinese Repository*] you will see what a field there is here for medical men. I have, in previous letters, said something on the subject; & now all of us are desirous that such a man should be here. He should be a first rate oculist, & understand all cutaneous diseases. While he heals the sick, & opens the eyes of the blind, he will find plenty of opportunities for distributing books.[17]

Bridgman and his colleagues in Canton had become increasingly convinced of the tremendous potential of a missionary hospital for disseminating knowledge of Christianity in China. After all, all other forms of intimate contact with the Chinese were formally forbidden by the regulations of the Canton system, and although the missionaries had found other means to distribute the religious tracts that they produced, it was always done at the risk of antagonizing the Chinese authorities and thus endangering the safety and interests of their mission. This need for a more secure and sustainable strategy for 'spreading the Gospel' in China became even more urgent and evident following the 'Napier Incident' of 1834.

The Napier Incident and the missionary crisis in Canton

Following the suspension of the British East India Company's monopoly of English trade in China in 1833, William John Napier (Lord Napier) was sent to Canton as the newly designated Chief Superintendent of British Trade to attempt to negotiate a more satisfactory set of arrangements with Chinese officials. Merchants and missionaries in China had long resented the restrictions of the Canton system and were hopeful that the new circumstances of trade would provide the British representative with a convincing justification for his appeal. In an article published in the *Chinese Repository*, Bridgman declared optimistically that:

> [T]he train of events now in progress must sooner or later, and perhaps within a very short period, introduce here a new order of things – overcoming ancient prejudices, breaking down misanthropic and antinational antipathies, and laying the foundations of an unrestricted intercourse between the people of China and the enlightened states of Christendom.[18]

Unfortunately, Lord Napier's attempt to open a dialogue on the subject with the Chinese authorities proved to be an unmitigated failure. Soon after arriving in Canton, he made a brash attempt to contact the governor of Canton, Lu Kun, by delivering a letter directly to the city gates. This was an explicit violation of Chinese regulations regarding official communications, and Lu Kun reacted angrily by expelling Napier from Canton and suspending British trading rights. As tensions escalated, Napier took his argument to the Chinese people by publicly posting a statement in Chinese that blamed the 'ignorance and obstinacy' of the Chinese governor for the current disturbance and insisted that the British intended 'to trade with China on principles of mutual benefit' and would continue to pursue this end until they gained this 'point of equal importance to both countries'.[19] To demonstrate his resolve, Napier ordered the British frigates *Andromache* and *Imogene* up the Pearl River as far as the port facilities at Whampoa, a short distance from Canton. If the Chinese failed to respond more positively to his demands, he was prepared to press the issue with military force.

But Lord Napier would not live long enough to carry out his threat, for he became desperately ill with malarial fever and passed away in Macao on October 11, 1834. Tragically, Robert Morrison, who had befriended Napier and had agreed to serve as his translator, also died earlier that summer after a rainy, night-time journey upriver from his home in Macao to join the

British Superintendent in Canton. Thus, in the end, Napier's mission had not only failed to achieve its original objective of re-adjusting relations with the Chinese, but had robbed the missionaries of their most experienced member and, even more disastrously, had intensified the suspicion and hostility of Chinese officials towards the Western residents of Canton.

With the authorities now on the alert for what they considered heterodox or seditious publications by the foreigners, Bridgman and the others could no longer print religious tracts in Chinese as they had been doing in the shop operated by their native convert Liang Afah; nor could they as openly or easily distribute such materials among the residents of Canton. In fact, a public decree issued by the 'Chief Magistrate of Nanhae' ordered the seizure and destruction of all the 'evil and obscene books of the foreign barbarians', threatening that any Chinese printers found assisting the missionaries would be 'immediately seized and punished with severity'.[20]

The new restrictions imposed on the foreigners by the Chinese forced the missionaries to seek viable alternatives to their former evangelical strategy. Prior to this unfortunate episode, the emphasis had been on the printing and distribution of religious tracts such as Liang Afah's famed 'Good Words to Admonish the Age' (*Quanshi liangyan*).[21] This activity had been generously supported by the various Bible and tract societies in England and America.[22] But with this avenue of access to the Chinese now strictly cut off, the establishment of a missionary-operated hospital became of paramount importance as it became the only feasible means for carrying on their work. Fortunately, Bridgman's hopes for a medical missionary were soon fulfilled by the arrival of Dr Peter Parker on 26 October 1834.

Dr Peter Parker: the first medical missionary to China

Parker was a graduate of both the Medical and Theological Departments of Yale College. He was ordained as a missionary in Philadelphia on 16 May 1834. His medical training, as described by E.V. Gulick, consisted of 'attending two years of lectures; it was academic, nonclinical, nonlaboratory and thus in line with the standard practices of good medical schools of that day.'[23] In addition, he spent a short but very useful period of practical training in an eye infirmary and hospital in New York City.[24] Although he was sent to China by the American Board largely in response to Bridgman's appeals for a medical missionary in Canton, Parker was given the latitude to settle wherever conditions proved favourable.[25]

Inasmuch as Parker had arrived in Canton during the darkest days immediately following the Lord Napier incident, it is not surprising that he decided that his prospects for establishing a medical practice, preaching the Gospel, and studying Chinese were, for the time being, better in Singapore at the station recently established by Ira Tracy. Therefore, in December

Figure 2.1

Dr Peter Parker by the Western trained Chinese painter Lam Qua, *c.*1840. Courtesy Yale University, Harvey Cushing/John Hay Whitney Medical Library.

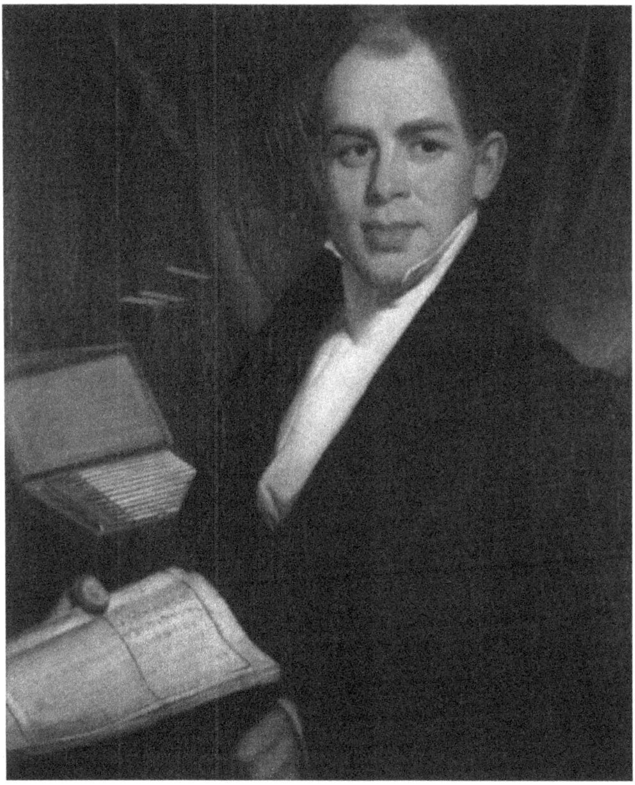

1834, he departed for his new post with the intention of returning to Canton after conditions had settled and he had acquired some mastery of the Chinese language. Not surprisingly, Bridgman was very unhappy with Parker's decision and continued to insist that Canton have its physician. Writing to the American Board in December, he remarked:

> Br Parker has given you fully the reasons for going to Singapore. But we want a physician here – & as you have elsewhere stronger demands for preachers immediately – one not a clergyman perhaps would be best for this place. Pray for us.[26]

Bridgman further publicised the importance of establishing a medical clinic in China by printing in the *Chinese Repository* a pamphlet written by an unnamed 'Philanthropist' which recounted the history and manifold benefits of Dr Colledge's former hospital in Macao. The author of this pamphlet applauded the spirit of benevolence that inspired Colledge's efforts, noting, 'a skillful and experienced surgeon or physician is everywhere hailed and welcomed by suffering humanity as the harbinger of hope and comfort.'[27] Elaborating upon this theme, the author described the introduction of vaccination into China by Dr Pearson and the operation of Colledge's Ophthalmic Hospital as 'the fountain from whence will spring the peaceable, gentle, and humane influence, that will open the Chinese empire to free and friendly intercourse with Europeans.'[28] Given the recent crisis in Sino–foreign relations, this additional positive consequence of medical work in China assumed even greater importance than it had previously.

Ironically, not long after his arrival in Singapore, Parker discovered that opportunities for learning the language were even fewer there than in Canton, and his time became quickly consumed by the flood of patients who sought medical treatment. In an entry in his journal dated 22 February 1835, Parker remarked:

> As it respects my intercourse with the Chinese, and my medical and surgical practice among them, it far exceeds all of which I ever thought, but in relation to the language, if I except the speaking of it, I am very far in the rear of what I hoped to have accomplished before the expiration of two months.[29]

As he told his sister Maria in a letter written home around this time:

> ...it is usual to receive about fifty patients at my house every morning, besides those whom I visit; and as my house is spacious and rice is cheap, I take patients to my house as I think expedient.[30]

In addition to the burden of his busy practice and great disappointment over his inability to devote sufficient time to language study, Parker's health steadily declined and he began to suffer from a variety of symptoms that he attributed to the tropical climate.[31] Therefore, after prayerfully contemplating his prospects in Singapore and concluding that they were highly unfavourable, Parker accepted an offer of passage aboard the *Fort William*, which was en route from Calcutta to Whampoa, and returned to Canton on 4 September 1835. Parker's few months in Singapore were not spent in vain, however, for he had acquired a great deal of experience treating the various illnesses and disorders that he would soon encounter in Canton.

The ophthalmic hospital in Canton

Unfortunately, the tense situation in Canton had improved little since the time of Parker's departure, and the activities of the missionaries remained under the strictest scrutiny as the Chinese authorities maintained their vigilance following their encounter with Lord Napier the year before. Indeed, virtually all contact with the Chinese residents of the city had been cut off, and the missionaries were confined to their residences in the foreign factories. Under these severe constraints, establishing a missionary hospital presented itself as the only means to reopen those channels of contact with the Chinese necessary for fulfilling their larger religious objectives. So, warmly welcoming Parker back into their community, the missionaries immediately turned their efforts in this direction; and within a couple of months, they arranged to rent a location for a hospital in the factories – at the greatly reduced rate of US$500 *per annum* – from a wealthy Cohong merchant named Howqua (Wu Chongyao).[32]

The site chosen was factory Number Seven of the Fungtai Hong. According to Parker:

> [I]ts retired situation and direct communication with a street, so that patients could come and go without annoying foreigners by passing through their hongs, or excite the observations of natives by being seen to resort to a foreigner's house, rendered it most suitable for the purpose.[33]

Furthermore, a large room on the second story made it possible to temporarily lodge at least forty patients and to provide seating for many more.

It was decided that the hospital would devote itself primarily to treatment of diseases of the eye. This was because such disorders were very common in China, and their treatment, as they knew from Colledge's experience, required relatively little time and attention and yet was perhaps the most appreciated because it was beyond the skill of native practitioners. Although Parker would by no means confine his practice exclusively to the treatment of eye disease, the treatment of this type of disorder held the highest promise for success, and would thus enable the missionaries to process the largest number of patients, to whom the missionaries could then distribute religious tracts and convey their evangelical message.

Parker began practicing medicine out of his new hospital in Canton on 4 November 1835, and as news spread among the Chinese of his great skill and success, he was flooded with patients.[34] As he reported to the American Board after only a few weeks of operation:

> I have now three hundred patients, who, with few exceptions, have been afflicted with ophthalmic diseases. Of this number, as large a portion have been discharged convalescent, as from the time and nature of their cases, could be expected. Unqualified confidence is manifested by those who have applied, and numbers have been put off whom I could not receive. Indeed we have put up a notice today, that no new patients can be received until fifteen days. Much gratitude is manifested by those who have benefited by the means used.[35]

This report was later printed in the *Missionary Herald,* a popular journal published by the American Board and distributed throughout New England. As subsequent reports were similarly publicised, Parker's benevolent accomplishments become widely known and admired by many in the United States who intently followed the affairs of America's small band of missionaries in China.

Indeed, within a short time, Parker became a celebrity among both Chinese and foreigners for his philanthropic labours and achievements. Although Bridgman was concerned about Parker's inability to find sufficient time to devote to improving his Chinese language skills, he was overjoyed at the positive influence the project had over the affairs of the Mission. In his letters to the American Board, Bridgman called upon the directors to increase their efforts to recruit more men able to serve in this capacity:

> Many able physicians should be sent. I am more and more in favor of such men being connected with all our missions. They are powerful auxiliaries – good pioneers. At every new station formed, I should be glad to see one of these men, to give his time – his whole time – after learning the language – to this branch of labor.[36]

Emphasising the importance of their own efforts to the larger mission of spreading the Gospel, Bridgman later wrote: 'The hospital not only affords opportunity for doing much good to the bodies, & thereby to show the skill and good-will of "distant barbarians", but it presents many and very excellent occasions to prescribe for moral maladies.'[37]

Dr Colledge was also impressed with the positive impact of Parker's hospital and, while not a missionary himself, wrote an article for the *Chinese Repository* that acclaimed such efforts as an invaluable accompaniment to missionary work. Sharing his own knowledge of the character of the Chinese people and their response to Western evangelism, Colledge wrote:

> Observation has convinced me that the only way by which they will be led into the course of reflection which shall result in the end so much desired by all who have their interest at heart, will be by exhibiting among them the

> virtues of charity and humanity, then leading them gradually to the comprehension of the motives and principles from which these virtues spring. Those who seek to convert, must first gain their confidence by rendering themselves useful.[38]

In order to accomplish this, Colledge suggested:

> [T]hose societies that now send missionaries should also send physicians, ...who on their arrival in China should commence by making themselves acquainted with the language; and in place of attempting any regular system of teaching or preaching, let them heal the sick and administer to their wants, mingling with their medical practice such instructions either in religion, philosophy, medicine, chemistry, & c., as the minds of individuals may have been gradually prepared to receive.[39]

Bridgman and Colledge were both of the opinion that for any medical missionary to be successful, he must be freed from the obligation of devoting too much of his time to the duties of preaching. Although Colledge admired Parker for 'having qualified himself to labor in this field both as a physician and minister of the gospel', he emphasised the point that 'more may be accomplished by keeping the two professions distinct.'[40] The editor's introduction to Colledge's article, probably written by Bridgman, also argued that:

> [A] division of labor is required, for when an individual undertakes the two, he will always be under the temptation of neglecting one of them, there being in either enough and more than enough to occupy all his time and strength.[41]

Parker's own experience undertaking the myriad responsibilities associated with the hospital seemed to verify this, for after only a few months of its opening, missionary reports to the American Board began to express concern that Parker's duties, while of inestimable value to the mission, threatened to overwhelm him.[42]

Parker had indeed become entirely absorbed by the work of the hospital. By the time of his 'Second Quarterly Report' on the hospital issued in May 1836, the facility had already treated a total of 1,283 patients. According to Parker, the number could have been much higher 'were the strength of an individual sufficient for the task of an adequate attendance.'[43] For nearly a month, however, he reported that:

> [T]he doors were nominally closed against new applicants, and at least one third of the new patients have gained admittance by importunity and the

> combined influence of their friends, when there were already as many in the hospital as could faithfully be attended.[44]

Parker even began to treat those who might have been expected to be the most hostile to the enterprise, noting how ten government officials, and more than twice that number of their clerks and private secretaries, had visited the hospital as patients. In all of these cases, Parker proclaimed, 'their grateful acknowledgement of benefits received have exhibited no less warmth than their countrymen, in the humble walks of life, whom they have met in large numbers upon the same floor.'[45]

The quarterly reports that Parker issued for publication in the *Chinese Repository* provided a detailed record of the hospital's services and achievements during the opening years of its operation. As originally intended, the majority of cases that Parker selected for treatment were disorders of the eye, which he listed under more than thirty categories. Cataracts, chronic ophthalmia, and 'opacity and vascularity of the cornea' were recorded as the most common of these aliments. Parker found that the oblique curvature of the upper eyelid peculiar to the Chinese, occasionally allowed the upper lid to fold under, 'occasioning the loss of many eyes, and the opacity and vascularity of the cornea in a still greater number.'[46] Parker was able to correct this condition with a simple surgical procedure pioneered by Dr Colledge, who had invented a pair of forceps specifically for this purpose. Parker also used the 'couching' technique for the treatment of cataracts with great success, restoring the eyesight of hundreds of grateful patients who had given up hope of correcting their condition through traditional Chinese medical practices.

While disorders of the eye thus continued to comprise the majority of the cases that Parker treated, in time he was increasingly called upon to apply his talents to other conditions and injuries as well. In each quarterly report, Parker would select some of the more interesting or unusual of these cases and provide a relatively detailed description of the patient's circumstances and treatment. In one report, for example, he described the case of a woman who had fallen nearly twelve feet off a ladder while taking in some clothes from an upper loft.[47] She had impaled herself on a piece of bamboo that passed through her right armpit and exited through her upper shoulder, fracturing her clavicle. Parker carefully cleaned and dressed the wounds, injecting them with a solution of nitrate of silver, and took measures to restrict any unnecessary movement of the injury for several days. While Parker was not very hopeful at first, within nine days the patient had recovered enough to return home.

In time, Parker also treated a large number of patients afflicted with tumours of various sorts. These cases proved to be the most challenging, and yet the most interesting, of those accepted for treatment. As Parker's skill as a surgeon became more practised and refined, his handling of these cases became more daring. In one report he describes the case of Chin Aying, a girl of thirteen years of age, who had become nearly incapacitated by three large sarcomatous tumors situated together between her shoulders and above the spine.[48] According to Parker, 'the largest of the cluster was firmly united to one of the spinous processes by a semi-cartilaginous or bony union.'[49] Not long after they were extirpated – a process that required some very delicate surgery – Parker was pleased to report that 'no unpleasant consequences have followed... and the wound is kindly healing up by granulations.'[50]

Some of the tumor cases treated by Parker were exceedingly grotesque, such as the man of twenty-seven whose facial tumour was eighteen and a half inches in circumference, or the 20-year-old female who had a pendulous tumour hanging from the chin and larynx that 'centrally measured 2 feet, 3 inches and vertically 3 feet, 2 inches.'[51] These 'new and anomalous diseases,' of course, brought even greater public attention to the missionary hospital in Canton and led Parker to call for not only the continuation of efforts already begun in his eye infirmary, 'but also of establishing other departments, and of supplying them with men of requisite qualifications.'[52]

The Formation of the Medical Missionary Society in China

As the operations of the missionary hospital in Canton expanded and diversified, the need for an administrative apparatus to manage the facility's business and finances became ever more apparent. As Bridgman explained in a report to the American Board in May 1836, while financial contributions for the hospital were generously forthcoming from both the Chinese and foreign residents of Canton, the absence of an executive organisation to attend to its management meant that 'the hand to prescribe and administer what is requisite, cannot be so readily supplied.'[53] Indeed, the money needed to sustain the hospital's operations was more than adequately supplied by the British and American merchants at Macao and Canton. As Parker had reported to the American Board within a few months after the hospital had opened: 'the hospital has received liberal, voluntary patronage from benevolent residents here and at Macao – $1,050 have already been subscribed. These donations are uniformly accompanied with kindest wishes for the success of the undertaking.'[54] By May, that amount had increased to $1400, which Parker graciously welcomed as 'an encouragement, a generosity, the more sensibly appreciated as it has been unexpected.'[55] It seems that Westerners doing business in China were more than willing to contribute to a cause that, unlike some of the other missionary enterprises, rendered such palpable benefits to the Chinese people.

Another need that Parker faced as the flood of patients to his hospital increased was well-trained and responsible helpers. While he occasionally received a few days of voluntary assistance from trained physicians who were then or previously connected with the British East India Company, such as William Jardine, the British merchant who had formerly served as a ship's surgeon, or Dr R.H. Cox, who at that time served as surgeon to the Company in Canton, there was a growing need for Chinese-speaking assistants with some rudimentary medical skills. As Parker declared in his Second Quarterly Report:

> [I]t would add much to the efficiency of the institution, if the constant services of a few well-educated native youth, anxious to become masters of the healing art, and prepared to go through a thorough course of instruction, could be secured; and the benefits, which would accrue to such young men, would by no means be inconsiderable.[56]

Pleased with the success of the hospital in Canton, and yet increasingly conscious of its growing needs, Parker, Bridgman, and Colledge issued a circular calling for the formation of a 'Medical Missionary Society in China' in order both to establish a permanent basis for the continued operation of Parker's hospital and to initiate similar projects elsewhere.[57] In the opening passage of the circular the men announced:

> Viewing with peculiar interest the good effects that seem likely to be produced by medical practice among the Chinese, especially as tending to bring about a more social and friendly intercourse between them and foreigners, as well as to diffuse the arts and sciences of Europe and America, and in the end to introduce the Gospel of our Savior in place of the pitiable superstitions by which their minds are now governed, we have resolved to attempt the foundation of a society to be called the 'Medical Missionary Society in China'.[58]

It is impossible to fully understand the motives declared in this introductory statement without taking into consideration the full range of activities undertaken by the missionaries at this time. Bridgman and the other missionaries who began to arrive in China in the early nineteenth century were motivated by the conviction that they were serving the cause of Christianity at the dawn of the prophesied Christian millennium.[59] Among the various signs of the advent of this era was the vast expansion of human knowledge that was establishing the conditions for universal prosperity and spiritual rejuvenation. Particularly inspired by the millennial vision of the evangelical theoretician Samuel Hopkins, the American missionaries believed that 'there will be a great increase of light and knowledge to a degree vastly beyond what has been before.'[60] Indeed, Hopkins saw the expansion of the religious spirit and the human quest for understanding as a dynamically integrated process of spiritual and intellectual perfection.[61]

Thus convinced that the spread of Christianity was inextricably bound with the spread of all forms of knowledge, the missionaries were committed to conveying both religious and non-religious – scientific, historical, etc. – truths and information to the Chinese. Therefore, around the same time that the missionaries were calling for the formation of a Medical Missionary Society they also established a Society for the Diffusion of Useful Knowledge in China. The chief function of this organisation was 'to prepare and publish, in a cheap form, plain and easy treatises in the Chinese language, on such branches of useful knowledge as are suited to the existing state and condition of the Chinese empire.'[62] In fact, the missionaries had begun to produce an increasing number of tracts in Chinese that introduced Western science, history, and literature – along with religion – to their Chinese readers. It is not surprising, therefore, that the circular calling for the Medical Missionary Society spoke in millenarian terms of the power of truth, even medical truth, as a revolutionising force capable of ushering in the higher truth of Christianity:

> In the vast conflict which is to revolutionize the intellectual and moral world, we may not underrate the value of any weapon. As a means, then, to waken the dormant mind of China, may we not place a high value upon medical truth, and seek its introduction with the good hope of its becoming the handmaid of religious truth? If an inquiry after truth on any subject is elicited, is there not a great point gained?[63]

Thus, given the crisis with the Chinese authorities regarding the distribution of foreign publications following the Lord Napier incident, the success of Parker's hospital in providing virtually the only means for distributing both religious and non-religious tracts to the residents of Canton assumed paramount importance. Bridgman's letters to the American Board at this time frequently noted this important use of the facility by those missionaries who assisted with its operation. Indeed, the materials that were now being produced at Ira Tracy's printing establishment in Singapore were to be distributed to the Chinese primarily through the channel provided by Parker's hospital in Canton. The hospital had therefore become an indispensable part of the larger missionary enterprise. That the hospital also enjoyed the enthusiastic support of the other foreign residents of China who applauded its purely philanthropic function was an added advantage that could hardly be overlooked.

In practical terms, the Medical Missionary Society was thus intended to provide permanent foundations for the continuation and expansion of the hospital in Canton while at the same time promoting the establishment of similar institutions elsewhere. In their circular, Parker, Bridgman, and Colledge listed four primary objectives necessary for achieving this goal. The first was to serve as a base of support so 'that those who come out as medical missionaries to China, may find here those to whom they can apply for assistance and information.'[64] Secondly:

> [T]hat by this means their services may be made immediately available, while, at the same time, they may be put in the way of learning the language for the purpose of fitting themselves to practice in parts of the country to which foreigners have not hitherto gained free access.[65]

The various grammars and dictionaries produced by the missionaries provided the most effective means for undertaking a study of the various dialects of Chinese. A primary function of the Medical Missionary Society would therefore be to co-ordinate and direct the placement and language training of those who sought to become medical missionaries in China.

The third objective of the Society would be to promote the recruitment of new medical missionaries to China by the various missionary societies of England and America, and inasmuch as they considered themselves 'acquainted with the peculiarities of the case', the men expressed their 'desire to draw attention to the selection of men of suitable qualifications'.[66] In other words, they would assist in identifying individuals who had the personal characteristics and educational training most conducive to success. Describing some of the personal characteristics of an ideal candidate, they wrote:

> It is indispensable that the men who shall conduct the institution be not only masters of their profession, and conciliating in their manners towards all classes, but *judicious* men – men thoroughly imbued with the spirit of *genuine piety*, ready to endure hardships, and to sacrifice personal comfort, that they may commend the gospel of our Lord and Savior, and so cooperate in its introduction among the millions of this partially civilized yet, *mysterious* and idolatrous empire – men willing to suffer the loss of all things for joys that await those who f*or Christ's sake* do good on earth.[67]

Lastly, and perhaps most importantly, the men proposed 'to receive any sums of money which may be given in aid of this object, and to disburse them as shall be deemed expedient, until the Society be formed, so that the labors of those who engage in the cause shall not be retarded.'[68] These funds were not, however, to be used to pay any form of salary to those who wished to become medical missionaries. Indeed, the men emphasised that 'in order to the success of the object contemplated, [*sic*] those who engage in it must not receive any pecuniary *remuneration*: the work throughout must be, and appear to be, one of *disinterested benevolence*.'[69]

In a final appeal for aid from the 'pious and benevolent', the men concluded their circular by reiterating the millenarian theme that lent such symbolic importance to medical institutions as the primary agency for disseminating Christianity to the Chinese:

> [W]hen the millions which compose this mighty empire shall feel the influence of true religion and civilization, when the light of Christianity shall take the place of the dark cloud of paganism, which now envelopes [*sic*] them, then will be fulfilled, in its spiritual sense, the prophecy of Isaiah: 'The eyes of the blind shall be opened, and the ears of the deaf shall be unstopped; the lame shall leap as an hart, and the tongue of the dumb sing.'[70]

Although the Medical Missionary Society would not become formally established until more than a year following the issuing of the circular by Parker, Bridgman, and Colledge, the three men undertook a number of preliminary steps to fulfil the objectives they had outlined. Parker's hospital continued to flourish as donations, now managed by the group as a whole, increasingly flowed in. In a report to the American Board dated 7 March 1837, the missionaries of Canton wrote:

> The Author of Mercies has continued his smiles upon the Ophthalmic Hospital. Of 2,800 patients, by the means employed, many enjoy sight, hearing, and health of which they were deprived. A considerable number also enjoy life who otherwise had been dead. The institution is every month becoming more & more extensively known & appreciated, as the cases from Nanking show. In neighboring villages he [Parker] is often recognized & invited into the household of his patients. The expenses of the Hospital have been less than the subscriptions & donations for its support the last year.[71]

Colledge had also started once again to devote more of his time to Chinese patients in Macao. In May 1837, Bridgman had even helped him procure a house that the men hoped to turn into a hospital similar to the one in Canton, personally journeying to Macao in August to close the deal and take possession of the facility.[72] In a joint letter dated 12 September 1837, that was later printed in the *Missionary Herald*, the Canton mission informed the American Board that 'the proposed Medical Missionary Society' had purchased a house in Macao for US$2,000 that was suitable for upwards of one hundred and fifty patients.[73] Over the next several months, Colledge undertook the responsibility of refurbishing the building in preparation for its opening under the auspices of the Medical Missionary Society.

Ironically, around this time, the directors of the American Board began complaining that its representatives were becoming pre-occupied with such ancillary projects while neglecting their primary duty to preach the Gospel. By the end of 1837, they had even begun pressuring the missionaries to curtail their involvement in all non-religious enterprises. The American Board insisted that the primary task of their missionaries was to preach the Gospel to the native people in their own language. In the report of its Twenty-Eighth Annual Meeting, it was stated that:

> [T]he leading object of the missions of the Board among the heathen is, with the blessing of God, to rear up native churches, place them under the care and instruction of competent native elders ordained over them, and furnish them with ample, self-propagating gospel instrumentalities.[74]

The missionaries were ordered to expend their time and resources in the most efficient manner possible, and inasmuch as 'the preaching of the gospel' was 'the most essential and least expensive of all the agencies', it 'should be supported, if necessary, by the sacrifice of all agencies not essentially connected with the conversion of the heathen and the permanent influence of the Christian religion.'[75]

This policy of the American Board conformed closely to the views of its Corresponding Secretary, Rufus Anderson. Anderson had long been wary of organisations such as the Medical Missionary Society and had begun to speak out more strongly against such undertakings. He urged all representatives of the American Board to focus exclusively upon their 'sublime spiritual object' and give up their vain pursuit of 'reorganizing, by various direct means …the structure of that social system, of which their converts form a part.'[76] It is not surprising therefore, that Parker's reports respecting the hospital became more defensive in tone, conceding, 'the danger should be guarded against of these becoming institutions for the relief of bodily evils merely, & not tributary to the good of the soul as they ought to be.'[77] But Parker also attempted to convince Anderson of the important role of medical men in conveying Christianity to the Chinese, arguing that 'pious men who are physicians merely… have a peculiar advantage in imparting instruction to the heathen,' for such a man has 'in his own person, opened the eye of the long blind, and removed the limb or administered the medicine with his own hand....'[78]

It becomes clear from their correspondence that Bridgman and Parker resented Anderson's suggestion that the missionaries were neglecting their ultimate purpose. When the American Board directed the Mission to go on a 'retrenchment system' in order to limit its expenditures of time and money to nothing other than their primary religious tasks, Bridgman told Anderson that 'I fear you do not understand things here so fully as it is desirable you should… were you here, you would have impressions, & different views, from what you now have.'[79] In the end, Bridgman and Parker resisted the efforts of the American Board to halt their involvement in the Medical Missionary Society, and although bitter differences of opinion over this issue would eventually cause Parker to sever his relationship with the American Board, the hospital in Canton and the work of the Medical Missionary Society would continue to benefit from the enthusiastic support of both Bridgman and Parker.[80]

The circular issued by Parker, Bridgman, and Colledge calling for an effective administrative organisation to facilitate the propagation of Western-style medical establishments finally came to fruition in February 1838, when a public meeting was convened in Canton for the formation of the 'Medical Missionary Society in China.' The first meeting was held in the rooms of the General Chamber of Commerce in Canton, where the group reviewed and adopted a constitution and designated an executive committee. Dr T.R. Colledge was elected as president; Dr Parker, William Jardine, Robert Inglis, Alexander Anderson, G. Tradescant Lay, and E.C. Bridgman were designated as vice-presidents. Unfortunately, Colledge, who was unable to attend this first meeting, was compelled by personal circumstances to leave China at the very time that the Medical Missionary Society was formally established; however, his prestige and experience as a pioneering physician in China meant that he would continue as the President of the Society until his death in 1879.

Reiterating most of the goals and themes addressed in the original circular of October 1836, the constitution of the Society declared the intention of its members to 'encourage the practice of medicine among the Chinese, to extend them some of those benefits which science, patient investigation, and the ever-kindling light of discussion have conferred upon ourselves.'[81] To achieve this end, the Society was to provide inducements for 'gentlemen of the medical profession to come and practice gratuitously among the Chinese, by affording the usual aid of hospitals, medicine, and attendants.'[82] Carefully delineating the range of authority that the Society intended to retain over those physicians who accepted its patronage, the men resolved that the Society will:

> [E]xpect a strict observance of any general regulations for the management of its institutions, and a diligent study of some one dialect of the Chinese tongue… and that it will reserve to itself the right of withdrawing its patronage, at the discretion of the committee of management, from any

individual who may, from non-compliance with its regulations, or from other causes, incur its displeasure.[83]

At the second meeting of the Medical Missionary Society held on 24 April 1838, Parker was asked to temporarily operate the newly prepared hospital in Macao that was left unattended with Colledge's departure. The occasion for this brief transfer of Parker's services was the need for improvements and repairs to the building housing the infirmary in Canton – repairs that were entirely paid for by the hospital's generous Chinese benefactor, Howqua. Parker opened the hospital in Macao on 5 July 1838, and during the three months that he worked there, he managed to treat 700 patients, mostly for diseases of the eye. Unfortunately, there was no qualified physician able to replace Dr Parker when he returned to Canton and the facility in Macao was temporarily forced to close.

Fortunately, however, appeals by the Medical Missionary Society for a qualified physician to serve in Macao were met in early 1839 by the arrival of Dr William Lockhart, a representative of the London Missionary Society. Lockhart, who was the first medical missionary drawn to China specifically to associate himself with the Medical Missionary Society, received his medical training at Meath Hospital in Dublin and Guy's Hospital in London.[84] Soon after arriving in China, he spent several months in Canton observing the operation of Parker's hospital and studying the Chinese language, and on 1 July 1839 he reopened the hospital in Macao. Unfortunately, the advent of the opium crisis that summer between the British and the Chinese forced him to leave Macao in August and take up temporary residence in Batavia, the Dutch colonial capital of the East Indies. In time, however, Lockhart would return to Macao to become one of the most influential figures in the medical missionary movement.

Conclusion

The Opium War between China and Great Britain marked an important turning point in Sino–Western relations by bringing an end to the Canton system of trade that had so restricted the activities of both merchants and missionaries in China. A major attempt by the Chinese government to stem the smuggling of opium into China by Western traders resulted in a humiliating military defeat for China's Qing dynasty rulers. The 1842 Treaty of Nanjing that ended the conflict forced the Chinese to cede Hong Kong to British control and entitled English merchants to set up operations in five new 'treaty ports'. By 1844, a series of additional treaties signed with the other major Western powers not only extended to them the privileges granted to the British but won the foreign merchants and missionaries a range of other concessions as well.[85]

While the war itself forced the temporary disruption of the operations of the Medical Missionary Society's hospitals in Canton and Macao, the new advantages gained with the establishment of the 'treaty port system' opened a broad range of new opportunities for the medical missionaries. Among these was the privilege of missionaries to purchase property in the treaty ports for the construction of churches and hospitals. Indeed, Article Seventeen of the American Treaty of Wangxia that allowed Westerners to 'enjoy all proper accommodation in obtaining houses and places of business, ...and also hospitals, churches and cemeteries,' was formulated by Bridgman and Parker who were hired to serve as translators and advisors for the American emissary to China, Caleb Cushing.[86]

The years following the Opium War thus witnessed a vast expansion of the projects undertaken by the Medical Missionary Society. At the annual meeting of the Society held on 28 September 1842, it was resolved that 'an Abstract of the history of the Society, from its commencement to the present time, with the prospects that are now opening for an extension of its sphere of usefulness, be drawn up and published.'[87] Published in the April 1843 issue of the *Chinese Repository,* the authors of this abstract triumphantly declared their aspirations:

> The prospects now opening, encourage us in the highest degree to persevere in the same course which has already proved to be so successful. Peace has been established with China, and upon terms that promise enlarged facilities for the prosecution of the labors of the medical missionary, as well as of others interested in the temporal and spiritual welfare of this large portion of their fellow men. Access is now given to five of the principle seaports of the empire – Canton, Amoy, Fuchau, Ningpo and Shanghai; and in these we have the best grounds for believing that a free intercourse with the people will be available; and it is with the liveliest gratitude to the Almighty, that we are enabled to state, that the Medical Missionary Society is in some measure prepared to take advantage of these new openings.[88]

Indeed, the Medical Missionary Society would succeed in establishing many new hospitals throughout China as the country was forced to open its doors ever more widely to Westerners, and although the proceedings of the Society would occasionally be marred by factional disputes among its leading members, no other Western organisation in China would win the same measure of esteem and support from philanthropists in both China and the West. Peter Parker would eventually leave his hospital in Canton to serve as a diplomatic representative of the United States Government in east Asia;

and while his accomplishments in this new career were significantly less successful than those he enjoyed as a physician, his personal example as a healer in China would remain the model for the Medical Missionary Society as it rapidly expanded its range of activities during the second half of the nineteenth century.[89]

Notes

1. W. Hunter describes these regulations as they were understood by the Westerners residing in Canton in *The 'Fan Kwae' at Canton, Before Treaty Days 1825–1844* (London: Kegan Paul, Trench, & Co., 1855; repr. Taipei: Ch'eng-wen Publishing Company, 1965), 28.
2. Letter of Instructions issued to E.C. Bridgman from the Prudential Committee of the American Board, signed by Jeremiah Evarts, Clerk, 7 October 1829, cited by E. Bridgman in *The Life and Labors of Elijah Coleman Bridgman* (New York: Anson DF Randolph, 1864), 20–27.
3. *Ibid.*, 25.
4. A. Pearson, 'Report submitted to the Board of the National Vaccine Establishment, respecting the introduction of the practice of vaccine inoculation into China, AD 1805', reprinted in the *Chinese Repository*, 2 (May 1833), 35–41.
5. Because of its relatively moderate climate, Macao was also used as a base of operations for non-Portuguese Westerners during the summer when most trade in Canton was suspended.
6. See A. Pearson, 'Report Submitted to the Board of the National Vaccine Establishment, Respecting the Introduction of the Practice of Vaccine Inoculation into China, AD 1805', *Chinese Repository*, 2 (May 1833), 40.
7. See E.V. Gulick, *Peter Parker and the Opening of China* (Cambridge: Harvard University Press, 1973), 45.
8. T.R. Colledge, 'Ophthalmic Hospital at Macao', *Chinese Repository*, 2 (October 1833), 272.
9. *Ibid.*, 272.
10. *Ibid.*, 271. In 1833, S. Wells Williams was sent to Canton as a representative of the American Board in China. He and Bridgman would serve as co-editors of the *Chinese Repository* over the nearly two decades of its publication.
11. *Ibid.*
12. *Ibid.*
13. Dr James H. Bradford, who received his MD from the University of Pennsylvania in 1823, served as a surgeon aboard American merchant vessels prior to becoming the physician for the American community at Canton.
14. E.C. Bridgman, 'Canton Dispensary', *Chinese Repository*, 2 (October 1833), 276.

15. *Ibid.*, 277.
16. *Ibid.*
17. E.C. Bridgman to R. Anderson, Canton, 26 December 1833, Papers of the American Board of Commissioners for Foreign Missions (ABCFM), Missions to China (ABC 16.3), reel 256.
18. E.C. Bridgman, 'The Chinese Language', *Chinese Repository*, 3 (May 1834), 13.
19. Cited by S.W. Williams in *The Middle Kingdom* (New York: John Wiley, 1847), 473.
20. This edict was translated by E.C. Bridgman and J.R. Morrison (son of Robert) and distributed in a circular letter dated 20 January 1835, ABCFM, reel 256.
21. First published in Canton by the Christian Union in China, 1832.
22. These included the American Bible Society, the British and Foreign Bible Society, and the American Tract Society.
23. Gulick, *op. cit.* (note 7), 15.
24. *Ibid.*, 17.
25. See 'Instructions of the Prudential Committee to Dr Peter Parker', *The Life, Letters, and Journals of the Rev. and Hon. Peter Parker, MD*, by G.B. Stevens (Wilmington, Delaware: Scholarly Resources Inc., 1972), 82–3. Originally published in 1896 by the Congregational Sunday School and Publishing Society, Boston and Chicago.
26. E.C. Bridgman to R. Anderson, Canton, 20 December 1834, ABCFM, reel 256.
27. E.C. Bridgman (ed.), 'An Opthalmic Hospital at Macao', *Chinese Repository*, 3 (December 1834), 364.
28. *Ibid.*, 366.
29. P. Parker's journal, cited by Stevens in *op. cit.* (note 25), 111.
30. P. Parker to Maria, 9 March 1835, cited by Stevens, *ibid.*, 114. During his seven months in Singapore, Parker would receive over one thousand patients.
31. See Stevens, *op. cit.* (note 25), 116.
32. D.W.C. Olyphant, a wealthy New York merchant who had long been a generous benefactor of the missionaries, undertook the financial arrangements for this facility.
33. P. Parker, 'First Quarterly Report of Ophthalmic Hospital at Canton', *Chinese Repository*, 4 (February 1836), 461.
34. A.W. Hummel, *Eminent Chinese of the Ch'ing Period* (Washington: United States Government Printing Office, 1943), 867.
35. P. Parker to American Board, Canton, 28 November 1835, reel 256, ABCFM.
36. E.C. Bridgman to R. Anderson, Canton, 8 February 1836, reel 256, ABCFM.

37. E.C. Bridgman to R. Anderson, Canton, 2 May 1836, reel 256, ABCFM
38. T.R. Colledge, 'Suggestions with regard to employing medical practitioners as missionaries to China', *Chinese Repository*, 4 (December 1835), 387.
39. *Ibid.*, 388.
40. *Ibid.*
41. *Ibid.*, 386–7.
42. See, for example, E.C. Bridgman to R. Anderson, Whampoa, 7 April 1836, reel 256, ABCFM.
43. P. Parker, 'Ophthalmic Hospital at Canton: Second Quarterly Report', *Chinese Repository*, 5 (May 1836), 32–3.
44. *Ibid.*, 33.
45. *Ibid.* This initially warm response of China's gentry towards Western medicine would change dramatically following the Opium War. As Western merchants and missionaries became increasingly perceived as enemies, China's upper classes began to regard it a treasonous to resort to Westerners for medical treatment. Thus, during the treaty port era the vast majority of Chinese who visited missionary hospitals came from the lower rungs of Chinese society.
46. Cited by Gulick in *op. cit.* (note 7), 146.
47. P. Parker, 'Second Quarterly Report', *Chinese Repository*, 5 (May 1836), 40.
48. P. Parker, 'Third Quarterly Report', *Chinese Repository*, 5 (August 1836), 188.
49. *Ibid.*
50. *Ibid.*
51. See P. Parker, 'Fourth Quarterly Report', *Chinese Repository*, 5 (November 1836), 325; 'Seventh Quarterly Report', *Chinese Repository*, 6 (January 1838), 438–39.
52. P. Parker, 'Fourth Quarterly Report', *Chinese Repository*, 5 (November 1836), 332.
53. E.C. Bridgman to R. Anderson, Canton, 2 May 1836, reel 256, *ABCFM.*
54. P. Parker to R. Anderson, Canton, 27 March 1836, *ibid.*
55. P. Parker, 'Second Quarterly Report', *Chinese Repository*, 5 (May 1836), 42.
56. *Ibid.*, 33.
57. This circular was issued on 5 October 1836 and later printed in the *Chinese Repository*, 5 (December 1836), 370–3.
58. *Ibid.*
59. See M.C. Lazich, *E.C. Bridgman (1801–1861), America's First Missionary to China* (Lewiston, NY: The Edwin Mellen Press, 2000), 11–59.
60. S. Hopkins, *Treatise on the Millennium* (Boston: Isaiah Thomas and Ebenezer T. Andrews, 1793; repr., New York: Arno Press, 1972), 57.
61. According to Hopkins, 'knowledge, mental light, and holiness, are inseparably connected: and are, in some respects, the same. Holiness is true light and discerning, so far as it depends upon a right taste, and consists in

it; and it is a thirst after every kind and degree of useful knowledge; and this desire and thirst for knowledge, will be great and strong, in proportion to the degree of holiness exercised: and forms the mind to constant attention, and to make swift advances in understanding and knowledge; and becomes a strong guard against mistakes, error and delusion. Therefore, a time of eminent holiness, must be a time of proportionately great light and knowledge,' *ibid.*, 57.

62. See minutes of the organisational meeting of the Society for the Diffusion of Useful Knowledge in China, *Chinese Repository*, 3 (December 1834), 380. Also published in the *Missionary Herald* (July 1835), 383.
63. *Ibid.*
64. P. Parker and E.C. Bridgman, 'Suggestions for the Formation of a Medical Missionary Society', *Chinese Repository*, 5 (December 1836), 370.
65. *Ibid.*
66. *Ibid.*
67. *Ibid.*, 371.
68. *Ibid.*
69. *Ibid.*
70. *Ibid.*, 373.
71. Canton Mission to Anderson, Canton, 7 March 1837, reel 257, ABCFM.
72. See E.C. Bridgman Journal, 28 August 1837.
73. Canton Mission to Anderson, 12 September 1837, reel 257, ABCFM.
74. See 'Twenty-Eighth Annual Meeting of the Board', *Missionary Herald* (November 1837), 473.
75. *Ibid.*, 472.
76. From a sermon by R. Anderson entitled, 'The Theory of Missions to the Heathen', cited by W.R. Hutchison in *Errand to the World: American Protestant Thought and Foreign Missions* (Chicago: Chicago University Press, 1987), 82.
77. P. Parker to Anderson, Canton, 7 March 1837, reel 257, ABCFM.
78. *Ibid.*
79. E.C. Bridgman to R. Anderson, Canton, 28 January 1837, *ibid.*
80. Following a long and contentious exchange of views over this matter with the American Board, Parker's connection with the organisation was permanently severed in 1847.
81. 'Constitution of the Medical Missionary Society', cited in Stevens, *op. cit.* (note 25), 135.
82. *Ibid.*
83. *Ibid.*, 136
84. See A. Wylie, *Memorials of Protestant Missionaries to the Chinese* (Shanghai: American Presbyterian Mission Press, 1867; repr. Taipei: Ch'eng-wen Publishing Co., 1967), 112.

85. The 'most favoured nation' clause included in the treaties that China was coerced to sign stipulated that any privileges granted to one nation would be automatically extended to all.
86. See Lazich, *op. cit.* (note 59), 233.
87. This Abstract was published in the 'Report of the Medical Missionary Society for 1841–42', *Chinese Repository*, 12 (April 1843), 189–91.
88. 'Report of the Medical Missionary Society', *Chinese Repository*, 12 (April 1843), 190.
89. J. Spence provides some interesting commentary on Parker's career as both a diplomat and a medical missionary in *To Change China, Western Advisors in China 1620–1960* (Boston: Little, Brown and Company, 1969), 34–56.

3

Local Voluntarism: The Medical Mission of the London Missionary Society in Hong Kong, 1842–1923[1]

Timothy Man-kong Wong

The chapter examines the genesis and development of the medical mission of the London Missionary Society in Hong Kong. It is divided chronologically into three major sections; namely the initial period during the 1840s to 1850s, the revival in the 1880s, and the subsequent consolidation of the mission after 1900. It argues that local voluntarism through the support of missionaries, affluent merchants, social leaders and senior government officials provides the key to understanding why and how the medical mission prospered from the 1880s onwards, and it examines the ways in which its independence became possible in the 1920s.

In its medical work in Hong Kong, the London Missionary Society (LMS) depended very strongly on local voluntarism. Its medical mission was inaugurated in Hong Kong in 1842, languished in 1853, restarted in the 1880s, and from 1924 began to be handed over to a local committee. By the latter date, the Hong Kong mission was considered one of the most successful of all of the LMS medical missions. Local voluntarism was the key to this success.

The LMS, which was established in 1795, was an interdenominational organisation supported by the Church of England and by Methodists, Presbyterians, Independents and other Protestant bodies.[2] Being interdenominational, the LMS recruited its missionaries from various denominations.[3] The drawback was that it lacked any persistent denominational support. It was therefore necessary for it to seek as many sources of support as possible. As the scale of its work expanded, the number of directors increased from thirty-four in 1796 to three hundred (excluding honorary directors) in 1890.[4] This in itself created administrative problems. There were also inevitable differences between the directors, who were anxious about expenditure – between 1796 and 1895 the LMS experienced forty-six years of budget deficits[5] – and the missionaries in the field who demanded better funding for their various local needs. Disputes between the two could sometimes be very bitter.

The LMS always evinced a keen interest in its work in China, but its actual support varied considerably over time. In 1844, for instance, John Morison (1791–1859), a board member of the LMS, stressed that the wrongs that the British did in the Opium War (1839–42) might be redeemed in part through the activities of the LMS China missionaries. He stated: 'The war with China, in itself a great evil, has been overruled for much good, in opening portions of that vast Empire to the labours of missionaries.'[6] Its funding for this work was, however, circumscribed by continuing financial deficits. Many LMS missionaries complained that they received inadequate financial support from the society. As Frederick Storrs Turner (1834–1916) – an LMS missionary in Canton and later in Hong Kong – lamented:

> I am not alone in feeling very serious dissatisfaction with your management of the great concerns committed to your charge. Your proceedings in respect to our Chinese Mission have been long characterised by painful inefficiency.[7]

This led to pressures from the LMS on its missionaries to develop local sources of funding as much as possible. In a major LMS text – titled *Missionary Principles and Plans*, Joseph Mullen (1820–79) – cited a resolution adopted by the Board of Directors on 11 November 1867 that focused on the need to reduce the budgets of its 'Eastern Missions'. Mullen had been an LMS missionary in India for twenty-one years before he became the foreign secretary of the LMS, and well knew the consequences of financial cuts for local work.[8] Only because the deficits were so serious at that time did the directors demand such cuts. They encouraged the missionaries to seek support from British administrators and local well-wishers. Mullen cited cases of local support in China, writing that the LMS 'has met with many similar friends, and especially in Hong Kong, Amoy, Shanghai, and Hankow, our missionaries speak with gratitude and affection of the help and sympathy they have received in their labours.'[9] Merchants and professionals – both British and non-British – as well as military officers had provided such support in the British colony of Hong Kong, and in treaty ports such as Shanghai and Hankow.

As a result of such voluntary support, 'China quickly became the most widespread medical field of the Society [LMS].'[10] By 1915, there were already fourteen LMS hospitals in China, four of which were in Hong Kong.[11] These were the Alice Memorial Hospital (founded in 1887), the Nethersole Hospital (founded in 1893), the Alice Memorial Maternity

Hospital (founded in 1904), and the Ho Miu Ling Hospital (founded in 1906). Given that Hong Kong had a relatively small population, the fact that there were four LMS hospitals revealed the importance of LMS medical mission work there. Of the different LMS missions in China, the Hong Kong station was probably the most successful in obtaining local money to support its work. One reason for this was that it had the largest foreign community resident in China. Another was that the colonial government supported the work of missionaries there in both the educational and medical fields. For example, starting in 1873, the government provided grants-in-aid to mission schools, and by the 1880s, the LMS had become a major partner of the Hong Kong government in education.

The key concept in this paper is local voluntarism and a word about it is necessary. A major connotation of 'voluntarism' is 'the involvement of voluntary organisations in social welfare.'[12] The term 'local voluntarism' is thus used here to refer to the voluntary assistance given by the people in Hong Kong – Westerners and Chinese alike – in a number of ways. It ranged from donating money to providing leadership for the medical mission. It varied in extent at different times, depending, for example, on the support extended by the colonial government and the performance of the economy in Hong Kong. The idea of 'local voluntarism', as applied here, does not exclude government involvement. In fact, the government subtly promoted the work in a number of ways. It must also be emphasised that many people provided voluntary support for the medical missions for secular rather than religious reasons, believing that doing so provided a means towards the popularisation of Western medicine as against Chinese medicine.

The initial phase: 1842–58

Benjamin Hobson (1816–73), the eighth medical missionary to arrive in China, was an important pioneer of such work.[13] He established a missionary strategy of preaching the Christian messages while healing. The preaching was mainly performed by his Chinese colleagues. Moreover, he sought to disseminate greater knowledge about Western medicine by writing and publishing books in Chinese on the subject. He also tried to establish a local medical school. His work provided a model for later medical missionaries in China.

Hobson was a qualified medical practitioner,[14] and had some brief training in the Chinese language.[15] He joined the Medical Missionary Society (MMS), arriving in Macao in December 1839 to serve in the MMS hospital there. After the Opium War, Hong Kong was ceded to Britain under the treaty of Nanjing in 1842. In the same year, William Lockhart (1811–96), an LMS medical missionary, supervised the construction of a missionary hospital in Hong Kong. According to Lockhart, 'it was thought more desirable to have the hospital in a British colony than in the Portuguese settlement of Macao.'[16] This hospital was on Morrison Hill, and began its service in June 1843.[17] Hobson took charge of the hospital between June 1843 and July 1845. He proved a capable manager as well as an excellent healer. In these two years, the total number of patients being treated in the mission hospital reached 7,221.[18] This number should be taken as a very positive figure, for the entire population of Hong Kong was only 16,000 in 1843, increasing to 19,500 in 1844 and 24,200 in 1845.[19] A Chinese preacher, Keuh A-gong (1785–1867), provided religious instruction for Hobson's patients.[20] There were regular religious meetings in different dialects. As a rule, the Cantonese meeting took place in the morning and was attended by around forty people. About twenty came to the Chaozhou meeting in the evening.[21]

Hobson left Hong Kong for England in 1845 as his wife had suffered poor health. As it happened, she passed away on the last stop of their voyage. Rather than return immediately to China, Hobson spent fifteen months in England seeking support for his work in Hong Kong. During his long absence, the work was continued through a rudimentary form of local voluntarism, with his Chinese apprentice, Chan A-poon (b.1822),[22] providing treatment for the sick. Three physicians supervised Chan's work, namely Alfred Tucker, the surgeon of the naval hospital ship, Francis Dill, the colonial surgeon, and A. Balfour, a private practitioner in Hong Kong. The management of the hospital was taken over by the colonial chaplain, Vincent Stanton.[23]

While in England, Hobson raised funds to open a medical school in Hong Kong to train Chinese doctors. During the time he was in Hong Kong, between 1843 and 1845, he had already apprenticed his Chinese assistants in Western medicine. Hobson remarked in 1846:

> I am making arrangements to establish a Medical School in Hong Kong, with a view not only to give to China a rational system of medicine, but raise up, and form a peculiar kind and fitness, a Native Agency of pious Medical Practitioners.... There will be a department wholly in the Chinese language for the instruction and improvement of Native Physicians in China[24]

His scheme failed to materialise in the 1840s, despite some official support, such as the promise from the Governor that land would be provided on an inexpensive lease. Although there is no statement in the records to explain why he gave up the idea, it might well be due to the conflicts that he had with Peter Parker (1804–88), a prominent medical missionary from the USA who was opposed to having Hong Kong as the base for such an institution. As it was, Hobson resigned from the MMS to avoid further conflict with Parker, and moved to Canton.[25] In the writings left by Hobson and Lockhart, it is stated that this shift took place as the LMS wanted to renew its work in Canton.[26] It took place at a time of economic crisis in Hong Kong, when merchants - Western and Chinese alike - were either leaving Hong Kong or withdrawing their capital from the territory.

After his medical school project failed, Hobson began to produce Chinese books on various aspects of Western medicine. He wrote five between 1851 and 1858: *Chuanti Xinlun* (Treatise on Physiology, 1851), *Xiyi Luelun* (First Lines of the Practices of Surgery in the West, 1857), *Fuying Xinshou* (Treatise on Midwifery and Diseases of Children, 1858), *Nieke Xinshou* (Practice of Medicine and *Materia Medica*, 1858), and *A Medical Vocabulary in English and Chinese* (1858).[27] His works were highly regarded, and, in the words of one observer, served to 'transform China's native doctors into an intelligent, progressive, and scientific medical profession by furnishing them with a scientific background.'[28] Hobson also sought to use his medical texts to propagate Christianity, particularly among educated Chinese. In the preface of *Chuanti Xinlun*, he wrote 'The last paper contains a short account of the history of man, varieties of colour, height, & c., and concludes with remarks upon his moral nature, and proofs of the unity, wisdom, and design of God in creation.'[29] His texts were highly regarded by contemporary medical missionaries and they had a far-reaching impact on the introduction of Western medicine, not only in China but also in Japan.[30]

Hobson was replaced as LMS medical missionary in Hong Kong in 1848 by Henri Hirschberg (1814–74).[31] Hirschberg had an entrepreneurial bent, and the hospital on Morrison Hill flourished under his management. He opened two new dispensaries, one at the Bazaar chapel of the LMS, the other on the Kowloon Peninsular, which was a part of Chinese territory.[32] He received evangelical assistance from Ho Tsun-sheen (1817–71), the only ordained Chinese pastor of the LMS mission, and Ng Mun-sow (d.1890), a theological student of the LMS mission.[33] The former preached in the hospital twice a week while the latter preached alternately in the morning.[34]

Although Hobson appears to have resigned from the MMS so as to avoid any further conflicts between the LMS and MMS, the friction, in fact, continued. The British-based LMS tended to be prejudiced against the American-based MMS. After Hobson's departure, there were almost no annual meetings of the Hong Kong branch of the MMS, and by 1852 it had ceased to function.[35] The MMS had provided matching grants for LMS medical work, and these funds dried up. The medical work now had to compete for scarce funds with other LMS projects, such as James Legge's highly successful Anglo-Chinese College and its preparatory school.[36] Legge (1815–97) was the foremost LMS missionary in Hong Kong at the time, and his work tended to get priority. In 1851, the LMS relinquished its hospital on Morrison Hill, turning it over to the navy, so that it became known as a naval hospital.[37] As a whole, the salaries of the LMS missionaries were cut, causing resentment and tension within the mission. Hirschberg, for example, complained that he had insufficient funds to cover his expenses and debts.[38] The fire that destroyed most parts of the city on 28 January 1852 provided a further blow, as the LMS could not afford to rebuild the facilities that were destroyed. Both Legge and Hirschberg raised funds privately to support their respective work. This in turn led to controversy between the two, as Legge accused Hirschberg of using the funds improperly.

Legge was in fact prejudiced against Hirschberg, a German Jew who had converted to Protestantism and had chosen to serve in the LMS because of its interdenominational character. Although Legge had interviewed him in 1846 and had raised no objections to his appointment to the LMS at that time, he and Hobson disliked the man on ethnic and racial grounds. Hobson once remarked: 'his [Hirschberg's] mind so very un-English and thoroughly German, and… [illegibly] expresses himself in our tongue.'[39] Richard Cole, an American from Indiana who worked in the LMS printing press, added fuel to the flames by telling Hirschberg that 'I have heard Dr Legge say, "there goes our friend the Jew, I am afraid that we shall find him to be a Jew before we are done with him. He is a half-educated man, and without any sense of propriety."'[40] Besides accusing him of financial impropriety, Legge criticised Hirschberg for carrying on a private medical practice in Hong Kong. Furthermore, he raised doubts about his faith, pointing out that he rarely showed up for Holy Communion and prayer meetings. In the face of such hostility, Hirschberg left Hong Kong for Amoy in 1853. The LMS failed to find a replacement for him, which brought an end to a decade of medical missionary activity in Hong Kong.

An opportunity arose in 1857 to revive the medical mission, when Wong Fun (1827–79),[41] a qualified practitioner of Western medicine and an LMS medical missionary, offered a year of medical service in Hong Kong. Wong was originally sent to Canton to take over Hobson's work in the Wei-Ai Hospital while Hobson was asked to take over the Lester Hospital in Shanghai. Because of the Second Opium War, Wong could not proceed to Canton. Instead, he stayed in Hong Kong and began his medical mission work. He made progress in his work and established a reputation – the number of patients per day rising from about sixty in early 1857 to 109 by the end of the year. Like other medical missionaries, he focused on healing the sick, and a Chinese preacher assisted him in preaching. Wong received the assistance from Hong Ren-gan (1822–64), a cherished assistant in the LMS Hong Kong mission who later turned out to be the Shield King in the

Taiping Kingdom.[42] Wong left for Canton in 1858. Though he returned in December 1860, he had by then resigned from the LMS in protest at not being treated on an equal footing with his British counterparts.[43] He was a superintendent of the Government Hospital in Hong Kong for a brief period before he left for Canton, where he set up in private practice. His knowledge in Western medicine became highly regarded.[44]

Nobody else of Wong Fun's calibre came forward within the LMS, and there was no medical work carried out under its auspices in Hong Kong until 1881, two decades later. The LMS missionaries appear to have been happy with what they had accomplished in their evangelical and educational work in the colony. The medical work was revived in the 1880s, largely because of a growing demand for Western medicine and because of government encouragement for mission involvement.

The revival of the 1880s

The revival of the LMS medical mission was brought about in Hong Kong in the 1880s, largely through local popular voluntarism. Three figures stand out: Emmanuel Raphael Belilios, Ho Kai, and Patrick Manson. Belilios (1837–1905) was from an Indian-Sephardic Jewish family of Calcutta. He was educated in that city, and then moved to Hong Kong in 1862. After enriching himself through opium trading, he turned to property development and other forms of business, and was at one time the Chairman of the Hong Kong and Shanghai Banking Corporation. He became a philanthropist who was keen to promote education and introduce Western medicine, offering two full scholarships for the Chinese to study Western medicine abroad. Nobody, however, took up his offer.[45] He supported public education in Hong Kong by donating money to build a girl's school. For this public work, he was awarded the Companion of the Order of St Michael and St George.[46]

Ho Kai (1859–1914) was the son of Ho Tsun-sheen, the first ordained Chinese pastor in the LMS Hong Kong mission, and was himself a member of the LMS church. He travelled to Britain to study medicine, graduating with the degrees of Bachelor of Medicine and Master of Surgery from the University of Aberdeen. He carried out his practical work at St Thomas' Hospital and became a member of the Royal College of Surgeons. He also studied law at Lincoln's Inn, London, where he was called to the bar. His achievement in his law exams attracted the attention of John Pope Hennessy (1834–91), the Governor of Hong Kong from 1878 to 1882, who wrote:

> Last year a young Chinaman born under the British flag in this Colony succeeded at that examination in defeating his competitors from the English, Scotch, and Irish universities, and in three of the subjects of examination he

> obtained the first place. This was Mr Ho Kai, one of the numerous Anglo-Chinese subjects that Her Majesty now has in this Colony. I think it is a matter we may all congregate ourselves upon. That young gentleman, who has been called to the English bar, will return, I think, this month to the Colony, and I am sure you will all join with me in welcoming him back.[47]

After his return to Hong Kong in 1882, Ho Kai was soon established as a leading public figure in the colony. He served as a member of the Sanitary Board from 1886 to 1896, and was a member of the Legislative Council from 1890 to 1914. He was knighted in 1912.[48]

Patrick Manson (1844–1922) received his medical education from the University of Aberdeen where he was awarded the degrees of Doctor of Medicine and Master of Surgery in 1866. Soon afterwards, he left for China, where he was appointed a medical officer for the Chinese Customs. During this service, he began to research into 'the role of bloodsucking insects in the transmission of disease.'[49] He took up private practice in Hong Kong in 1883, and was there until 1889. He subsequently founded the London School of Tropical Medicine.

In 1881, E.P. Belilios offered HK$5,000 as a matching grant for any hospital project. His aim was to promote secular Western medicine; as a Jew he held no brief for the Christian missionaries. Although the LMS missionaries appear to have disliked him for his religion, they were willing to compete for the grant, as it appeared to provide a means to restart their medical mission in Hong Kong. They set up an *ad hoc* committee to work out how to take advantage of the proposal and applied to the directors in London for a medical missionary.

Meanwhile, Kwong Yat-sau (1840–1921), a Chinese Christian, had taken the initiative in establishing a dispensary at the Taipingshan Chapel. Born in China, Kwong had accompanied his father to Australia, where he was educated and converted to Christianity. After his return to China, he became a self-supporting itinerant preacher who combined medicine and preaching. He moved to Hong Kong, where he began preaching and dispensing medicine at the Taipingshan Chapel.[50] He managed to persuade William Young (d.1888), a medical practitioner in Hong Kong,[51] to offer free consultation in the dispensary from 7am to 9am everyday. The dispensary was named Nethersole, in honour of the mother of the major sponsor, Henry William Davis, an affluent merchant in Hong Kong. Davis, however, left Hong Kong soon after, and the dispensary closed in 1882.

Although the LMS directors had by now approved of the proposal to establish a mission hospital, there were as yet insufficient funds to match Belilios' offer of HK$5,000. The foreign secretary of the LMS visited Hong Kong in April 1883 and after discussions it was agreed that the hospital would have to be established in an area of low property prices and that the Queen's Road Chapel might be sold to provide the cash to buy a site on Hollywood Road. An organising committee was established in February 1884, of several eminent social leaders including current members of the Legislative Council. Four out of the six unofficial members of the Legislative Council were involved, namely, Francis Bulkeley Johnson (d.1887),[52] Thomas Jackson (1841–1915),[53] Wong Shing (1825–1902),[54] and Frederick Stewart (1836–89).[55] Other committee members included: E.P. Belilios, Ho Kai, Patrick Manson, Wei Yuk (1849–1922),[56] Wong Wing-Sheung (1860–97),[57] John Chalmers (1825–99),[58] among others. The LMS was not altogether happy with the composition of this committee as it was felt that it might exercise too much control over the hospital. The committee had, for example, taken upon itself the power to appoint and remove the medical officers.[59] Some of the practitioners of Western medicine in Hong Kong also threatened to withdraw from the project if they were not given sufficient representation on the Hospital Management Board. The LMS was thus worried about losing control. Another problem was that the sale of the Queen's Road Chapel had raised only $8000, an insufficient sum for what was turning out to be an expensive project.

The impasse was overcome through the intervention of Ho Kai, who promised to cover the cost of the construction of the hospital if it was named after his recently deceased wife, Alice Walkden. Alice Walkden (1852-1884) was from an upper-class British family, her father a Member of Parliament. She was, according to a LMS source, 'an excellent Christian lady',[60] and the LMS had no reason to object to Ho Kai's proposal.[61] A pious Chinese Christian, Chan Ayow, also known as Ko Chan-shi or simply Mrs. Caldwell, agreed to sell some of her land for the hospital site. Although the plot was worth, in her estimation, some HK$70,000, she asked for only HK$14,000 for it from the LMS.[62] Her only condition was that a part of the land be used for building a chapel, later known as the To Tsai Church. The project now became a viable one. There was a high-profile public fundraising campaign, with a two-night alfresco fete that attracted 12,000 participants.[63] The acting governor, William H. Marsh (1827–1906) laid the foundation stone in June 1886, providing more publicity for the project. As John Chalmers noted:

> With very few exceptions, the community of Hong Kong, from the Governor downwards, have always been heartily in their support of the Hospital, and it has never had any lack of funds. Sometimes, the local papers were inclined to throw cold water on it, but that was before our success was established.[64]

The Alice Memorial Hospital began its work in 1887.[65]

The LMS medical mission in Hong Kong was reinforced through the opening of the Hong Kong College of Medicine for Chinese in 1887.[66] Ho Kai, Patrick Manson and James Cantlie (1851–1926) provided the driving force behind this college. Cantlie, who had arrived in Hong Kong only that year, had recent teaching experience in London and provided 'solid underpinning and organisation which a medical school required.'[67] The medical college used the premises of the Alice Memorial Hospital for its teaching, and some doctors in the hospital were at the same time teachers in the medical college. The medical college was, however, a secular undertaking, even though many of its students were Christians or from Christian families. Notable examples included Sun Yat-sen (1866–1925), Kwan King-leung (1869–1945), Wong Sai-yan (1870–1928), and Wong Chung Yik (1889–1930).[68] After finishing his further education at Edinburgh and Cambridge, Wong Chung Yik returned to Hong Kong to practise medicine and later became the first Chinese professor at the University of Hong Kong, when he was appointed Professor of Pathology in 1920.[69]

Meanwhile, Patrick Manson had become a major reason for H.W. Davis to take a fresh interest in the Nethersole Dispensary. He agreed in 1887 to donate $7,000 to revive this institution, stating: 'I hope the project may prove useful for the Chinese and work well possibly in aid of Dr Manson's scheme.'[70] Although Davis was well aware that this was an LMS venture, he appeared to have been encouraged to make his donation because Manson, a doctor with a high reputation, was supporting it. In this way, the voluntary service of such public figures could be a critical component in the building up and consolidation of the medical mission of the LMS in Hong Kong. It was seen, above all, as a matter of general public interest. As it was, the greater part of the money for these projects came from the public rather than from the LMS. Whereas the LMS contributed $14,000 for the Alice Memorial Hospital project, the public donated $34,500.[71] The Nethersole dispensary later attracted a donation of $12,000 in the will of Richard Young, brother of William Young – the doctor who had worked there in 1881–2.[72] By such means, the LMS medical mission picked up new momentum during the 1880s, providing a firm base for its notable success in the ensuing decades.

Chinese pastors and Chinese church leaders also played an important role in the development of the LMS medical mission in Hong Kong. As mentioned earlier in this chapter, Kwong Yat-sau played a key role in opening the Nethersole Dispensary at the Taiping Shan chapel. Two other church leaders, Wong Uen Sham and Lai Fuk-chi, were instrumental in establishing dispensaries in 1884 in the Taiping Shan and the Sai Ying Poon areas. William Young worked in these two dispensaries after his return to

Hong Kong in 1884. Both Wong and Lai had experience of medical work. Wong Uen-sham had been an assistant to some German medical missionaries in the Guangdong area before he was ordained as a Rhenish pastor. Lai Fuk-chi, his son-in-law, was hired by the LMS as a local preacher. Lai had received training in Western medicine while he had been assisting John Glasgow Kerr (1824–1901), an American medical missionary in Canton. Lai's work was highly regarded within the LMS, and he was even allowed to run the dispensary he had established, when the medical missionary was absent.[73] Chinese preachers and church leaders were also active in evangelical work among the patients who attended the Alice Memorial Hospital and Nethersole Dispensary. Wong Uen-Sham's son, Wong Yuk-cho (1845–1903), the Chinese pastor of the newly founded To Tsai Church, started a training class for evangelists, which Wong Fuk-yue attended and became committed in preaching in Chinese to medical patients for a long period of time.[74]

The success of this revival of medical mission work was made possible through a combination of religious commitment and secular philanthropy. The missionaries were prepared to accept help from all quarters, even from non-Christians, such as E.P. Belilios. People such as Belilios, in turn, had no objection to their donations being used for work that was partly evangelical. As John Chalmers remarked:

> [S]hall we not thank E.P. Belilios the Jew for $5,000? Indeed I think it is a good way of connecting him. And so Mr Belilios is now about to give five times that sum for the erection of a Medical College affiliated with the Hospital which he has not the slightest objection to Dr Thomson's evangelistic work in the Hospital.[75]

Through such philanthropic work, Belilios and other public figures were able to enhance their reputation in the colony and gain public honours. Ho Kai was another such figure. He almost certainly held political ambitions that were reinforced through his public service.[76] His work in bringing the Alice Memorial Hospital into being revealed him as a diligent organiser and able mediator between the different parties, including the medical professionals, who were often in disagreement. As a Hong Kong Chinese who had received both medical and legal training in Britain, he was able to relate to and bring together a wide range of people. In particular, he was an alumnus of Aberdeen University, the same identity that Patrick Mansion, James Cantlie, and Frederick Stewart commonly shared. Stewart became the first rector of the medical college. Ho Kai is generally considered to have been the single most important figure behind the inauguration of the Alice Memorial Hospital.[77] The fact that figures such as Belilios, an Indian business magnate, and Ho Kai, a Chinese Christian, were able to play such important roles in the public life of Hong Kong also indicates that it was a more liberal and, in certain respects, less racist society than it had been during the 1840s. This was probably critical in providing the space within which both Western-educated Asian philanthropists and the revived medical mission could thrive.

The consolidation of the LMS medical mission after 1900

By 1911, a LMS report was able to claim: 'The Medical work of the LMS in Hongkong is one of the most important and well developed branches of its endeavour in the South of China.'[78] By then, there were two more LMS hospitals and the society had also become involved in the training of doctors and nurses. Again, this was all due to a flourishing local voluntarism.

The Alice Memorial Maternity Hospital came into being because of new ideas about midwifery. The Government of Hong Kong had already criticised Chinese practices surrounding childbirth, seeing them as causes of high infant mortality. By the beginning of the twentieth century, many Chinese social leaders and affluent merchants were coming round to this view and were seeking means to change the situation.[79] The new maternity hospital was founded in 1904 as a result of generous support from the public. The Chinese sponsors placed a condition on their provision of $2,000 annually to cover the salary of a female medical missionary. She was required, 'to treat the women of subscriber's family in their own houses... [and] to mix with the Chinese ladies and introduce to them Western hygiene and health care.'[80] This condition sheds a revealing light on some of their motives for providing the funding. During its first decade, two LMS women medical missionaries ran the new maternity hospital. The first, who was in charge from 1904 to 1909, was Alice Deborah Sibree (1876–1928). She had studied medicine at the London School of Medicine, qualifying in 1901, and had taken further training in Edinburgh and Glasgow.[81] The second, from 1910 to 1913, was Eleanor Whitworth Perkins (b.1882). She had trained at the Royal Free Hospital, London, qualifying as Doctor of Medicine and Bachelor of Surgery of the University of London in 1906.[82] The LMS did not send any replacement between 1913 and 1920. The vacancy was filled eventually in 1921 by Gladys Mande Turner (b.1887), who had received her medical education at the University of Birmingham where she had been awarded Bachelor of Medicine and Bachelor of Surgery in 1916.[83] Turner continued in the post for two years; she resigned in 1923 on marrying John Fraser, then head of the Hong Kong Sanitary Department. During the period after Perkins' departure, the maternity work was largely in the hands of Lavinia Kate Rayner (b.1880), a missionary nurse who had trained as a nurse and midwife at the Middlesex Hospital in London and who was registered as a midwife in Hong Kong.[84] She played a key role in assisting medical missionaries and doctors in the provision of maternity service.

The Ho Miu Ling Hospital was established by the LMS in 1906 on a piece of land that was provided by the Government adjacent to the Alice Memorial Hospital. Ho Miu Ling (1847–1937), Ho Kai's sister, financed this project. Like her brother, she was a Christian with strong connections to the LMS. Her husband was Ng Ting-fang (1842–1922), the first Chinese member of the Legislative Council in Hong Kong and later a prominent politician in China. She was a prominent public benefactor, having already provided an unconditional loan to cover the construction cost of the Anglo-Chinese Ying-Wa College.[85]

The LMS also continued to maintain close links with the Hong Kong Medical College for the Chinese.[86] For example, Thomas Burton (b.1862), who had trained in Edinburgh and Vienna and served as an LMS medical missionary in Hong Kong in 1893–4, taught chemistry there. He resigned from the LMS in 1894 to work as the Secretary of the college. John Christopher Thomson (b.1863), another Edinburgh medical graduate (1888) was sent by the LMS to Hong Kong in 1889 to superintend the Alice Memorial Hospital. He was appointed a Senate member of the medical college in 1890, a position he held until 1909. He became the Director of Studies and Secretary of the College in 1895. He resigned from the LMS the following year, and was appointed as an assistant surgeon by the government so that he could concentrate on his medical college work. He taught pathology (1889–91), midwifery and diseases of women (1891–3 and 1897–1901), clinical surgery (1892), materia medica and therapeutics (1892–4), physiology (1895–6), chemistry (1896–7), surgery (1896–7), diseases of tropical climates (1901–9), fevers (1908), and clinical medicine (1909). He finally left Hong Kong in 1909.[87] Robert McLean Gibson (1870–1935), also an Edinburgh medical graduate (1896), was sent by the LMS to replace Thomson as superintendent of the Alice Memorial Hospital in 1896. While he continued in this post until 1918, he taught at the medical college, in physiology (1899–1901), midwifery and diseases of women (1901–2), anatomy (1902–9), the practice of medicine (1903–5), and clinical surgery (1902–9). On the administrative side, he served as court member (1909–15), the Director of Studies (1902–9), and Secretary and Treasurer (1909–15). Later, when the college became a part of the University of Hong Kong, he became a founding life member of the university court, and lecturer in clinical surgery (1912–15), and operative surgery (1916–20).[88] Non-medical LMS missionaries such as John Chalmers lectured at the college in subsidiary subjects – in his case, teaching physics between 1887 and 1898. Ho Kai taught medical jurisprudence. Wan Man

Kai (1870–27), alias Wan Tun Mo, a tutor in medicine, physiology and surgery, was well connected with the LMS. His father was a LMS preacher in Bolou of Guangdong Province and later in Hong Kong. He received medical training under John Kenneth Mackenize (1850–88), a LMS medical missionary in Tientsin. Before he returned to Hong Kong, he worked at John Kerr's mission hospital.[89]

As the reputation of the college spread beyond Hong Kong, students were attracted from other regions of southeast Asia, and even from India. Due to this new demand, it was decided in 1907 to drop the two words 'for Chinese' from the name of the medical college. In 1909, the government complemented the college for its work in the following terms:

> Most of the licentiates have settled in the Colony, and are exerting a most useful influence in the direction of displacing the native medical methods and popularising Western medical and sanitary knowledge, while a considerable number of them are employed as resident surgeons in the hospitals for Chinese, as medical officers in charge of the Public Dispensaries, and as assistant medical officers on the railway works.[90]

By popularising and raising the demand for Western medicine in the colony, the college reinforced the medical work of the LMS there. It also helped the more general work of the society, as it aligned the mission with what were seen as the progressive forces of science and technology, as well as providing another example of its public service.

From the 1880s onward, the LMS played a major role in popularising Western medicine among the Chinese of Hong Kong. This was in part because it attracted many Chinese patients to its hospitals, but also because it employed some talented Chinese doctors and surgeons who gained a high reputation for their healing among the general public. It publicised the work of these Chinese doctors in newspapers during its fundraising drives, which raised their public profile and helped to establish confidence in them.[91] The government noticed this, and drew on the mission resources to implement its own health programme.[92] For example, it managed to recruit Chung King Ue (d.1903), alias Chung Boon Chor, the first Chinese house surgeon at the Alice Memorial Hospital. Appointed to the mission hospital after being trained by John Kenneth Mackenzie in Tianjin, Chung was soon being praised by its administrators:

> [H]is kindliness and tact in dealing with the patients is most commendable while his fluency in speaking English, Cantonese, and Mandarin, and his knowledge of several minor dialects of Chinese are of great advantage in a Hospital where such a large variety of nationalities meet.[93]

After a severe outbreak of plague in Hong Kong, Chung was appointed by the government in 1898 to take charge of the Tung Wah Hospital. His remit was to introduce Western medicine into this hospital for the Chinese.[94] After five years of work there, he was commended by the Inspecting Medical Officer: 'His kindness, courtesy, tact, and professional skill combined to enable him to effect the very great improvements that were made during this tenure of office, and for which the credit is practically entirely to him.'[95]

Chung's successor as the house surgeon at the Alice Memorial Hospital was Wan Man Kai, a fellow graduate from the same Viceroy's Medical College in Tianjin. He was praised in the annual reports of the LMS for his knowledge and his skill in Western medicine.[96] Later, he performed surgical operations along with Chung at the Tung Wah Hospital. He was known as a skilled anaesthetist, and it was reported that there had been no deaths under his care and that all of his patients had recovered well.[97] Another Chinese doctor was To Ying Fan, alias Coxion To, who served at the Alice Memorial Hospital for twenty-three years. His wife and son were also employed in this hospital in different capacities.[98] Other Chinese doctors who worked for the LMS for some time before then establishing themselves in private practice were Wan Man Kai, Kwan King-leung, Ho Ko Tsun, Lee Ying Yau and Benjamin Cheonglam Wong. Their prior affiliation with the LMS hospitals was one of their cherished assets, but their success in private practice in return helped boost public confidence in the LMS hospitals.

Although the involvement of the LMS in the training of doctors decreased after the University of Hong Kong took over the medical college, the LMS continued to play a leading role in the training of nurses and midwives. There was a continuing strong demand for nurses. As the matron of the Nethersole Hospital commented in 1910: 'We have work for more nurses if we could accommodate them.'[99] A decade later, it was reported:

> Every year the standard of nursing seems to be improving; the nurses of today can scarcely be compared with those of a few years ago, when only those of the servant class could be secured to look after the sick; now the Chinese women are looking upon nursing as a profession, and are taking it up with a higher motive.[100]

The midwives training program at the Alice Memorial Maternity hospital also established a good reputation, as was recognised by the government.[101] All nurses at the mission hospitals were Christians, and it was expected that they would be actively involved in evangelical work.[102] Bible classes were held for the nurses, run by Chinese pastors such as Cheung Chuk Ling (1877–1966) of the To Tsai Church.[103]

There was continuing voluntary support for the medical work of the LMS during the first two decades of the twentieth century, and if anything it became more extensive. Several prominent social leaders served on the finance committee of the LMS hospitals, and thus became involved in their management.[104] Notable in this respect were Francis Henry May (1860–1922) and Arthur Wimbolt Brewin (1867–1946). Both held important government positions, the former the Captain Superintendent of Police; the latter, the Registrar-General. Their duties required them to keep close contact with the Chinese population of Hong Kong, and one way they managed to do this was through their connection with the LMS hospitals. Both were promoted to the rank of Colonial Secretary and both served as members of the Legislative and Executive Councils. May became the Governor of Hong Kong between 1912 and 1919. Some of the other committee members were at one stage or other also members of the Legislative Council, such as Wei Yuk (1849–1921), Chau Siu Ki (1863–1925), Ho Fook (1863–1926), Lau Chu Pak (1867–1922), Tso Seen Wan (1868–1953) and Ng Hon Tsz (1877–1923). Others had a big reputation in Hong Kong, such as Au Tak (1840–1920) and Sin Tak Fun (1856–1924). These Chinese leaders were leading professionals or affluent merchants who were involved in property development, banking, trading, and other forms of business enterprise. In brief, they were symbols of wealth and power. Given their status and power in society, their participation in the management of the hospitals, though nominal in reality, helped build up the LMS medical mission into a well-received social institution. In doing so, they induced further local voluntarism.

Conclusion

Through local voluntarism, the LMS medical mission in Hong Kong was able to be largely self-supporting. The work was supported in part by the government of the colony, but this covered only a small part of the total costs. At the beginning of the twentieth century the annual grant was only HK$ 300, rising to HK$ 2,300 by the late-1910s. In 1909 the total cost of the medical mission was HK$ 12,600, rising to HK$ 17,938 in 1914, HK$ 27,570 in 1919, and HK $ 57,934 in 1923.[105] With such costs, and their rapid escalation, there was no way in which adequate funding could be obtained either from the government or from donations from Britain. This was particularly the case in the period after the first world war, when there was great economic hardship in Britain. Without large voluntary sector subscriptions, the medical mission would have been unsustainable.

This was despite the fact that the mission health services did not focus on healing members of the more affluent classes of Hong Kong. Their targets were the general public and poor. As one missionary stated in 1921:

> Many both rich and poor have been admitted, the majority being from the poorer class, this is due to the fact that there is very little accommodation for the wealthier Chinese women in the Nethersole Hospital... Private patients are financially a help to the Hospital as each patient pays $2.5 per day, whereas the general ward patients pay only twenty-three cents per day, the poor nothing, and the hundreds of women and children who come to treated as out-patients pay nothing at all for medicine and treatment... They cannot understand either why the Mission Hospital should require so little money from them, while the native doctors demand nearly all their money. There are so many practical illustrations in a Mission Hospital that can be given to these poor ignorant people to help them to understand the meaning of the Gospel.[106]

It was clear that many in Hong Kong appreciated the help that was given to the needy in this respect, and this created a good impression of the mission and of Christianity more generally. This helped to gain funding from affluent well-wishers of all sorts.

The logic of this process was that this class gradually became more and more actively involved in the running of these establishments. In 1923, the LMS hospitals were placed under the management of a local committee, which consisted of eminent social leaders and wealthy merchants. The LMS reduced its commitments by covering only the salaries of a medical missionary and a matron. This move towards greater local independence was in part a response to attacks on Christian missionaries for being too complicit with colonial rule. Despite this, the LMS did not withdraw from medical work in Hong Kong. The reasons for this, which are a subject of another study, include the great influx of population from China and the changing situation in China in the ensuing decades that led to a fresh influx of foreign missionaries into the territory.

Notes

1. The author wishes to acknowledge many useful comments from Ka-che Yip and David Hardiman. Besides, a note of romanisation on Chinese names seems necessary. Instead of converting every name in Pinyin, I follow a person's English name that appears in either missionary archives or governmental records.
2. S. Neill, *A History of Christian Missions* (London: Penguin Books, 1990), 213–14; A.F. Perry, 'The American Board of Commissioners for Foreign

Missions and The London Missionary Society in the Nineteenth Century: A Study of Ideas' (PhD thesis, Washington University, 1974), 468.

3. During the early history of the LMS, it established a close connection with the Anglicans, the Independents, and Scottish Presbyterians. Perry comments that the LMS was 'a good example of the evangelical united front in operations.' For an in-depth discussion, see *ibid.*, 2–37.
4. *Ibid.*, 39.
5. The sources of incomes were mainly four: subscriptions and donations, special objects (such as centenary fund, contributions for Female Missions), legacies, and dividends. Expenditures include two major items: the accounts of missionaries and missions, as well as the account of its administration. For details, 'Appendix III: Analysis of the Income and Expenditure of the London Missionary Society from 1796 to 1895', R. Lovett, *A History of the London Missionary Society,* Vol. 2 (London: Henry Frowde, 1899), 750–5.
6. J. Morison, *The Fathers and Founders of the London Missionary Society: A Jubilee Memorial; Including A Sketch of the Origin, Progress, and Prospects of the London Missionary Society,* new edn, (London: Fisher, Son & Co., 1844), xxxi.
7. *A Letter to the Directors of the London Missionary Society* (Norwich: Henry Pigg, 1865), 5–6.
8. G. Anderson (ed.), *Biographical Dictionary of Christian Missions* (New York: Macmillan Reference USA, 1998), s.v. 'Joseph Mullen and Hannah Lacroix', 408.
9. J. Mullen, *Missionary Principles and Plans: As Illustrated by Letters Recently addressed by the Directors to the Missionaries of the Society* (London: London Missionary Society, 1869), 35.
10. C. Northcott, *Glorious Company: One Hundred and Fifty Years Life and Work of the London Missionary Society* (London: London Missionary Society, 1945), 157.
11. *Ibid.*, 158.
12. *Oxford English Dictionary,* Internet edition, 2002, s.v. "Voluntarism."
13. E. Gulick, *Peter Parker and the Opening of China* (Cambridge: Harvard University Press, 1973), 75.
14. He received medical education at the University of London where he was awarded Bachelor of Medicine. He was a member of the Royal College of Surgeons.
15. He had a brief training in the Chinese language with James Legge and William C. Milne at the University College under Samuel Kidd. M.K. Wong, *James Legge: A Pioneer at Crossroads of East and West* (Hong Kong: Hong Kong Educational Publishing Company, 1996), 15.
16. W. Lockhart, *The Medical Missionary in China: A Narrative of Twenty Years' Experience* (London: Hurst and Blackett, 1861), 126.

17. E.J. Eitel, *Europe in China: The History of Hong Kong from the Beginning to the Year 1882* (Hong Kong: Kelly & Walsh, 1895), 191.
18. Lockhart, *op. cit.* (note 16), 203
19. Y.T. Ng, *The Early Population of Hong Kong: Growth, Distribution, and Structural Change, 1841–1931* (Hong Kong: Department of Geography, The Chinese University of Hong Kong, 1984), 4.
20. Robert Morrison, the LMS pioneer missionary, baptised Kueh A-gong in Macao in 1830. After baptism, Kueh worked as an assistant in the mission first in Malacca and then in Hong Kong. He was also a preacher in the LMS Chinese churches. See C.T. Smith, *Chinese Christians: Elites, Middlemen, and the Church in Hong Kong* (Hong Kong: Oxford University Press, 1985), 7 and 213.
21. B. Hobson, *A General Report of the Hospital at Kum-Le-Fau, in Canton from April 1848 to November 1849* (Canton: S. Wells William, 1850), 6.
22. Not much background about Chan Apoon is known. In 1841, he began as an apprentice in Western medicine under Hobson. By 1844, as claimed by Hobson, Chan Apoon had already achieved certain fluency in English, he did well in anatomy, diseases and operations on eyes, *Chinese Repository*, 14 (1844), 380–1. Later, he left the mission hospital to take up a better-paid job as an interpreter in a Chinese firm. Hobson, *op. cit.* (note 21), 36–7.
23. Lockhart, *op. cit.* (note 16), 207.
24. *Substance of an Address; Delivered by Benjamin Hobson, Esq., M.B. at a Meeting of the Friends of the Chinese Association, in aid of the Medical Missionary Society in China* (Hackney: n.p., 1846), 6–7.
25. For the details of his conflicts with Parker, see Gulick, *op. cit.* (note 13), 125–31.
26. Hobson, *op. cit.* (note 21), 7–8, and Lockhart, *op. cit.* (note 16), 208.
27. The English titles are from A. Wylie, *Memorials of Protestant Missionaries to the Chinese: Giving a List of Their Publications, and Obituary Notices of the Deceased* (Shanghai: American Presbyterian Mission Press, 1867), 126–8.
28. C.B. Whitmore, 'A History of the Development of Western Medicine in China' (PhD thesis, University of Southern California, 1934), 155–6.
29. Cited in *Chinese Repository*, 20 (1851), 381–2.
30. G.H. Choa, *'Heal the Sick' was their Motto: The Protestant Medical Missions in China* (Hong Kong: Chinese University Press, 1990), 72. For a brief study of the impact of the medical texts that Hobson produced, see Zhao Pushan, 'On The Five Texts on Western Medicines by Benjamin Hobson and Their Impact in China', *Modern Historical Studies*, 2 (1991), 67–83, 100 [in Chinese].
31. He received his medical training at Berlin University, and he was a member of the London College of Surgeons; see Hobson, *op. cit.* (note 21), 8.
32. Lockhart, *op. cit.* (note 16), 208–10.

33. Ho Tsun-sheen, who was ordained in 1846, was the key person in the LMS Chinese church. He studied the Bible and wrote commentaries to the Gospel according to L. Pfister, 'A Transmitter but not a Creator: Ho Tsun-sheen (1817–1871), the First Modern Chinese Protestant Theologian', in I. Eber, S.K. Wan and K. Walf (eds), *Bible in Modern China; The Literary and Intellectual Impact* (Sankt Augustin: Institute Monumenta Serica, 1999), 165–97. Ng Mun-sow studied theology at the Anglo-Chinese college and was one of three Chinese boys invited to Buckingham Palace. Later, he left the LMS mission and joined the Hong Kong Police as an interpreter and later the Chinese Maritime Office. See, Y.S. Leung, 'Some Found It, Some Lost It: James Legge and the Three Chinese Boys from Malacca', *Asian Culture,* 1 (February 1983), 55–9.
34. A Letter to the LMS by Hirschberg, dated 28 January 1851. London Missionary Society Archives, Incoming Letters, South China, 5/2/A.
35. Gulick, *op. cit.* (note 13), 130.
36. Three Chinese boys from the Anglo-Chinese College and James Legge were invited to the Buckingham Palace where they had an interview with Queen Victoria and Prince Albert. They were of course capable of attracting much publicity in the media not only in Hong Kong but also Britain. The preparatory school attached to the Anglo-Chinese College became a popular school in Hong Kong. The number of students reached 83 in 1856. For details, see M.K. Wong, 'The Historical Significance of the Anglo-Chinese College in Sino-Western Cultural Exchange', *On Problems of Asian History: The Collection of Essays in Honour of Professor Hideo Fukazawa's Retirement* (Morioka: Centre of Asian History, Iwate University, 2000), 23–39 [in Chinese].
37. Minutes of the LMS Hong Kong Missions, 8 and 16 September 1851. London Missionary Society Archives.
38. J. Paquette, 'An Uncompromising Land: The London Missionary Society in China, 1807–1860', (PhD thesis, University of California, Los Angeles, 1987), 258–9.
39. *Ibid.*, 260
40. Cole, who had been appointed to work in the LMS Hong Kong mission in 1847, was dismissed by the LMS directors in 1852 largely, it seems, because of their anti-American prejudices. They consistently undervalued his contribution, even though his colleagues in Hong Kong appreciated his work, see C. Su, 'The Printing Press of the London Missionary Society among the Chinese', (PhD thesis, University of London, 1996), 350–2; Paquette, *op. cit.* (note 38), 259–68.
41. Wong Fun was a student of the Morrison Education Society school in Hong Kong. Samuel Brown took him, along with two more Chinese boys, to Massachusetts where he had his education in Monson Academy, and he

furthered his education at the University of Edinburgh where he obtained the degree of Doctor of Medicine. After he finished his medical education, his application to be a China medical missionary was accepted. Smith, *op. cit.* (note 20), 159–60.

42. K.W. So, E.P. Boardman and P. Ch'iu, 'Hung Jen-kan, Taiping Prime Minister, 1859–1964', *Harvard Journal of Asiatic Studies* 20: 1 and 2 (June 1957): 262–94; see also F. Michael and C.L. Chang, *The Taiping Rebellion: History and Documents*, Vol. 1 (Seattle: University of Washington Press, 1966), 134–68.
43. C. Su, 'Wong Fun and the London Missionary Society' *Journal of the History of Christianity in Modern China*, 3 (2000), 21–30 [in Chinese].
44. Whitmore, *op. cit.* (note 28), 182 and 218.
45. E.H. Paterson, *A Hospital for Hong Kong: The Centenary History of the Alice Ho Miu Ling Nethersole Hospital* (Hong Kong: Alice Ho Miu Ling Nethersole Hospital, 1987), 13.
46. S. Bard, *Traders of Hong Kong: Some Foreign Merchant Houses, 1841–1899* (Hong Kong: Urban Council, 1993), 92–3.
47. A report written by John Pope Hennessy to the Earl of Kimberley, dated 8 February 1882, reprinted in *Hongkong Annual Administration Reports*, Vol. 1, 1841–1886 (London: Archive Edition, 1996), 657.
48. G.H. Choa, *The Life and Times of Sir Kai Ho Kai: A Prominent Figure in Nineteenth Century Hong Kong*, 2nd edn (Hong Kong: The Chinese University Press, 2000).
49. Whitmore, *op. cit.* (note 28), 223–6; see also *Hong Kong Government Gazette* (9 May 1891), 405.
50. Kwong later joined St. Stephen's Church, where he was ordained. Ko Cheuk-shing, 'A History of the To Tsai Church', in C.M. Lee (ed.), *The Silver Jubilee of the Hop Yat Church of the Church for Christ in China* (Hong Kong: Hop Yat Church, 1957), 33 [in Chinese]. See also, Y.S. Lau, *A History of Christianity in Hong Kong* (Hong Kong: Chinese Churches Union, 1941), 270–3 [in Chinese].
51. He obtained the degrees of Doctor of Medicine and Master of Surgery, and he received his education from a medical school in Montreal, Canada. See C.T. Smith, *A Sense of History: Studies in the Social and Urban History of Hong Kong* (Hong Kong: Hong Kong Educational Pub. Co., 1995), 322.
52. He was a senior partner of the Jardine and Matheson Company. Before he came to Hong Kong, he worked in Shanghai. He was appointed by the Governor of Hong Kong to serve as a member of the Legislative Council of Hong Kong in 1878 and from 1881 to 1884. G.B. Endacott, *Government and People in Hong Kong: A Constitutional History* (Hong Kong: Hong Kong University Press, 1964), 251; and C. Criswell, *The Taipan: Hong Kong's Merchant Princes* (Hong Kong: Oxford University Press, 1981), 151.

53. Thomas Jackson was the chief manager of the Hong Kong and Shanghai Banking Corporation between 1876 and 1902. He was elected by the General Chamber of Commerce to be a member of the Legislative Council from 1884 to 1886. After his term of service at the Legislative Council, he served in some other committees of public interest. On the occasion of his death, F.H. May, the governor, highly regarded his character and contribution and put it in the records of the Legislative Council. See *Hong Kong Hansard* (23 December 1915); see also, Endacott, *op. cit.* (note 52), and Criswell, *op. cit.* (note 52), 147–8.
54. Wong Shing had an English education in Hong Kong in the 1840s and had a brief sojourn in the USA. He was a pious Christian, and worked for the LMS Press. He also worked for Li Hung-chang, a reformer official, and later worked in the Chinese legation in Washington. In Hong Kong, he was a well-respected figure. He was one of the founding directors of the Tung Wah Hospital. He was appointed by the Governor of Hong Kong to be a member of the Legislative Council between 1884 and 1890. See Endacott, *op. cit.* (note 52), 100.
55. After graduation from the University of Aberdeen, Frederick Stewart was recruited to be the first principal of the Central School, the first government fully funded school. He was shifted to head the office of the Registrar-General, a position that mostly handled the well-being of the Chinese in Hong Kong. Also in this capacity, he was appointed as an unofficial member of the Legislative Council between 1883 and 1884. Endacott, *op. cit.* (note 52); see also G. Bickley, *The Golden Needle: The Biography of Frederick Stewart (1836–1889)* (Hong Kong: The David C. Lam Institute for East–West Studies, Hong Kong Baptist University, 2000).
56. Wei Yuk's father, Wei Kwong, was an adopted son of an American missionary, and he became an affluent merchant thanks to his Western education. Wei Kwong sent Wei Yuk to have his university education in Scotland. The Wei family extended its familial network through marriage with Wong Shing's family. Like Ho Kai, Wei was active in public service. He was a member of the significant social institutions in Hong Kong, such as the Tung Wah Hospital, the Po Leung Kuk, and the District Watchmen Committee. Notably, he was a member of the Legislative Council from 1896 to 1914. He was knighted in 1919.
57. Wong Wing-sheung's father was Wong Shing. From 1895 onwards, Wong Wing-sheung was involved in the revolutionary activities overthrowing the Qing court. E.J.M. Rhoads, *China's Republican Revolution: The Case of Kwangtung, 1895–1913* (Cambridge, MA: Harvard University Press, 1975), 39–41.
58. John Chalmers received his education from the University of Aberdeen and Cheshunt College. In 1852, he came to Hong Kong where he had worked

for seven years, and then transferred to take charge of the Canton mission. From 1879, he concurrently took charge of the Canton and Hong Kong missions. He achieved a good standard in the Chinese language. He was the author of the following books: *The Origin of the Chinese* (Hong Kong: De Souza & Co., 1866); *Lau-tsze* (London: Trübner, 1868); *The Question of Terms Simplified* (Canton: E-Shing, 1876); and *An Account of the Structure of Chinese Characters under 300 Primary Forms* (London: Trübner, 1882).

59. J. Chalmers, 'The Decennial Report for Hong Kong, 1880–1890', London Missionary Society Archives.
60. *Ibid.*
61. Alice Walkden had a considerable fortune, but after her death Ho Kai gave most of it to her siblings who, had come with her to Hong Kong so that they could return to Britain. Walkden and Ho Kai had a daughter, but he believed that it was best that her maternal family bring her up in Britain, in part using the money he had donated to them. He used the residue of the inheritance to help cover the cost of establishing the Alice Memorial Hospital and the Hong Kong College of Medicine. T.Y. Kuo, Y.L. Shen and W. Hsieh, *The Reminiscences of Mr. Fu Ping-chang* (Taipei: Institute of Modern History, Academia Sinica, 1993), 10 [in Chinese].
62. Ko, *op. cit.* (note 50), 33.
63. 'Report of Botanical and Afforestation Department for 1886', Sessional Papers for the Legislative Council, Hong Kong Government, 1887, 328.
64. Chalmers, *op. cit.* (note 59).
65. There are three major scholarly accounts for the establishment of the Alice Memorial Hospital. Paterson, *op. cit.* (note 45); C.T. Smith, 'Sun Yat Sen's Middle School Days in Hong Kong and the Establishment of Alice Memorial Hospital', in *op. cit.* (note 51), 320–38; and Choa, *op. cit.* (note 48).
66. D.E. Evans, *Constancy of Purpose: Faculty of Medicine, University of Hong Kong* (Hong Kong: Hong Kong University Press, 1987); N.H.L. Ng, *Interactions of East and West: Development of Public Education in Early Hong Kong* (Hong Kong: The Chinese University Press, 1984), 121–4; Choa, *op. cit.* (note 48), 57–78.
67. Evans, *op. cit.* (note 66), 29. James Cantlie qualified in 1875 as a Bachelor of Medicine and Master of Surgery of the University of Aberdeen. He was also a Fellow of the Royal College of Surgeons of England and he held a Certificate of Health, Royal College of Physicians. See, *Hong Kong Government Gazette* (9 May 1891): 405. He went to Hong Kong in 1887, where he had a brief yet remarkable career. He was responsible for rescuing the captured Sun Yat-sen in London. This event made Sun the focus of international media and the most well-known revolutionary in China.
68. It is well known that Sun Yat-sen was a Christian. Kwan King-leung was a

Christian and his family was deeply rooted in the LMS Hong Kong mission. Wong Sai-yan was a Christian, and his father was Wong Him-yue, a pastor of the Rhenish Mission. Wong Chung Yik was a Christian, and his father was Wong Yuk-cho, the Chinese pastor of the To Tsai Church. It may be noted that Wong Him-yue and Wong Yuk-cho were brothers. Wong Tze-fu, *The Wong's Family.* (Hong Kong, 1954); Lau, *op. cit* (note 50), and C.S. Wong, *History of To Tsai Church: The First Independent Church of China* (Hong Kong: Chinese Christian Literature Council, 1986). [In Chinese]

69. S.F. Li, *Hong Kong Surgeon* (New York: E.P. Dutton & Co., Inc, 1964), 25–31.
70. Chalmers, *op. cit.* (note 59).
71. J. Chalmers, 'Report on Hong Kong Station for 1886', Reports: South China, London Missionary Society Archives. See also, Smith, *op. cit.* (note 51), 328.
72. Smith, *op. cit.* (note 51), 322–3.
73. J. Chalmers, 'Report on Hong Kong Station for 1888', Reports: South China London Missionary Society Archives.
74. Chalmers, *op. cit.* (note 59), and Wong, *op. cit.* (note 68), 20–2. Wong Yuk-cho was the pastor of the To Tsai Church, a Chinese church that became independent of the LMS.
75. Chalmers, *op. cit.* (note 59).
76. Smith, *op. cit.* (note 51), 325.
77. In the centennial history of the London Missionary Society, it was remarked that 'a large hospital, containing ninety beds, was erected by Dr Ho Kai, the son of an early convert, in 1886', Lovett, *op. cit.* (note 5), 464. Although this is an exaggeration, it is a view that was often repeated. See, *The London Missionary Society Decennial Report, 1910–1911,* London Missionary Society Archives, South China, Reports, 20; and N. Bitton, *Our Heritage in China* (London: London Missionary Society, 1913), 53.
78. *London Missionary Society Decennial Report 1901–1911: Hongkong, Canton & Poklo* (Hong Kong: Hong Kong Printing Press, 1911), 20.
79. For details, see J. George, 'Moving with Chinese Opinions: Hong Kong's Maternity Service, 1881–1941', (PhD thesis, University of Sydney, 1992), 98–130.
80. *Ibid.*, 103.
81. 'Register of Medical and Surgical Practitioners', *Hong Kong Gazette* (5 May 1905), 637; see also J. Sibree, *London Missionary Society: A Register of Missionaries, Deputations, etc., from 1796–1923* (London: London Missionary Society, 1923), 148. For the background of this newly founded hospital and the problems that Sibree faced, see J. George, 'The Lady Doctor's "Warm Welcome": Dr Alice Sibree and the Early Years of Hong Kong's Maternity Service 1903–1909', *Journal of the Hong Kong Branch of*

the Royal Asiatic Society, 33 (1993), 81–109. She returned to Hong Kong after her brief stay in Britain, where she continued to work to improve maternity services. She was later appointed as a medical officer of the Hong Kong Government and her work in this post came to be highly regarded. It was for example recorded that: 'Of pre-eminent value are her efforts to create for the Colony an adequate supply of Chinese midwives and nurses fully trained according to Western standards'; 'Report of the Secretary for Chinese Affairs for the year 1925', *Administrative Report for 1925,* C12. She was awarded an MBE by the government and was also made a Sister of the Order of St. John of Jerusalem. *Register of the LMS Missionaries, idem.,* 148.

82. *Hong Kong Government Gazette* (16 December 1910), 547. She resigned in 1913 and left for Britain to marry Isaia Edward Mitchell, an LMS medical missionary in Hong Kong. He received his medical training from the University of Montreal where he was awarded Bachelor of Arts, Doctor of Medicine, and Master of Surgery. He registered as a medical practitioner in Britain in 1903. *Hong Kong Government Gazette* (10 June 1910), and Sibree, *op. cit.* (note 81), 150. He came to serve as an LMS missionary in Hong Kong in 1904, but moved to Macao in 1906, Canton in 1907, and Poklo between 1908–10. He moved back to Hong Kong and worked there between 1910 and 1913. After his marriage with E. W. Perkins in 1913, the LMS sent the Mitchell family to Tingchowfu and Hankow in China. They returned to work as medical missionaries in Hong Kong in 1920.
83. *Hong Kong Government Gazette* (28 October 1921), 453.
84. Sibree, *op. cit.* (note 81), 160; *The Hong Kong Government Gazette* (2 January 1914), 3.
85. S.L. Lau, *Sanctuary of Excellence: The History of Ying Wa College* (Hong Kong: Ying Wa College Old Boys' Association Limited, 2001), 126 [in Chinese].
86. *Decennial Report, 1901–1911, op. cit.* (note 77), 23.
87. *Hong Kong Government Gazette* (18 December 1897), 1093; Sibree, *op. cit.* (note 81), 120; *The Government Gazette* (16 October 1897 and 5 November 1898); Evans, *op. cit.* (note 66), 263–4.
88. *Hong Kong Gazette* (18 December 1897), 1093; Sibree, *op. cit.* (note 81), 137; Evans, *op. cit.* (note 66), 260.
89. His father was Wan Wai-Ching, a pastor in the LMS Poklo mission. The Wan family later moved to Hong Kong.
90. 'Institutions not supported by the Government', Hong Kong Administrative Report for 1909, Hong Kong Government publication, 18.
91. The meeting with Dr Chung, Medical Committee meeting, 29 January 1895, in 'Medical Committee Report', Sessional Papers for the Legislative Council, Hong Kong Government publication (1895).
92. *Ibid.*

93. *Report of the Alice Memorial Hospital Hong Kong in Connection with the London Missionary Society* (Hong Kong: n.p., 1890), 7; 'Report of the Principal Civil Medical Officer for 1897', *The Hongkong Government Gazette* (24 September 1898), 980. Apparently, he was a well-respected practitioner. The Inspecting Medical Officer acknowledged that 'His kindness, courtesy, tact, and professional skill combined to enable him to effect the very great improvements that were made during this tenure of office, and for which the credit is practically entirely to him', in 'Report of the Principal Civil Medical Officer for the year 1902', Sessional Papers for the Legislative Council, Hong Kong Government publication (1903), 273.
94. 'The Report of the Principal Civil Medical Officer for the 1897', *Hong Kong Government Gazette* (24 September 1898). For an excellent study, see E. Sinn, *Power and Charity: The Early History of the Tung Wah Hospital, Hong Kong* (Hong Kong: Oxford University Press, 1989).
95. 'Report of the Principal Civil Medical Officer for 1897', *The Hong Kong Government Gazette* (24 September 1898), 980; 'Report of the Principal Civil Medical Officer for the year 1902', Sessional Papers for the Legislative Council, Hong Kong Government publication (1903), 273.
96. A. Wright (ed.), *Twentieth Century Impressions of Hong Kong: History, People, Commerce, Industries and Resources* (London: Lloyds Greater Britain Publishing Company, 1908; reprint, Singapore: Graham Brash, 1990), 178–80; *The One Hundred and Third Report of the London Missionary Society* (London: London Missionary Society, 1898), 31.
97. 'Report of the Principal Civil Medical Officer for 1898', Sessional Papers for the Legislative Council, Hong Kong Government publication (1899).
98. Paterson, *op. cit.* (note 45), 58 and 70.
99. J. Stewart, 'Report of Hong Kong Mission for the Year of 1910', [n.d.], London Missionary Society Archives, South China, Reports.
100. L.K. Rayner, 'Alice Memorial and Affiliated Hospital for the year of 1921', [December 1921] London Missionary Society Archives, South China, Reports.
101. Midwives trained in the Alice Memorial Maternity Hospital were exempted from taking the written examination and some clauses that were required for those who wanted to obtain a government certificate. For details see 'Rules framed by the Midwives Board under Section 4 of the Midwives Ordinance, 1910', *Hong Kong Government Gazette* (22 September 1911), 400–3.
102. J. Stewart, 'Report of Hong Kong Mission for the Year of 1910', [n.d.], and J. Stewart, 'Report of Hong Kong Mission for the year of 1909', 26 June 1910, both are available at the London Missionary Society Archives, South China, Reports.
103. L.K. Rayner, 'Report for 1917 [on the nurses]' London Missionary Society Archives, South China, Reports. Report for 1921.

104. The house committee was abolished in 1898. The finance committee played a significant role. Of course, the *de facto* control was still with the LMS and its medical missionaries in Hong Kong. A major move for change was installed under the new constitution in 1924.
105. The expenditure was recorded in *Hong Kong Administrative Reports* for the respective years.
106. L.K. Rayner, 'Alice Memorial and Affiliated Hospitals for 1921', [December 1921], London Missionary Society Archives, South China, Reports.

4

Professionalising the Rural Medical Mission in Weixian, 1890–1925

John R. Stanley

During the nineteenth century, medical missionary work was very strongly associated with evangelising, and medical missionaries were expected also to take part in evangelising activities. In the early-twentieth century there was an influx of more experienced doctors who were concerned first and foremost with the medical side to their work. Another important development was an opening up of funding for this medical work by the Rockefeller Foundation. This chapter examines these issues in the context of the mission station at Weixian in China. It looks at problems that the professional staff at the hospital experienced in establishing modern and professional medical care, examines the role of the Rockefeller Foundation in the establishment of the Shadyside Hospital, and considers issues raised when secular medical concerns gained a greater weight within missions. Finally, it reflects on the importance of these changes for rural hospitals.

Whereas there has been considerable research and writing on mission-based systems of education in China, medical mission work has remained a neglected field of study. It is generally agreed that missionary work in education had a deep impact on China, as it provided a new model for primary, secondary, and university education that was widely extended in the post-1911 period. Missionaries also promoted education for women in both urban and rural areas, and they took part in the movement against foot binding. By contrast, we know little about the impact of the medical missionaries. It has been argued that this was greatest in the rural areas where there were little or no alternative forms of medical treatment available to the people. This is, however, disputed by C.C. Chen (Chen Zhiqian), who argues that their greatest influence was in the treaty ports and large urban areas.[1] This study will seek to shed light on the matter through a study of the medical work of the American Presbyterian Mission at Weixian, in the interior of the Shandong province. It will focus on the conflicts and problems encountered by these medical missionaries in this rural setting between 1890 and 1920.

The American Presbyterians in China and Shandong

The American Presbyterians eventually became one of the largest mission groups active in China, and their methods had a profound impact on those adopted by other societies. In the beginning, however, their work was very uncertain. G. Thompson Brown has analysed the debates between two main Presbyterian tendencies. On the one hand, there was what he defines as the 'Old School', which believed that it was the responsibility of the Church to organize and support foreign missions; on the other, there was the 'New School' that believed motivated individuals should organise the necessary work without any formal backing from the Church. Several attempts were made by the Old School between 1812 and 1831 to establish a Foreign Missions Board under the General Assembly. After one such effort had failed in 1831, some of its supporters set about establishing their own board called the Western Foreign Missionary Society. Between 1832 and 1837 this society sent out sixty missionaries to work among native americans in the United States, to Liberia, and to India. The General Assembly of the Presbyterian Church formally approved the establishment of a Foreign Missions Board and incorporated the organisation and missionaries of the breakaway group in 1837.[2]

The first decision the Board made was to concentrate its efforts in China. China was seen to be a large and important area for mission work that had the advantage of having a single written language, with a people who were considered to be ignorant of the 'true God', and ready and willing – so it was believed – to accept Christianity.[3] In December 1837 the Board appointed Reverend John A. Mitchell, and Reverend Robert and Mrs Eliza Carter Orr to open the mission. Their initial job was to locate an area for a base of operations. According to G. Thompson Brown they 'desired…a place that was healthy, where people and property would be protected and where there was a goodly number of Chinese.'[4] As part of their work they were to establish schools, begin printing Christian literature, and spread the word of God.[5] As was the case with other missionary groups at that time, the first missionaries did not settle in the Chinese Empire.[6] Rather, they established a residence in Singapore and began to work among the local Chinese. The early pioneers were plagued by ill health. Mitchell developed a fever and died in October 1838, and in 1841 Orr was forced through illness to return to the United States. In 1840, Reverend Thomas L. McBryde, Dr J.C. Hepburn, and their wives reinforced the group. However, the climate was not suitable for their health and the mission could not be put on a stable footing.

By 1843, conditions in China had changed as a result of the First Opium War.[7] The ensuing treaties allowed the missionaries to relocate to the new treaty ports. The Presbyterians chose the treaty port of Xiamen (Amoy), which was approximately four hundred miles north of Guangzhou (Canton) and was said to have a healthier environment for foreigners. Xiamen was abandoned in 1848, with Ningbo becoming the chief centre. The missionaries in this latter place had already opened a boys' boarding school in 1845, with twenty-three students who studied Chinese classics, geography, Western history, arithmetic and the Bible.[8] Another station was opened in 1850 in Shanghai.[9] Dr John G. Kerr established the first dispensary to be run by this mission – in Guangzhou in 1854. In 1856, he reported that he had treated 20,000 patients there.[10] New areas of China were opened up to the missions after the Second Opium War (1856–60). The American Presbyterians established a new mission for Peking (Beijing) and Shandong.[11] In May 1861 Reverend Samuel Gayley and Reverend J.A. Danforth moved from Shanghai to the newly designated open port of Dengzhou[12] in the Shandong Province.[13] British Baptists soon joined them there, and together the two missions would eventually establish the Shandong Christian University. The work of the American Presbyterians in Shandong was boosted by the arrival of three new missionaries between 1861 and 1863: John L. Nevius (1861), Calvin Mateer (1863), and Hunter Corbett (1863). These three pioneer missionaries – the 'Shantung Triumvirate'[14] – initiated a series of religious and secular ventures that became the trademark of the mission's work in Shandong.

From their stations at Chefoo and Dengzhou the Presbyterian missionaries went far into the countryside, sometimes travelling as much as two hundred and fifty miles into the hinterland of Shandong.[15] Hunter Corbett was particularly keen to open stations in the interior, even criticising John Nevius for confining his work to the areas around the provincial capital of Jinan, which was located in the extreme west of the province. Corbett argued that it was better to launch itinerating tours from the interior, obviating the need to make long trips from the coast that – considering the size of the province – had a negative effect on the health of the missionaries.[16] By the 1880s, with the number of communicants increasing rapidly – from, for example, 877 in 1881 to 1,149 in 1882[17] – the necessity for a new station in the interior became more apparent. Nevius opposed this, as he believed that all stations should be self-supporting. He was eventually overruled, and plans for opening a new station at Weixian were initiated.

In many respects, Weixian was ideally situated for such a mission station. An old and historic city, it was connected to Jinan – about 120 miles to the west – by an important trade road that ran across a broad plain. For many years a relatively minor centre, it had by the late-nineteenth century 'grown from a more modest level to become the centre of commerce in the eastern portion of Shantung.'[18] Whereas in 1573 it had a population of only 21,769, by 1672 the figure had increased to 143,120, and by 1906 it numbered 497,328.[19] The region around the city was also densely populated, with about four million people in all. Wealth was concentrated in the hands of a sizeable gentry class. In the words of Charles Roys: 'Centuries of wealth have made its people proud and conservative beyond measure, even for China.'[20] In this respect the place was less congenial for the missionaries, and they were to encounter considerable opposition from its conservative elite over the years.

As early as 1865 Calvin Mateer of the Dengzhou station and Hunter Corbett of the Chefoo station had toured the area. Although they did not enter the city at this time, they reported on its potential:

> The streets were full of people, and they were not sparing in their expressions of enmity and contempt. We saw a great number of elegant memorial arches near Wei Hsien and learned that it is a very wealthy place. This was indicated by the many elegant burying grounds around it, and by the good condition of the walls. The country all around, and indeed most we passed through to-day, was very rich.[21]

They were not the only missionaries to take an interest in the area. The Reverend Alexander Williamson of the United Presbyterian Church of Scotland and the National Bible Society of Scotland had worked there during 1867, and the Reverend MacIntyre, of the United Presbyterian Mission of Scotland, followed him in the next decade.[22] Neither of them was able to establish a permanent base in Weixian and they soon moved on. In 1872, the Reverend J.S. McIlvaine opened a mission station at Jinan, deep in the interior. In 1881 the American Presbyterians decided to open a permanent station in Weixian, which they considered an area of hope for mission work.[23] It was believed that there were several advantages in having a base in this city, as it was a major centre for trade that attracted large crowds of up to ten thousand people on market days.[24] Being at the heart of a densely populated area, it was easy for the missionaries to carry on their evangelical work without going on long itinerations into the countryside. Already, there was a nucleus of converts in the area. Hunter Corbett reported that there were at least three hundred within a 'radius of one day's journey' from Weixian.[25] Without a missionary base in the area, the converts lacked any regular contact with the Church and it was feared that they might waver in their new faith.[26] It was agreed that this could be remedied only if a new station was opened midway between the coastal cities and Jinan. The missionaries who were selected for this new post were the Reverend Robert

Mateer, the Reverend John Laughlin, Annie Laughlin, and Dr and Mrs Horace Smith. They sailed for China in the autumn of 1881 and on their arrival in Shandong began to study the language and made preparations for opening the Weixian station. Once funds were made available by the Foreign Board to purchase land, Robert Mateer, Laughlin and Hunter Corbett travelled there together – a journey of four days. As they began to enquire about buying a plot, prices began to increase exponentially. They therefore decided to search outside the city wall, being helped in this by a local preacher of the mission, Li Fu-yuan. Eventually, they managed to secure five *mu* of land from a local farmer that was ideally situated on a major road that led to the city, about one mile to the southeast. It was on the West bank of the Yu River, and adjoined the Li family village (*Li Jia Zhuang*). The missionaries insisted on erecting Western-style constructions, even though the local people would have preferred Chinese-style buildings.[27] From an initial simple house, the number of buildings increased in time to include two schools, a large three-storey hospital, a department of the Christian College, a Bible School, and residences for the missionaries and teachers. Other hospitals and schools were gradually established elsewhere in the region, covering an area of about five hundred square miles. A firm basis was thus established for educational, medical, and evangelical work, and this soon became one of the leading mission stations in all of Shandong.

Bringing medical personnel to the countryside

Many of the early mission doctors arrived full of faith, believing that their chief priority was evangelism. They tended to tolerate the fact that the amenities for their medical work left much to be desired. Attitudes began to change from around 1900, when they began to become increasingly frustrated with the low quality of the medical infrastructure. They held that they were there to heal bodies, not just save the souls of the patients. This – the idea of the Social Gospel – affected their relationship with the non-medical missionaries and it led, at times, to open conflicts within the Shandong Mission.

The first resident doctor in Weixian was Horace R. Smith, MD, and he was expected to begin medical work immediately upon his arrival in April 1883 as it was believed that this provided one of the best means to overcome the hostility of the urban population towards the foreign missionaries.[28] The doctor was required to build a bridge for the evangelists. There were, however, problems from the start. Smith had managed with some difficulty to rent a part of an inn within the city for his dispensary, but very soon pressure from the local population forced the landlord to break the agreement. As a result he had to conduct his work from outside the city in a cramped part of a house. It was clear that this arrangement would not enable him to carry on any long-term work.[29] In June 1883 Smith left Weixian for the summer and there is no further record of a doctor before 1884. There is no mention in the records of any of the evangelists of the mission writing on Smith's behalf for funds for a building, which suggests that they were not as committed to the medical work as they might have been. Nevertheless, they were vociferous in their letters to the Presbyterian Foreign Board in demanding a replacement for Smith.

The second mission doctor in Weixian was J.M. Matthewson. In describing him, Frank Ellinwood, Secretary of the Foreign Board, only stated that he was from California and that 'he will be able to meet in some degree the disappointment of the people'.[30] Although he apparently obtained a positive response from the local population, the other resident missionaries did not provide him with adequate backing. His sole supporter appears to have been Jennie Anderson (Chalfant), who wrote that the doctor was entirely overworked and lacked the facilities to make his work really effective. She suggested that another doctor be appointed to assist him.[31] Robert Mateer and other evangelists overruled her, arguing that an extra minister was needed more urgently than a doctor. For them, winning souls took precedent over saving lives. Mathewson had to return to the USA in 1886, once more leaving the station without a resident doctor.

The evangelists began to have second thoughts after the death that same year of Sadie Mateer, Robert Mateer's first wife. This led to some soul searching, and a new willingness to forego ministerial reinforcements in favour of medical personnel and facilities. Robert Mateer made the search for new medical personnel into something of a personal quest. He had his own definition of what constituted a good missionary doctor, and evangelism came high on his list of virtues. Although he was prepared to accept a female doctor, he preferred a male one if possible. He doubted the Board's ability to choose a doctor, arguing that conditions in the interior were such that only missionaries from that field could adequately judge the quality of an appointee. Writing to Frank Ellinwood, he stated that the Foreign Board had made mistakes in the station's appointments and that he wanted more control over appointments to the station. In common with many other missionaries at this time, Mateer was prepared to press his views on the Foreign Board in a much more assertive manner than had hitherto been the case. He was adamant that mission doctors should work within the guidelines set by the evangelists. Through his efforts Drs William Faries, Mary Brown, and Madge Dickson (Mateer) were eventually appointed in 1890.

A small hospital called the Mateer Memorial Hospital had been completed in 1889, and it was to serve as a base for the work of the new medical missionaries throughout the Weixian region. Working in tandem with the evangelists, they were expected to spend a lot of time itinerating in the surrounding region, using the hospital as a base. Although this brought the doctors closer to the rural population, it meant that the medical work in Weixian city tended to stagnate. The hospital facilities improved only slowly. Within a couple of decades, and with the arrival of new medical missionaries, it became apparent that the medical infrastructure was very inadequate. The new staff were also more prepared to assert themselves against the evangelical missionaries. They wanted to be able to make a real impact on the health of the population as a whole, and they demanded outstation dispensaries and the construction of a new hospital. They were, moreover, not willing to be treated by the evangelists as subordinates within the mission enterprise. In the process, they redefined the role of medical work within the missionary movement.

Dr Charles Roys and evangelistic apathy

The desire for new facilities went hand- in-hand with an increasing emphasis on public health and new developments in medical theory. The 'germ theory of disease' was beginning to take root in medical circles, leading to demands by foreign residents in China for sanitary and public health improvements in the localities they inhabited.[32] Colonial officers in Shanghai and Xiamen tried to improve the sanitation in their respective cities so as to prevent disease.[33] In 1886 an article was published in *The Chinese Recorder*, entitled 'Sanitary Salvation,' in which the author argued that ague and typhoid were common in China as a result of the 'sheer laziness' of the Chinese, who emptied their slops around their houses, the problem being compounded by 'narrow, overcrowded sleeping-rooms, dark, damp and filthy'.[34] The missionaries had done little in this area, in part because of a lack of staff, and in part because it was not work that was seen to be a vehicle for conversion.

The situation began to change in the early-twentieth century, as more missionaries understood the importance of such measures. Many felt that 'public health work would not only benefit the people the missionaries served, but would also reduce the medical missionaries' workload as a result of improvement of the health of the people.'[35] Articles and letters began to appear in *The China Medical Missionary Journal* – later *The China Medical Journal* – advocating public health improvements. Initially, the focus was on publishing leaflets to increase the general knowledge of the Chinese about these problems. Despite this, there were some areas that the *CMJ* tended to ignore, such as the increasing problem of tuberculosis. Many missionary doctors refused to treat this disease because of the high death rate. They felt that any benefit that might be gained by the Chinese would be outweighed by the harm that would be done to the missionary cause, given that the patients were likely to die anyway, and that their failure to bring about a cure might deter people from coming to their hospitals. A major breakthrough in public health work came about as a result of the Manchurian plague outbreak of 1911 that killed approximately 60,000 people. Although compared to some other Chinese epidemics the death rate was not so high; what was striking was that eighty traditional-medicine physicians sent to the plague area also succumbed to the disease, and it was not until Wu Lien-teh instituted effective sanitary and public hygiene measures that the plague was controlled.[36] In the words of the missionary journal *The Chinese Recorder:* 'This [was] the first time... in history, when the Chinese have attempted Western methods for combating the plague.'[37] From then on, a greater effort was made by both the Chinese and the missionaries to introduce public health issues into their medical and educational programs. There were public health campaigns with lectures, and a day-to-day inculcation of sanitary ideas amongst the students in mission schools. The missionaries also sought to improve conditions in their own hospitals, where overcrowding of patients tended to create unsanitary conditions. In some cases, particularly in the rural areas, the medical amenities had not been established with any view to expansion, and it proved hard to overcome this problem.

In Weixian, the most energetic proponent of this programme was Dr Charles Roys. A graduate of the Columbia University College of Surgeons and Physicians, he had been appointed to the mission in November 1903.[38] He belonged to a new generation that had higher ambitions for medical work than those who had preceded him. Keen to make use of his modern training, he wanted to experiment with new techniques, such as the creation of outstation dispensaries. When he reached Weixian, he found that conditions were very different from those he had experienced in the USA. He was particularly concerned at the overcrowding in the hospital wards. Although there were a total of thirty-five beds in the two hospitals – one for men and one for women – he reported six months after his arrival that between twenty-three and forty individuals were being treated in the men's hospital alone. Because there were no professional nurses, the relatives or friends of patients were allowed to remain on the premises to provide care, increasing the overcrowding even more. In 1906, he wrote that patients 'were sleeping on the floor, on benches in the waiting-room, and even on doors which had been taken off their hinges.'[39]

The evangelical missionaries were particularly worried that if an epidemic broke out in such unsanitary conditions within the mission compound, the students in their schools were likely to be infected. They therefore sought to raise funds for the construction of isolation wards accessible from the hospital yard, requesting US$450 to begin such works at the 1906 meeting of the Shandong Mission. Their chief concern was their educational work, rather than improving the hospital facilities as such. In response, the Minneapolis Presbyterial Society donated US$430 in the name of Robert F. Sample, their main aim being to protect the health of the increasing population of school students in the event of an epidemic.[40] Dr Roys continued to be dissatisfied with the work as it stood in Weixian. Although the work in the hospital was expanding rapidly, with 249 inpatients in 1907, he was eager to extend the medical facilities to a wider population. He opened a dispensary within the city walls where much of the minor outpatient work could be performed. This proved to be a successful move, with the number of patients attending the dispensary soon growing to nearly 6,000 each year. Roys was also concerned that only minor surgery could be performed in the main hospital, due to a lack of equipment and proper facilities for postoperative care. Much surgery, notably abdominal operations, could only be performed at a very high risk to the patient, and failure tended to undermine the reputation of the doctors in Weixian.[41] Between January and June 1907 Roys performed 120 operations, dealing with cases of cancer, various tumours and a range of minor complaints, but no abdominal cases that he refused to operate upon.[42] To overcome this problem, he requested funding for a sterile operating theatre, supplies of antiseptics and clean dressings. A Mr. Bristol eventually met his demand – in part – with a gift. Roys raised further money by taking some of the funds from the dispensary. From this, it is apparent that the other missionaries at Weixian were not willing to cover these costs, their chief priority being education. The Foreign Board also was not very helpful in this respect. In 1909, Roys reported that the lack of space for general inpatients was impinging on his ability to conduct surgical work. Only twelve beds were available for surgical cases when over forty were needed, particularly during the post-harvest rush each spring and autumn.[43]

Although the Shandong Mission approved funding for a new ward, the situation had still not been rectified by March 1910. One of the reasons for this appears to have been the lack of space the hospitals were given in the compound. Due to the increasing student population and the delay in moving the Point Breeze Academy, Arts College, and other teaching institutions, they were 'hemmed in on every side'.[44] Once again, educational work took priority. Despite this, in 1911 the mission approved a plan to alter the existing hospitals and forwarded a request for US$250.[45]

The medical staff was not the only group to complain about the condition of the hospitals. The Chinese members of the Cooperation Committee lodged a protest in this respect in 1912/3. However, they were forced to concede that little could be done without additional building work.[46] Writing to the Rockefeller Foundation's China Medical Board in 1914, Dr Roys noted that there were only twenty-six beds for fifty-nine patients in the men's hospital, and twenty beds for forty patients in the women's hospital. He attempted to solve the problem by pitching a tent in which fourteen beds were placed. This plan was abandoned after it was found that the tent could not be secured properly and patients were not willing to stay in it.[47] It is clear that the doctors were going to great lengths to improve conditions. In this, however, they received almost no recorded support from the evangelists and educational workers.

With new plans to remove the Arts College from the main premises by 1917, the way appeared clear for an expansion of the medical facilities. One of the top priorities was a new hospital that would combine the male and female sections. Because of years of neglect, simple improvements would not be adequate. By this time the general missionary body in Weixian was prepared to back the scheme, and a request was submitted for US$10,000. On receiving this request a committee was set up, and it concluded that there was a great need for the project.[48] Hearing this, Dr Roys immediately began looking for the best possible site for the new hospital, which he began to plan. His vision was for a two-storey hospital with two wings containing sixty-four beds in all, which would have increased the patient capacity by twenty beds. Additionally, he noted that the present location did not allow for proper enlargement and the ground it was located on was too low which made it vulnerable to dampness in the summer. He even foresaw its possible flooding by the Yu River, a premonition that became a reality only nine months later.[49]

Although the other missionaries appeared to be behind the project, the foot-dragging continued as the request trickled through the mission bureaucracy. In 1914, the request for funds was formally taken up by Oliver Crawford, of the China Council, and Dr James Lowrie. Following a request from the Shandong Mission Executive Committee, chaired by Dr Charles Johnson, another committee was set up to look into approving the funds before the next meeting of the Shandong Mission. Lowrie was sent to Weixian to investigate the conditions there. He found that the problems were as had been reported, and he agreed that funds needed to be raised quickly. Crawford endorsed this, noting in a letter the great importance of the Weixian station 'whose Christian constituency is nearly one-fifth of that of our entire China Mission.' He also stated that up to that time Weixian had maintained the 'poorest and cheapest plant' and that it needed a new 'first class hospital' to increase its standards in line with its importance in the China field.[50] To this end $32,500 Mexican Silver (Mex.) was approved for the project at a Mission meeting in July.[51] This included $22,000 for the hospital, $2,000 for equipment, $8,000 for a residence – assume for the doctor – and $500 for the land. This was despite the fact that the Foreign Board itself did not take any action on the demand for funds at this time.

Roys knew that very substantial funding would be required if his ambitious plans were to be realised. The general rule was for the mission doctors to first approach the mission boards for funds. However, as the boards were generally slow to respond and unwilling to fund projects in an adequate manner, the doctors also looked to sources outside their own organisation. One such source was the China Medical Board of the Rockefeller Foundation, established in 1914.[52] The founding of this body marked a new phase in medical work in China, allowing for medical work to be expanded on its own merit rather than for evangelical purposes primarily. Medical missionaries no longer had to justify their work in evangelical terms. With its financial resources the Board filled a void that no missionary group was able or willing to fill. The scope of the projects the Board was prepared to fund was enormous. Its main focus was on the Peking Union Medical College, founded by the Boards of the American Presbyterians, American Methodists, and the London Missionary Society.[53] Grants were also available for hospitals in individual stations. On 15 March 1915, John D. Rockefeller, Jr, wrote to the missionary bodies in the United States stating that one of the purposes of the Board was to give 'assistance in strengthening existing medical schools and hospitals and their personnel,' as well as 'to establish, equip and support new medical schools and hospitals.'[54] A hospital had to be inspected by the Resident Director of the China Medical Board, Mr Roger S. Greene, to determine the merit of its application for funding.

The China Medical Board also required that an enterprise be fully supported by the missionary organisation.[55] It did not take over the hospitals that it gave grants to – the mission boards remained the administrators of the hospitals, they were given the right to appoint additional medical personnel not funded by Rockefeller and were allowed to carry out evangelistic and philanthropic work in their hospitals and dispensaries. In effect, this gave the mission boards power to decide which of their hospitals would be funded. Without strong backing from the missionaries of a station as a whole, it was unlikely that an application would succeed. Dr Roys, however, tried to circumvent his own Foreign Board – which he appears to have believed was moving too slowly in the matter – and in the spring of 1914 approached the China Medical Board directly. In a 'Statement of Facts' on the history and present conditions of the hospital, he complained that the existing building had been planned only as a dispensary, and argued that a new building was urgently required. He outlined his plans for a two-storey building that would have two wings – one for men and one for women – containing sixty-four beds, and with special wards to be used for general inpatients and surgical treatment. He emphasised that the existing surgical equipment was in good condition, but the facilities in which to use it were very poor. He stated that so far he had raised only US$1,000 of the $10,600 needed for this purpose.[56]

In this statement, Roys alluded to his plan to introduce new treatment for tuberculosis. Ever since he had started work in Weixian he had been very concerned about the large numbers of pupils in the mission college and schools who suffered from this disease, noting that 'one sees many deformed children here, mostly from tuberculosis, but very few deformed men or women.'[57] He insinuated that these children were being allowed to die in part because the Chinese physicians were unable to treat the disease and in part because the missionary doctors had been lax in the matter. In 1906, he had forced twelve sick students to give up their studies, even though he knew that they were likely to suffer badly in their careers as a result.[58] For other pupils, he tried to catch the disease in its early stages, and then ensure that they lived in a healthy manner, spending plenty of time outdoors.[59] The idea was raised at the Shandong Mission's Annual Meeting in 1911 for a tuberculosis sanatorium connected to the Union Medical College in Jinan. The motion was passed, and for the first time tuberculosis came to the forefront of mission medical policy.[60] Dr Roys was appointed by the mission to solicit funds for this work. Between 1911 and 1914 he wrote to prominent anti-tuberculosis campaigners in the USA such as Dr Jacobs of Baltimore and Dr Otis of Boston. People were not, however, willing to give money to this cause in China at this time.

In his application to the China Medical Board, Roys argued that funds were required for facilities for tuberculosis patients, and that such work fit perfectly with the aims of the Foundation.[61] He stated that 'where so large a proportion of the population is actually succumbing to the scourge as here in China, it is idle to discuss prevention if curative measures are to be ignored; and the surest means of securing the respect of the Chinese for the preventive measures we advocate, is to show them that our curative measures are effective in at least some of the cases.'[62] Roys' plans in this respect included a building especially for tuberculosis patients with separate courts for men and women that could be 'thrown wide open'.[63] He also proposed an orthopaedic ward for treating patients with bone tuberculosis, which he found to be prevalent among Chinese children. They already, he said, had the residential staff to take up the work and just needed the funds, which he anticipated would run to US$5,000. The work in Weixian would serve as a model, he argued, encouraging other groups to raise funding for such projects from their own home boards.[64]

The Rockefeller Foundation sent George B. McKibbin in May 1914 as their representative to assess the situation. He reported:

> He [Dr Roys] is very much ashamed of his hospital but seemed to be doing the best he could under the circumstances. He has a few crowded buildings with about thirty beds, all Chinese style built about fifteen years ago. Patients furnish everything and everything was dirty.[65]

While the China Medical Board was considering Roys's application, disaster struck. The Yu River flooded the hospital on 8 September 1914, destroying much of the drug supply, the *kangs* (Chinese-style beds), and six wardrooms. The other buildings were coated with a deep layer of mud, their foundations sank and there was structural damage to their walls.[66] Discouraged by this setback, Dr Roys decided to leave for the new Medical School in Jinan that was a part of the newly consolidated Shandong Christian University.[67]

Dr LeRoy Heimburger and the Shadyside Hospital

After working for some years as the only foreign doctor at Weixian, Roys had been joined in 1913 by Dr LeRoy Heimburger. He was the person who eventually found the funding for a new hospital, one that still stands today. This was despite the continuing opposition from the Home Board to the direct fund-raising tactics that both Roys and Heimburger undertook. Heimberger scaled down Roys's overambitious plans so as to bring down costs, and set about acquiring cheap medical equipment and stores that became available after the first world war.[68] Even with these cost-cutting measures he still felt that he received no substantial support from the mission establishment.

In June 1915 the China Medical Board officially requested recommendations from the Foreign Board for hospitals requiring funding for 'additional medical and nursing staff'.[69] The Presbyterian's China Council recommended Weixian, Jinan, and Jining from the Shandong Mission. For Weixian, US$14,095.30 was requested for the purchase of land, the construction of a new hospital building and residences, and for new hospital equipment.[70] The application soon ran into difficulties. After an inspection of the Weixian and Jining hospitals, the Director of the China Medical Board, Greene, reported that:

> Neither institution has at present any accommodation worthy of the name of a hospital in any sense. The plant in each case consists of a dispensary building, which includes an operating room, and blocks of one-storey Chinese buildings opening directly on to the court yard, with brick floors in most cases. At Weihsien the Men's and Women's hospitals together cost only about $5,500 gold, including the walls around the compound. They were built in 1902.... The patients are accommodated partly on dirty k'angs (brick

> stove-beds) and partly on iron beds, on which are spread first some coarse kaoliang matting and then the patient's own bedding. There the patients lie unbathed, in their own clothing, attended by their own friends or servants who cook for them and even bring their own kaoliang stalks for fuel. There is practically no nursing in the ordinary routine, and the conditions are as nearly as possible what they would be if the patients were in their homes and there visited by the foreign doctor.... At both places the latrines were unprotected by doors or screens, and that at Weihsien was in filthy condition.... At neither Weihsien nor Tsiningchow was there any laboratory, and even the centrifuge at the former place was out of commission.[71]

Greene later noted that the funding requests were poorly planned. For example, staff residences had been requested even though there would be ample housing with the removal of the Arts College. He considered that the sum requested for building the hospital – US$10,340 – was 'insufficient,' and he was not satisfied that the Presbyterian Board had the funds to make up the extra amount needed.[72] The foot-dragging that had gone on for years now came back to bite the mission.

Greene was not entirely dismissive. He accepted that Dr Heimburger was doing good work in difficult circumstances. He praised his attempts to raise hygiene standards by reducing the number of beds from twenty-six to sixteen, severely limiting the number of patients, and introducing a kitchen and laundry. However, he also noted that the Mission did not give the doctor's work adequate support:

> He is not receiving, however, the sympathetic co-operation of his clerical associates, who have permitted the kitchen only as an experiment, and are inclined to criticize the reduction in the number of patients admitted. When added to this one considers that in spite of the pitiful shortage of equipment the doctor is given by the mission an annual grant of only about $1,200 Mex., or about $500 gold, to work with, one can realize how discouraging his position is. The total expenses, not including the foreigner's salaries, are only about $1,000 gold.[73]

To aid the doctor in his new efforts at the hospital Greene approved US$940 for the purchase of additional equipment. He was most insistent that this money be used to purchase bedding and clothing for the inpatients so as to improve conditions in the hospital.[74] Despite this small grant, the application was otherwise rejected. The deciding factor was the lack of support given to the medical work by the evangelists and the home board. They were allowed to re-apply for the funds in the future, but Greene warned that without a better plan and adequate funding from the Foreign

Board, it 'would be a waste of money for us [China Medical Board] to co-operate there.'[75]

The missionaries and Foreign Board were disappointed by the decision of the China Medical Board. However, it is important to note that they misunderstood its programme, being under the impression that money would be given to all hospitals listed by the China Council and Foreign Board.[76] The Rockefeller people, on the other hand, only intended to give funds to strengthen existing institutions that appeared to have an impressive future and that could provide a well-planned strategy for improvement. It was now clear to the Foreign Board that if they wanted to obtain funding from the China Medical Board they would have to provide more support and better funding for medical work, which eventually they did. The hand of the medical personnel within the mission organisation was strengthened, and they were allowed more say over the future form of the projected hospital.

The Presbyterian Church embarked on a big fundraising programme in the USA for a 'Million Dollar Campaign Fund'. The first large amount to be donated for the hospital fund was from the Shadyside Presbyterian Church in Pittsburgh, which had previously contributed generously to Weixian. After this church had raised a considerable sum in November 1916, its pastor, Hugh Kerr, announced in February 1917 that US$10,000 of this sum would be donated for the hospital. The amount was given in two phases, in March and June of that year.[77]

Plans for the new two-storey hospital were completed in August 1917 and an estimate of costs set out. The plans provided for two wards – men's and women's – containing thirty beds each, six private men's rooms, three private women's rooms, a chapel with seating for eighty people, a children's ward containing eight beds, operating rooms, a sterilising and instrument room, an examining room, a laboratory, and nurses quarters in the attic. The hospital was designed larger than required to allow for future expansion without the need for erecting more ward buildings. There was room for an additional sixteen beds in the attic if they were needed in the future.[78] Despite this, further funds were not forthcoming, leading to increasingly accusatory letters by Heimburger. In a letter of 1919 to the Secretary for Specific Work, George Trull, he noted with anger that the station had been trying to get a 'new modern hospital building with the proper equipment to carry on a modern scientific medical work.'[79] It seemed as if the hospital would never be built. He complained of the small level of support given to medical missionaries and their low status within the mission community and stated that medical men were no longer prepared to tolerate poor facilities and bad working conditions. The mission organisation was, he said, to blame for this state of affairs, and noted that if it continued in this vein they would be unable to obtain medical men in the future:

> Doctors will not be obtainable if they must become regular mission members unless a more liberal policy is maintained in the future. We medical missionaries feel that our work is not a substitute for the spread of the Gospel but an integral part of that work.... In consequence our mission is composed of several over-worked, busy from sun-up to sun-down and many times after that, with not time or too tired after the day's work is over to read and keep up with the times, and with hundreds of matters which come up in running a hospital, which could be handled by a man less professionally trained, to worry about, as bookkeeping, buying drugs, etc., and keep him on edge.[80]

Heimburger's outspokenness appears to have worked, as he managed to obtain the remaining funds soon after. The doctors were at last beginning to establish themselves as powerful figures within the mission community. In Weixian, this would continue to be the case for the rest of that station's history.

Heimburger argued that the plans, as they stood, would certainly bring great improvements in the hospital, but that medical standards were continually rising, and that much more was required. New equipment was needed to keep the hospital in line with hospital standards as set by the Medical Committee of the Eastern Asia Conference.[81] More nurses, improved wards, and better laboratories would be necessary. Otherwise, he stated, the new hospital would soon be obsolete.[82] Although the home churches donated more money over the following five years, the breakthrough came in 1923, when the Shadyside Presbyterian Church donated US$12,481.02. Building work started on what came to be called the 'Shadyside Presbyterian Hospital'.[83] The new hospital incorporated a number of sanitary features. For example, the entrance was placed in the basement so as to confine what Heimburger described as the 'filth' there:

> A patient entering will go to the steward or stewardess and receive his admission ticket, he will then be disrobed, his clothing taken to the fumigating closet and after disinfection stored until the patients discharge. The patient after a bath will be given hospital clothing and sent to his room in as clean a state as soap and water will make him. So in this way we will eliminate a lot of dirt and vermin from our wards. And we also hope to keep the dirt usually carried in by visitors shoes in the down stairs rooms by making them first go there, remove their shoes or put on cover-alls, and get a visiting card before going to the wards.[84]

Completed in 1925, the wards and operating rooms were named after people associated with both the Weixian mission and the Shadyside Church. There was an operating room dedicated to Charles K. Roys, a wardroom to Charlotte E. Hawes, and a small children's ward to Howard Heinz.[85] Unfortunately, Dr Roys did not live long enough to see the hospital that he and Dr Heimburger had worked so hard to establish.

Conclusion

The rural medical missionary enterprise went through prodigious change between the closing years of the nineteenth century and the 1920s. This process has been illustrated in this chapter through an examination of the case of the Weixian mission. Until the 1890s, the medical missionaries were prepared for the most part to accept the lead of the evangelists. After 1900, the general professionalisation of medicine and rising medical standards led to growing demands for better facilities and working conditions for the medical wing of the missions. Increasingly, medical work was being seen as an end in itself – as a Christian duty that went beyond evangelism and conversion alone. This led to growing tensions and conflict between the two mission groups. The entry of the Rockefeller Foundation into the medical mission field in China brought about a sea-change in attitudes, as the extra funding it could provide and its prestige as an institution meant that the evangelists and mission organisations were made to pay more heed to improving their medical standards. Initially, hospitals in the cities of China gained most from this change, but by the 1920s hospitals in the rural interior were also benefiting. In the case of Weixian, although no significant funding was forthcoming from the Rockefeller Foundation, the new situation led to a mission-led campaign to fund better medical care in the area, leading to the construction of an impressive new hospital. For the first time, the medical missionaries in Weixian had facilities that matched their professional expectations.

Notes

1. C.C. Chen, *Medicine in Rural China: A Personal Account* (Berkeley: University of California Press, 1989), 9, 15.
2. G. Brown, *Earthen Vessels and Transcendent Power: American Presbyterians in China, 1837–1952* (New York: Orbis Books, 1997), 11–13.
3. *Ibid*, 13.
4. *Ibid*, 14.
5. *Ibid*, 14 and 24.
6. Before the First Opium War opened China to foreign residence, many groups worked among the overseas Chinese populations in Singapore, Malacca, and other southeast Asian areas.

7. Brown, *op. cit.* (note 2), 24–5.
8. *Ibid*, 32–3.
9. *Ibid*, 27–38.
10. *Ibid*, 36.
11. In 1888 it was separated into the Shandong and Peking Missions.
12. Dengzhou (Penglai) was later replaced as the open port in Shandong by Yantai (Chefoo).
13. *Ibid*, 54.
14. *North China Herald*, cciii (1937), 3642: 321.
15. *43rd Annual Report of the Board of Foreign Missions, 1880,* Presbyterian Historical Society, Philadelphia (PHS hereafter), 65.
16. 'H. Corbett to F. Ellinwood', 1 June 1880, Chefoo, PHS. MF10.F761a.r203.
17. *44th Annual Report of the Board of Foreign Missions, 1881,* PHS, 79 and *45th Annual Report of the Board of Foreign Missions, 1882,* PHS, 85.
18. D. Buck, *Urban Change in China: Politics and Development in Tsinan, Shantung 1890–1949* (Madison: University of Wisconsin Press, 1978), 22.
19. 'H. Corbett to F. Ellinwood', 1 November 1881, Chefoo. PHS. MF10.F761a.r204; R. Forsyth, *Shantung* (Shanghai: The Christian Literature Society, 1912), 91; and *Wei Cheng Qu Zhi* (Jinan: Qi Lu Shu She Chu Ban, 1993), 133.
20. 'C. Roys to Friends', 8 October 1905, Weixian, PHS, MF10.F761a.r256.
21. D. Fisher, *Calvin Wilson Mateer* (Philadelphia: The Westminster Press, 1911), 119.
22. MacIntyre's mission to Weixian took place between 1873 and 1876. John Heeren states 'Timothy Richard says that in 1874 he spent a day in Weihsien with "the Reverend Mr. MacIntyre, of the United Presbyterian Mission of Scotland", and Nevius says that MacIntyre lived in the city of Weihsien for a period of two years.' However, the exact dates of his arrival and departure have not been located to this point. J. Heeren *On the Shantung Front* (New York: The Board of Foreign Missions of the Presbyterian Church in the USA, 1940), 74–5.
23. 'C. Mills, J. Leyenberger and H. Corbett to the Executive Committee of the Presbyterian Board of Foreign Missions', 17 January 1881, Dengzhou. PHS. MF10.F761a.r204.
24. 'Letter from J. Laughlin', *The Foreign Missionary,* xli, 12 (1883) 529.
25. 'H. Corbett to F. Ellinwood', 1 November 1881, Chefoo. PHS. MF10.F761a.r204.
26. Calvin Mateer argued that living in the coastal cities compromised their work. In his words: 'Living at an open port has some conveniences...but what are they when compared with the advantage of being near the people for whom you are laboring.' 'C. Mateer to the Board of Foreign Missions',

19 December 1881, Dengzhou. PHS. MF10.F761a.r204.
27. 'Letter from J. Laughlin', *The Foreign Missionary.* xlii, 4 (1883), 164.
28. *Ibid,* 165.
29. 'Letter from H. Smith', *The Foreign Missionary.* xlii, 5 (1883), 210–1.
30. 'F. Ellinwood to R. Mateer', 31 October 1883, New York. PHS. MF10.F761a.r233
31. 'J. Anderson to F. Ellinwood', 16 March 1886, Weixian, PHS, MF10.F761a.r206.
32. Snow's work on cholera (1854) demonstrated how the disease was spread by water supplies and poor sewage disposal; in 1876 Lister demonstrated 'the benefit of antisepsis and its application to surgery'; and in 1882 and 1895, respectively, Koch and Pasteur demonstrated that microorganisms were involved in disease. J. Jewell, 'Chinese and Western Medicine in China', in S.M. Hillier and J.A. Jewell (ed.) *Health Care and Traditional Medicine in China 1800–1982* (London: Routledge and Kegan Paul, 1983), 22.
33. *Ibid.*
34. 'Sanitary Salvation', *The Chinese Recorder,* xvii, 9 (1886), 353.
35. Y.-w. Cheung, *Missionary Medicine in China* (Lanham: University Press of America, 1988), 22.
36. R. Croizier, *Traditional Medicine in Modern China* (Cambridge: Harvard University Press, 1968), 46.
37. *The Chinese Recorder.* xlii, 4 (1911), 245.
38. Although appointed in November 1903, he did not depart from the USA until October 1904.
39. 'C. Roys to Mr. Wisner', 7 July 1907, Weixian, PHS, MF10.F761a.r257.
40. 'Minutes of the Twelfth Annual Meeting of The West Shantung Mission held at Ichowfu September 29 to October 10, 1906', PHS. MF10.F761a.r260; 'A Short Medical Chapter, 1908', *Woman's Work for Woman.* xxiv, 2 (1909), 37; 'Charles Roys, Personal Report for the Year 1907–1908', PHS. MF10.F761a.r261; and 'Personal Report of Margaret Bynon, 1908', PHS. MF10.F761a.r261.
41. 'C. Roys to Mr. Burrell', 24 March 1907, Weixian, PHS, MF10.F761a.r257 and 'C. Roys to Mr. Wisner', 7 July 1907, Weixian, PHS, MF10.F761a.r257.
42. 'C. Roys to Mr. Wisner', 7 July 1907, Weixian, PHS, MF10.F761a.r257.
43. 'Weihsien Station Report for the year 1 September 1908 to 31 August 1909', PHS. MF10.F761a.r261, 8.
44. 'R. Wells to A. Brown', 29 March 1910, Weixian, PHS, MF10.F761a.r258; 'Report of the Woman's Hospital, Weihsien, for the year ending August 31, 1910', PHS. MF10.F761a.r261; and 'Report of the Wei Hsien Men's Hospital for the year 1911–1912', PHS. RG82/4/2/20/2.
45. *Minutes of the Annual Meeting of the Shantung Mission, 1911*, PHS, 35.

46. It is likely that the Cooperation Committee conceded this point under pressure from the non-medical missionaries, though there is no clear evidence for this as such. 'Report of the Weihsien Station for the year ending August 20, 1913', PHS. RG82/6/2/20–2 and C. Roys, 'New Hospital for Wei hsien', 22 January 1914, Weixian, PHS, RG82/8/7/88.
47. 'Statement of facts relating to the Hospitals of the American Presbyterian Mission, Wei hsien, Shantung', 1914. Rockefeller Archive Center, Tarrytown (hereafter RAC). RG4/1.1/25/525/338 and *78th Annual Report of the Board of Foreign Missions, 1915*, PHS, 150.
48. The Committee consisted of Dr James B. Neal, William E. Winter, and Mrs W.B. Hamilton. The task of this Committee was not only to look into this one request, but to look into what to do with the entire Arts College property when it moved to Jinan. *Minutes of the Annual Meeting of the Shantung Mission, 1913*, PHS. 49.
49. 'C. Roys to A. Brown', 11 January 1914, Weixian, PHS, RG82/8/7/88; C. Roys, 'A New Hospital for Wei hsien', and 'Statement of Facts relating to the Hospitals of the American Presbyterian Mission, Wei hsien, Shantung', 1914. RAC. RG4/1.1/25/525/338.
50. 'O. Crawford to A. Brown', 31 March 1914, Shanghai, PHS. RG82/8/5/106-5.
51. The committee organised to investigate the proper placement of the hospital consisted of Mr Ralph Wells, Dr Charles Roys (Chairman), Mr Wang Yuen Tei and Reverend Li Tao Hwei. We also assume that $32,500 Mex. equalled approximately US$10,000 at the time of the meeting. 'Minutes of the Annual Meeting of the Shantung Mission of the Presbyterian Church in the United States of America', PHS. RG82/8/9/20– 1, 46 and 16.
52. M. Ferguson, *China Medical Board and Peking Union Medical College* (New York: China Medical Board of New York, 1970), 18, 20–1.
53. Here I have used 'Peking' rather than 'Beijing' as the work carried on by the Rockefeller Foundation was known as the Peking Union Medical College; *ibid*, 24; 'Rockefeller Fund Tells China Plans', PHS. RG 82/10/10/1057; and 'Editorial Notes', *Woman's Work for Woman*, xxx, 9 (1915), 194.
54. Quoted in Ferguson, *op. cit.* (note 52), 22.
55. 'Untitled' PHS. RG 82/10/10/1057.
56. 'Statement of Facts relating to the Hospitals of the American Presbyterian Mission, Wei hsien, Shantung' (1914), RAC, RG4/1.1/25/525/338.
57. 'C. Roys to A. Brown', 26 August 1906, Iltio Bay. PHS. MF10.F761a.r257.
58. 'Personal Report of C. Roys, MD', 16 September 1906, Weixian, PHS. MF10.F761a.r261 and 'Personal Report of Dr and Mrs C. Roys for the year 1904-1905', PHS. MF10.F761a.r261.
59. It was not until 1914 that the first connection between the tuberculosis epidemics and lack of ventilation in the missionary schools was given in *The*

Chinese Recorder, although the problem was likely to have been of general knowledge by this time. 'Personal Report of C. Roys, M.D', *ibid.*, and E. Judd, 'Ventilation in Schools – Letter to the Editor', *The Chinese Recorder*, xlv, 3 (1914), 185–6.

60. *Minutes of the Annual Meeting of the Shantung Mission, 1911*, PHS, 27.
61. 'C. Roys to the Medical Commission of the Rockefeller Foundation', 28 May 1914, Weixian, RAC, RG4/1.1/25/525.
62. 'An Open Letter to the China Medical Commission of the Rockefeller Foundation', *China Medical Journal*, xxviii, 4 (1914), 310.
63. Dr Roys noted that tuberculosis in children was becoming more of a problem with the establishment of government schools. He reported that the 'percentage of students in missionary and in Government schools who partly or completely finish their course only to die of tuberculosis, is appalling.' 'Statement of facts relating to the Hospitals of the American Presbyterian Mission, Wei hsien, Shantung', (1914) RAC, RG4/1.1/25/525/338.
64. *Ibid.*
65. 'Visit to the Hospital at Weihsien with Dr C. Roys, G.B. McK' (20 May 1914), RAC, RG4/1.1/25/525/338.
66. 'The Weixian Station to Dr Wm. Merrill', 10 September 1914, Weixian, PHS, RG82/8/7/90 and 'Annual Report of the Weihsien Station, Shantung Mission for the year ending July 1, 1915', PHS, RG82/10/7/20– 2.
67. The Shandong Mission of the American Presbyterians and the Baptist Missionary Society agreed upon the idea for a Medical School when the Union College was established.
68. He attempted this through obtaining cheaper labour and waiting until local prices went down.
69. 'Shantung Mission, Council Minute, June 29, 1915', PHS, RG82/10/7/20–1.
70. The sum of US$10,340 from the China Medical Board was to be put towards the new hospital building. The residences, land, and equipment requests were in addition to this. 'R. Greene to W. Buttrick', 12 May 1916, Beijing. RAC. RG4/1.1/25/525/338.
71. 'R. Greene to W. Buttrick', 17 March 1916, Beijing. RAC, RG4/1.1/25/525/338, 1.
72. 'R. Greene to W. Buttrick', 12 May 1916, Beijing, RAC, RG4/1.1/25/525/338.
73. 'R. Greene to W. Buttrick', 17 March 1916, Beijing, RAC, RG4/1.1/25/525/338, 3.
74. 'R. Greene to W. Buttrick', 12 May 1916, Beijing, RAC, RG4/1.1/25/525/338.
75. 'R. Greene to W. Buttrick', 17 March 1916, Beijing, RAC, RG4/1.1/25/525/338, 3–4 and 5.

76. 'A. Brown to W. Buttrick', 1 March 1916, New York, RAC, RG4/1.1/25/525/338 and 'W. Buttrick to S. White', 24 June 1916, RAC, RG4/1.1/25/525/338.
77. 'H. Kerr to A. Brown', 5 February 1917, Pittsburgh. PHS. RG82/11/21/1523; 'A. Brown to the Shantung Mission', 7 March 1917, New York. PHS. RG82/13/16; and 'A. Brown to the Shantung Mission', 19 June 1917, New York, PHS, RG82/13/16.
78. 'L. Heimburger to A. Brown', 5 August 1917, Weixian, PHS, RG82/13/7/45.
79. 'L. Heimburger to G. Trull', 2 March 1919, Weixian, PHS, RG82/17/15/46.
80. 'L. Heimburger to A. Brown', 19 October 1919, Weixian, PHS, RG82/17/15/48.
81. 'L. Heimburger to A. Brown', 14 January 1918, Weixian, PHS, RG82/15/22/35
82. 'L. Heimburger to A. Brown', 5 August 1917, Weixian, PHS, RG82/13/7/45 and 'L. Heimburger to A. Brown', 14 January 1918, Weixian, PHS, RG82/15/22/35.
83. On the cornerstone the Chinese name Ji Du Yi Yuan was given alongside it.
84. 'L. Heimburger to A. Brown', 7 June 1918, Weixian, PHS, RG82/15/2/36.
85. 'Letter to H. Kerr', 17 January 1923. PHS. RG82/15/20/2040; 'A. Brown to the Shantung Mission', 3 May 1920, New York. PHS. RG82/18/18; 'Untitled', 23 February 1923. PHS. RG82/15/20/2040; 'Untitled', 24 March 1923. PHS. RG82/15/20/2040; 'Appropriation Notice', 24 July 1923. PHS. RG82/15/20/2040; 'Untitled', 1 August 1923. PHS. RG82/15/20/2040; and *Wei Fang Shi Ren Min Yi Yuan Zhi* (Weifang: Wei Fang Shi Xin Wen Chu Ban, 1991), 2.

5

Christian Therapy: Medical Missionaries and the Adivasis of Western India, 1880–1930

David Hardiman

This chapter examines the work of medical missionaries amongst some of the poorest and most disadvantaged of peoples in India, the adivasis (indigenous peoples). Local healers had previously been the only significant providers of health care amongst them, but from the late-nineteenth century onwards, missionaries began to carry out medical work, generally with the intention of gaining legitimacy with a view to religious conversion. This process could at times give rise to tension and social conflict.

The adivasis of India – a disparate and scattered series of communities – were considered by the British to share a common 'primitivism'. Living for the most part in isolation in the hills and forest tracts, and surviving largely from hunting and gathering or rudimentary swidden agriculture, they were considered by the colonialists to be 'aboriginals' or 'early tribes'. They were characterised, amongst other things, by their 'clan'-based systems of kinship and their 'animistic' religious beliefs. Sometimes, they were defined in terms of their habitat, as 'jungle tribes'. In the twentieth century they were given the bureaucratic label of 'scheduled tribes'. In reaction to all of this, from the 1940s onwards many of them claimed, assertively, to be adivasis, or 'original inhabitants'. In this way, they came to be seen as a political constituency, with interests in common. A new all-India collectivity was thus forged.[1]

The British believed that they had a moral duty to 'civilise' these 'backward' people. They set about this through campaigns of military 'pacification'. In the process, they managed to recruit some of them to serve in British-officered militias that became responsible for maintaining 'law and order' in the forest and mountain tracts. Although most adivasis continued to live in remote areas and maintained a certain degree of independence, they experienced an increasingly oppressive control by colonial tax and forest officials as well as indigenous landlords and usurers. There were numerous revolts by these people during the colonial period, but, armed only with swords, axes, spears, and bows and arrows, they were no match for colonial troops and the local militias, and were quickly crushed, often with great bloodshed.

In India, the largest concentrations of such peoples were in the northeast. Elsewhere, many were found in the central-eastern region, in what is now the state of Jharkhand and areas adjoining to it in Bengal, Orissa, and Bastar, and in a belt of western India running over the four modern Indian states of Rajasthan, Gujarat, Madhya Pradesh, and Maharashtra.[2] In this latter area – which forms the subject of this paper – there were two main types of adivasi – the Bhils and the so-called 'Kaliparaj'. The Bhils, the largest, had in the past been organised in warlike kinship groups that had prevented outside rulers from extending their control over the mountains. The British had subjugated them – with considerable difficulty – during the first half of the nineteenth century. Even afterwards, there were several Bhil revolts. The 'Kaliparaj' were found only in the southern part of this area. The term, which meant 'the black people' was a derogatory one used by outsiders to describe members of a variety of local communities, such as the Chodhris, Dhodiyas, Gamits, Konkanas, and Varlis. They were considered to be less warlike than the Bhils.

The adivasis, who in the past had mostly lived from shifting cultivation, hunting and gathering, were encouraged by the British to practise a more settled and intensive agriculture. In many cases, they were excluded from large tracts of forest that they had previously controlled, so that state foresters could exploit the timber wealth of the woodlands.[3] Landlords, usurers and liquor dealers who were protected by the colonial and princely states ruthlessly exploited those who became settled.[4] A large proportion of the adivasi area of western India was ruled by Indian princes rather than directly by the British colonial state. Although nominally independent, these princes relied on British troops and British-run Bhil militias to maintain their control over their territories, and in important matters they had to follow the dictates of the colonial officials who resided in the capital cities of the princely states, who were known as 'Residents'.

Although there was no very pronounced hierarchy in adivasi society as compared to the caste-based society of the plains regions, there was a structure of power that was to be important so far as missionary work was concerned. A headman supported by a group of patriarchal elders normally controlled a 'village' – which in physical form was often no more than a collection of scattered huts. In the case of the Bhils, each such unit – called a *pal* – consisted generally of one exogamous patrilineal lineage, so that the headman and the elders were responsible for maintaining the solidarity of a kinship-based local community.[5] The prime responsibility of a member of such a 'village' was considered to be towards the community as a whole. The elders were considered to have a duty to insist that individual members conform to the ethos of the group. This involved enforcing a range of customs, beliefs, practices and rituals. Certain men were considered to be wise in healing and able to communicate with a world of spirits that was believed to exercise a direct daily control over the lives of all. These people – whom we may describe as 'exorcists' – were influential and respected figures. Without the support of the headmen, elders, and exorcists, the missionaries had little chance of winning converts from amongst the adivasis on any very significant scale.

It is generally considered that the position of adivasi women was better than that of Hindu and Muslim women. They did not have to observe purdah, and they had – it is claimed – greater economic independence.[6] Their society was, however, strongly patriarchal, so that these advantages were relative at best. Women were expected to marry into a different lineage, which meant normally outside their paternal village. A brideprice was paid that made them, in effect, the property of their husband. Adivasi wives were considered to have a right to leave their husband, but a repayment of the brideprice had to be negotiated with the woman's father or new husband. They were not considered to have any right of property in either their father or husband's families. In adivasi stories that were collected from the Dangs tract of South Gujarat in the 1940s, men were depicted as a matter of course as being in a dominant position, exercising political power and living an adventurous life, while women were shown as preparing food, sweeping floors, grinding grain, washing clothes, fetching water, collecting wood, and, above all, caring for their children.[7] Women's songs told of their fear of marriage into a strange household, the great 'force' used on a tender young girl, their desire to be loved and their fear that their husband would run off with another woman.[8] Women were considered to be particularly susceptible to possession by evil spirits and becoming witches, and were in consequence excluded from important ritual ceremonies. Women of subordinate families tended to be a target for accusations of witchcraft – an insidious device used often by the elders to settle scores and bring people into line. Christianity offered a possible escape for socially disadvantaged adivasis who were seeking a new dignity and independence in their lives, but their conversion was likely to be resisted strongly by the elders and the exorcists.

Indigenous systems of healing

Although the evidence relating to the health of these peoples in the pre-colonial period is sparse and needs investigation, it seems likely that they suffered from many of the diseases found in India in general. British reports written soon after their subjugation in the early-nineteenth century speak of their emaciation from poor and inadequate diet and the prevalence of 'fever' – by which it seems is meant malaria. Many were observed to suffer from a 'tumid spleen', which was seen to be a consequence of chronic 'fever'.[9] It is likely that many suffered also from sickle-cell anaemia, which, though debilitating, provided protection against malaria.[10] Dr Thomas Hendley, who ran a dispensary for Bhils employed by the British in the militia for the Rajasthan-Gujarat border region known as the Mewar Bhil Corps, wrote in 1875 that although generally healthy, they dreaded smallpox, which was for them a killer. Many suffered from guinea worm and skin disorders, two problems that were 'mainly due to the filthiness of the people, whose legs often remain coated for days with mud.' Venereal disease and goitre were however unknown among them. Also:

> Insanity is uncommon, perhaps unknown as we should expect in a savage race with the mind rude and uncultivated and little to excite it. I have never seen a case of mania, and only one or two of dementia in old age.[11]

Dr Jane Birkett, the first medical missionary of the Church Missionary Society (CMS) to work on a long-term basis in the Bhil area, had to deal with cases of diarrhoea, dysentery, 'fever' (probably malaria) and jaundice within days after her arrival in 1900. She stated that: 'Everybody in this valley seems to be down with fever, and almost everyone has a huge spleen.' She also mentioned a terrible epidemic of cholera that had killed large numbers in that year.[12] In a later report, she spoke of the high prevalence of eye diseases, which were easily treated, but could lead to blindness if neglected. Many also suffered from ulcers, itch and ringworm.[13] During a medical tour of late-1906, she found she had to treat cases 'chiefly of fever, enlarged spleen, ophthalmia, skin diseases and ulcers.'[14] Figures for diseases treated in dispensaries in Banswara State – a region with a large Bhil population – during the late nineteenth century show that on average each year seventeen per cent were cases of 'diseases of the eye', sixteen per cent 'malarial fevers, ague and remittent', ten per cent 'diseases of the skin', ten per cent 'ulcers and abscesses', eight per cent 'respiratory affections', four per cent 'diseases of the ear', three per cent 'diarrhoea,' two per cent 'worms', two per cent 'rheumatic affections', and two per cent 'dysentery.' The remaining twenty-six per cent of cases were for a variety of complaints that made up less than one percent of the total each.[15] These figures provide only a rough indication of some of the most common complaints, as most diseases went untreated in dispensaries, and the doctors there would have had a reputation for being able to cure particular problems. Taken, however, with the impressionistic accounts of Hendley and Birkett, they suggest that the disorders that the Bhils were most likely to seek a remedy for were eye disease, malaria, worms, skin complaints and abscesses.

They were not likely, however, to try to seek attention from a qualified medical practitioner in the first instance. Most treatments were carried out in the villages by indigenous healers. The same reports mention a range of remedies and treatments that the Bhils themselves applied. Hendley mentioned that they had their own inoculation against smallpox, which they preferred to western-style vaccination.[16] They did this by dipping a grain of dust into the pustule of a smallpox patient, and then inserting this into the skin of a healthy person with the help of a needle. While doing so they invoked the goddess Kanai.[17] As was common throughout India, the Bhils believed that in cases of smallpox the body of the sufferer was possessed by a goddess and thus made feverish. Helen Lambert has described how villagers in Rajasthan were still in the 1980s holding communal ceremonies of worship that were designed to placate such goddesses and thus protect themselves from the disease.[18] The invocation of Kanai by the Bhils during inoculation would seem to have had a similar aim.

Hendley also reported that the Bhils used various herbal remedies, such as the roots of certain plants or leaves of trees. Thus, a small shrub called *bhut bhangra* was dried and powdered and used to treat open wounds. If a purulent wound was caused by the bite of a tiger, a cure was obtained from the *kajera* tree. *Sat* or *Bara Mula* was used in cases of fever accompanied with dry swollen tongue and bad smell, and as a mouthwash. Hendley lists eight such herbal remedies.[19] There must have been many more, as studies by ethnobotanists have shown. Pal and Jain, for example, provide a descriptive catalogue of about 900 herbal remedies used by Indian adivasis.[20] Hendley also stated that the 'priests are the chief physicians, although most old men are supposed to know something about medicine.'[21] By this, he presumably meant medicines derived from herbs and tree products that were obtained locally.

Another popular remedy was that of cauterisation. This involved applying a heated iron to the body, causing a burn. Dr Jane Birkett commented on this in her first report from the Bhil area:

> One thing that catches the eye at once is the scars from burns that are seen on the abdomen and legs of every other man or woman you meet. They were inflicted during the cholera epidemic, and burning the skin over the seat of pain seems to be the only idea of treatment that the natives have.[22]

This was often done using a red-hot arrowhead. Healers in the Dangs also used this technique, using a hot iron to cure stomach complaints. In some cases, the iron was applied on the middle of the back below the neck.[23]

It was believed that many maladies and diseases were caused by the possession of the sufferer's body by deities and spirits, or caused by the glance of an evil eye. The forests were believed to harbour many malevolent spirits that were always waiting for a chance to possess a victim, and regular rituals were held to propitiate them. When a person or domestic animal fell ill or died, adivasis often abandoned their mud and straw home, which was now considered haunted. They would rebuild it elsewhere.[24] During epidemics of killer diseases, such as cholera, they frequently abandoned their villages, even leaving the corpses unburied for fear that they would be possessed if they handled them.[25] As District Collector J.B. Richey commented, this would have helped to protect them from the infection.[26] Their action was not, however, informed by any germ theory of disease, and the same logic could work to very different ends. For example, Mrs Berkebile, a missionary working with the adivasis of Vada, complained in 1909 that in cases of smallpox the people would flock to the house of the sufferer so as to worship the goddess, thus spreading the infection when they returned home.[27]

The foremost remedy for all forms of spirit possession was exorcism by a ritual specialist, known as a *bhagat* by the Kaliparaj and a *bhuvo* by the Bhils. They learnt their skills in a long apprenticeship with an older exorcist. Although they were paid in kind for their services, they earned their livelihood mainly through cultivation, in common with their fellows. During an epidemic of, for example, cholera, a *bhagat* would be called and would be possessed by the goddess responsible for the disease. Speaking through the exorcist, the deity would tell the villages what they should do to propitiate her. In one example cited in the literature, a goat was sacrificed at the shrine to the goddess and its head placed in a shallow bamboo basket on top of a mound of cooked rice, red powder and limes, all of which was taken in procession to the boundary of the village. The people of the neighbouring village buried this ritual paraphernalia, and then carried out a similar ceremony themselves, taking the goddess further and further away.[28]

In cases of non-epidemic disease, witchcraft was often suspected as a cause. It was believed that malevolent female spirits known as *joganis* haunted the forests. When they possessed an adivasi woman, she became a witch.[29] She was able to harm people through spells or a malevolent glance of her 'evil eye'. Many adivasis wore charms to protect them from witches. When a person fell ill, the first remedy was often the use of such a charm. It was, for example, reported in 1907 that in cases of sore eyes, Bhils would take a string and tie knots in it while throwing salt on a fire. As the salt spluttered, the charm was believed to enter into the string. It was then worn around the neck.[30] If such self-applied remedies against witchcraft failed and the person remained sick, an exorcist was called. His task was to use his powers to identify the supposed witch. Once 'discovered' the woman was tortured so as to drive the spirit from her body. Frequently, the alleged witch died as a result. The missionary Arthur Birkett reported in 1914 that in the past three years three women had been done to death in such a manner in the area around Kotada: 'One was killed with an axe and one had a red hot iron thrust into her…'[31]

Exorcism was considered a great skill and exorcists enjoyed a high reputation in their society. The village elders, and even the local ruling elites, such as the Rajput gentry, normally supported their prescriptions, however vicious they may have been. In cases of alleged witchcraft, weaker members of the society tended to the ones accused, such as old women, widows, or, in a few cases, subordinate males. There was a clear connection between local power and the resolution of such conflicts, the aim being to restore a social stability that was seen to be threatened by disruption from within. In this way, illness and the anxieties that it gave rise to provided a means by which the local elders and elites maintained their control. The British, after their conquest of India, sought to outlaw the persecution of witches, a practice seen as barbaric.[32] Those accused of killing witches were considered to have committed murder, and were punished accordingly. This was resented by the adivasi elites, and as the belief in sorcery continued to be maintained strongly, it tended to drive such practices underground rather than suppress them.

The coming of mission medicine

Because of the great difficulties involved in winning converts from among caste Hindus and Muslims, missionaries in India tended to focus their activities on the more marginal social groups, notably Untouchables and adivasis. These were people who had a low stake in maintaining the existing *status quo*, and it was anticipated that they would prove most amenable to proselytisation. On the whole, these expectations were fulfilled more in the case of Untouchables than adivasis, for most of the cases of mass conversion were among Untouchables. However, even though conversions were few, the missionaries had a strong presence in many adivasi areas, being particularly influential in the spheres of educational and medical work.

Although the colonial state sought to distance itself from missionaries as a matter of policy, colonial officials in adivasi tracts were often keen that missionaries should come to work there. There were pragmatic and instrumentalist reasons for this. Christianity, it was argued, could further the overall colonial 'civilising mission', which in this context involved the acculturation of adivasis into a peaceful and subordinate subjecthood.[33] As Sir Lepal Griffen stated in 1883 in regard to the Bhils of the princely states of southern Rajasthan:

> I believe that it would be an immense advantage if the Bhils could be converted to any form of Christianity by missionaries, either Catholic or

Protestant... It is obvious that the inconveniences and even danger which attend proselytising enterprises in Brahmanical and Muhammadan States, which possess a creed as dogmatic and systematic as Christianity itself, do not exist with reference to a people like the Bhils, who have no dogmatic theology, and who would accept with very little difficulty the civilising creed which would be offered to them.[34]

Under such pressure, the princes who ruled large tracts of the adivasi area agreed to allow missionaries to enter their territories. Their states were generally very deficient in modern forms of education, and they were prepared even to provide subsidies if the missionaries opened schools in adivasi villages.[35] They also valued access to modern forms of medical treatment.[36]

The missionaries who came in response were moved by a belief that their own path to salvation lay through dedicated social work that would pave the way for the saving of 'heathen' souls. Their efforts in India towards this end had involved a hard struggle, which had frequently yielded poor results. Often, the dominant castes would refuse even to allow subordinate caste people to attend mission meetings. I.S. Long found this when he tried to preach in the area around Jalalpur in South Gujarat, where Anavil Brahmans treated the subordinate Dubla agricultural labourers like serfs:

[T]he caste people are like the dog in the manger. They will not accept themselves nor will they let the common people, who would gladly take to something better and nobler, even congregate to listen long enough to get an idea of what Christianity is.[37]

Adivasi society, by contrast, was seen as being free from the stranglehold of caste. As one missionary wrote in 1906: 'Caste has not found its way into the Dangs as yet, and if we get in before caste ideas do, we do well.'[38] Encouraged by such sentiments, the missionaries entered these areas confident that their labours would bring a swift reward. They saw the adivasis as a kind of *tabula rasa*, so-called 'lost souls' mired in primitive beliefs, who would respond with enthusiasm to their preaching once they understood the superiority of the Word of the Lord. In common with so-called 'animists' all over the globe, the adivasis were seen as ripe candidates for successful proselytisation.

Dr James Shepherd of the United Presbyterian Church of Scotland was the first to begin such work. Shepherd (1847–1926), who was trained in medicine in his hometown of Aberdeen and then Berlin, and in theology in Edinburgh, established a practice in Udaipur city in 1877. On his preliminary tour of the state in that year, he visited Kherwara, the headquarters of the Mewar Bhil Corps, where the Commander of this

Figure 5.1

'Shepherd with some Bhil friends.'
George Carstairs, *Shepherd of Udaipur and the Land he Loved* (London: Hodder and Stroughton, 1926), facing p.241.

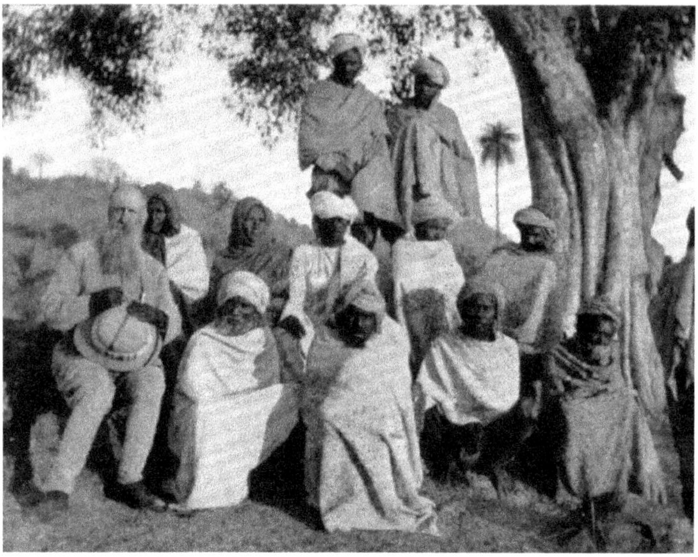

militia, Colonel Gordon, received him with warm hospitality. Gordon introduced Shepherd to three of the principle headmen of the Bhils of the area, and the missionary was able to preach to some Bhils. He felt from the response 'that the Master was with us, and would cause the seed which had been sown that morning to spring up and bear abundant fruit to His praise and glory.'[39] Shepherd's main work over the next forty-three years was carried out in the capital city of Mewar State, Udaipur, where he established a highly successful hospital. He often, however, treated Bhils who came to the city to sell forest produce. They came to him suffering from complaints such as malaria, dysentery, rheumatism, tuberculosis, infected sores, and broken bones. According to his biographer: 'When it became known that eyes could be given to the blind, old men would occasionally be led in to be operated on for cataract.' In this way the name of the 'Padre Saheb' was known in the Bhil tracts even before he started undertaking regular preaching and healing tours there.[40]

Figure 5.2

'Missionaries and Missioner at Lusadia.'
The Church Missionary Gleaner, October 1911, p154.

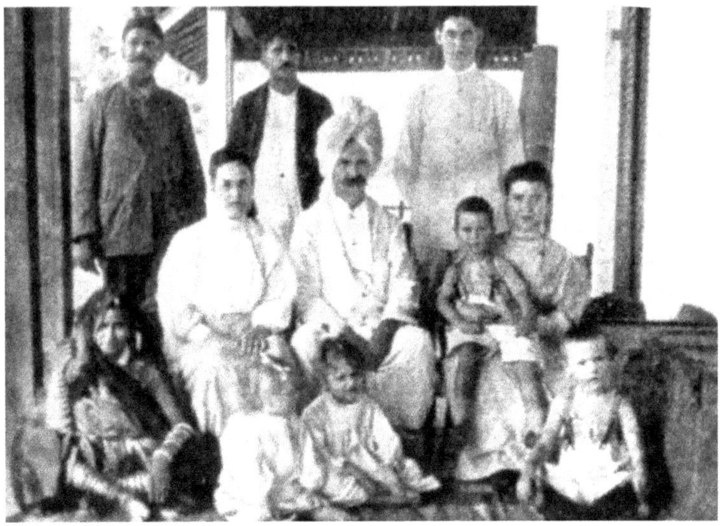

Arthur Birkett is in the centre, with Jane Birkett on his right. Birkett was considered unusual amongst missionaries of his time, as he adopted Indian dress.

Soon after Shepherd began work in Udaipur, the Church Missionary Society established a base in the heart of the Bhil tract, at Kherwara. The wife of a junior officer of the Mewar Bhil Corps was the daughter of the Bishop of Exeter, and after she wrote to him of the need for missionaries to the Bhils, he agreed to finance such a person. The Reverend C.S. Thompson arrived there in 1880, and established a mission station. He was to stay there until his death from cholera in the epidemic of 1900.[41] Although he was not trained as a doctor, he had observed Shepherd at work in Udaipur, and believed that medical work provided the best means for gaining the confidence of the Bhils. Just before he arrived, however, the government doctor attached to the Mewar Bhil Corps had cajoled some Bhils with the help of money-payments to come to his hospital to be operated on. Other Bhils had been terrified, believing that the doctor was trying to murder them. Thompson reported that as a result, 'it is a very rare thing indeed to see a Bhil man, woman, or child, near the dispensary.'[42] When he went to their villages, they hid or fled. It was only after he decided to camp in one village and wait for the people to come that he began to get a few patients. In the words of the missionary:

> On the Tuesday we had fifteen visits for medicine or treatment; on Wednesday, thirty; on Thursday, forty-five; on Friday, fifty-nine; and on Saturday, fifty-eight; total, 207. Among the number was the headman of the village. On the Wednesday, Thursday, and Friday we held little meetings to make known the Saviour. We did not think it advisable to say too much in this way on our first prolonged visit.[43]

By focusing on medical work during the early years of his mission, Thompson gradually allayed the fears of the Bhils; though he failed to win a single actual convert before 1889.

Other CMS mission stations were established in the Bhil region in the following years – at Kotada, also in Mewar State, and at Lusadiya and Biladia in Idar state in what is now northeastern Gujarat. Although there was a strong focus on medical work, none of the early missionaries were doctors as such. The first qualified person to work with this mission was Dr A.H. Browne, who was sent immediately after Thompson died. Dr Jane Birkett was sent to replace him after a few months. As Jane Haskew, she had gone to India in 1888 to work as a doctor for the CMS Zenana Mission at Lucknow. While working there, she had married a fellow CMS missionary, the Reverend Arthur Birkett. They were transferred to the Bhil mission together in November 1900. Jane Birkett found that the medical facilities at Lusadiya were rudimentary in the extreme – the 'dispensary' consisting of a small one-roomed shed of wattle and daub.[44] While she examined patients on one side of the room, her Indian assistant administered dressings and medicine on the other. She demanded that the CMS provide something better, and in 1905 it was agreed that a new three-roomed dispensary and a 'hospital' that consisted of two separate one-roomed buildings for three male and three female inpatients would be built. A separate house for the Indian assistant was also sanctioned.[45] In 1906, a total of thirty-two inpatients and 11,878 outpatients were treated in the new buildings.[46]

Patient numbers increased gradually over the next decade. In 1911 new wards were built at Lusadiya, increasing the beds for inpatients to twenty-eight. In 1914, 312 inpatients were treated. Outpatient numbers rose from 15,331 in 1910 to 20,953 in 1914. However, besides Jane Birkett and her assistant from 1902, John Brand, who was an Indian Christian who had been trained at the Agra Medical Missionary Training Institute,[47] there was only one other member of staff, a dresser whom Brand himself had taught. There were no nurses, so that the care of inpatients had to be carried out by relatives or friends who lived in rudimentary huts next to the wards. When the Birketts were away for extended periods on visits to hill stations or on furlough in Britain, Brand ran the dispensary and hospital by himself. Touring was out of the question at such times.[48] With no improvement in the facilities or new staff, there was no significant increase in patients, and in several years the numbers treated were below the above figures. With Dr Birkett's retirement in 1922, followed by John Brand, in 1923, and without any adequate replacement for either until the late-1920s, the work declined badly. During the mid-1920s there were no inpatients at all, and hardly three thousand outpatients were being treated each year.[49] Mrs Lily Shaw, a trained nurse who was the wife of the missionary-in-charge at Lusadiya, the Reverend C.L. Shaw, carried on the work virtually single-handed.[50]

During the 1890s two more missionary organisations started work amongst the adivasis of western India. The Jungle Tribes Mission of the Irish Presbyterian Church opened a mission in the eastern Panchmahals in 1892 – a Bhil area – with bases at Dahod, Jhalod and Sunth. The Church of the Brethren, an American organisation, established its first mission in South Gujarat at Valsad in 1895, moving inland from there to the adivasi areas over the next decade, with bases at places such as Rajpipla, Jhagadia, Sagbara, Vuli and Umalla (Rajpipla State), Vyara (Baroda State), Dahanu and Vada (Thana District), and Ahwa (the Dangs). The adivasis in this area were largely of the 'Kaliparaj' communities, such as the Chodhras, Gamits, and Konkanas, though there were also some Bhils. Neither of these missions employed qualified doctors during the early years, though most of the missionaries turned their hand to healing. For example, the first missionary in the Dangs was J.M. Pittenger. Immediately after his arrival in 1907 he toured the tract handing out medicine and preaching. He treated many cases of scabies, malaria, and eye diseases such as conjunctivitis.[51]

As soon as resources were available, the missionaries constructed substantial mission buildings in their centres, clustered around a church, which they sought to make as imposing as possible. It was believed by missionaries that a grand church raised their status in an area.[52] These buildings included schools, often with boarding facilities for pupils who came from a distance, and a dispensary or – in the cases of Udaipur and Lusadiya – a hospital where outpatients and possibly a few inpatients could be treated. Surgery was considered to be of specific benefit, as it was believed to provide the most dramatic proof of the superiority of Western medical technique. In particular: 'The treatment of cataracts has seemed to many to be almost miraculous, and has opened many a closed door to missionary influence.'[53] Shepherd in Udaipur carried out regular surgery of all sorts, ranging from cataract removal, to amputations, and abdominal operations.[54] In Lusadiya, on the other hand, Jane Birkett lacked any proper facilities and carried out only a few minor operations. In 1914, Arthur Birkett complained that his wife had been unable to practice any real surgery for eight years, 'and it is surgery which tells most'.[55]

Locally employed evangelists preached to the patients as they waited, often for hours, for treatment at these dispensaries and hospitals. Inpatients received regular visits from such evangelists, and the literate were given religious tracts to read. Prayers for recovery were held at the bedsides of patients. The Bhil patients do not on the whole seem to have resented such activity, as it provided a diversion while they waited or lay in bed, and many appear to have seen it as a part of the conditions of treatment. This did not mean that they were for the most part much influenced. As Jane Birkett complained in 1907: 'One can *feel* the words rebounding like a ball against a stone wall, and one realises one's impotence and the incessant need of the Holy Spirit's personal work in these hearts of stone.'[56]

In addition to their work at the centres, the missionaries undertook periodic tours – known as 'itineration' – normally during the cold season from November to March. They would establish a camp, and go out to nearby villages each day preaching and encouraging people to come forward for medical treatment. A medicine chest equipped with instruments and a range of drugs had to be carried on the tour. The aim was to win the confidence of the people in Western medicine so that they would be encouraged to bring their sick to the dispensary or hospital in the future.[57] There was also more regular medical visiting, as at Lusadiya, where Dr Jane Birkett established a system of bi-weekly medical itineration, covering forty-nine surrounding villages, each of which was visited on a regular basis. In this way, many neglected medical cases were discovered and some patients were persuaded to come to the main hospital for extended treatment.[58]

In their reports home, the missionaries often claimed remarkable results for such medical work. It was, for example, stated in an account of a tour of a Bhil area in 1914 that: 'As soon as the news spread that we had come, we were simply besieged on all sides for medical help, and sicknesses of all kinds were brought to us.' Although the medicine provided was rudimentary, and the missionaries concerned were without any formal medical training, their treatments were reported to have cured many.[59] By this means, according to one Irish Presbyterian missionary, they acquired a reputation amongst Bhils as *akkalwala*, or men of wisdom.[60] A study of the mission archives shows, however, that their success was in fact contingent and limited, as we shall see later.

Christian healing

The system of medicine practised by the missionaries was known locally as *Angrezi Dawa*, or 'English medicine'.[61] This term covered both the use of biomedical drugs, inoculation through injections and the use of surgery and hospital-based treatment. The figure of the European-style doctor was important in this, and in some parts of northern India this medical system was known as 'Doctory', for, in the words of Neshat Quaiser:

> The doctor was one of the most visible representatives of European knowledge. He looked, dressed and spoke differently... The doctor with his stethoscope created an aura and mystery around himself; he symbolised 'modern' medicine.[62]

Despite its claims to be in 'advance' of other forms of therapy, it was seen popularly in India to be just one system among many, and was not initially accepted as being superior as such. In time, it developed a certain amount of prestige, as it was associated with the British rulers, the missionaries and the local Indian elites. This, however, took time.[63]

Another novelty of mission medicine was that it was moved by a desire to provide access to this 'English medicine' for the poor and disadvantaged through dispensaries and hospitals. During the first half of the nineteenth century, missionaries had begun to extend their work in a medical direction both at home and abroad. The Edinburgh Medical Missionary Society, founded in 1841, in part sought to provide support for medical missionaries to overseas territories, but also ran a dispensary for the Irish workers of the city. Similar 'medical mission' dispensaries were established in many British cities during the nineteenth century.[64] This was all carried out against a background of governmental 'sanitary' initiatives, designed to raise the general health of the population. Because they saw themselves as being in a medical vanguard, charitably-minded physicians were often intolerant of what they saw as antiquated forms of therapy or folk-superstition. At times, their initiatives could become coercive, particularly in a colonial context. They believed very strongly, however, that they were acting for the good of all.

There were traditions in India of providing charitable medical facilities. Jain merchants had for many centuries distributed medicine and financed dispensaries for the poor in the cities – a tradition that was carried forward in the nineteenth century into a medical philanthropy that provided access for the poor to biomedical treatment.[65] These activities were however almost entirely confined to the cities. The foremost Ayurvedic text, the *Charaka Samhita*, considered charitable work to be the best form of medical practice of all: 'He who practices medicine out of compassion for all creatures rather than for gain or for gratification of the senses surpasses all.'[66] The adivasis would have had some contact with Aryurvedic doctors who came to their hills and forests in search of herbs, and may sometimes have taken treatment from them.[67] Such doctors did not, however, establish rural clinics to treat forest-dwellers on a regular basis.

Medical missionaries were also distinctive in being evangelical Christians who saw their form of medicine as being blessed by God. Healing was, they believed, brought about in part through their medical skill and knowledge, and in part through prayer. They saw no contradiction in this, for medical science was but one expression of God's great power. As Christians, they had a duty to apply the benefits of Western science, which was God-given, to alleviate misery, wretchedness, pain and disease.[68] They recognised that people were often cured as much through faith as by the doctor's skill. The medical missionary Arthur Neve thus recognised that even the best medical knowledge applied by the ablest of physicians was inadequate to the task of curing many ailments. He argued that: 'It is God who heals, but He works through means, and where the means fail He may work in other not understood ways.'[69]

A statement made by C.L. Shaw, a CMS missionary to the Bhils, is illuminating in this respect. In a report of 1913, he argued that a strong reason for the popularity of the charismatic religious leader of the Bhils, Govind, was that it was believed that he had the ability to cure disease supernaturally. He noted that Govind had converted far more Bhils to his brand of Hinduism than the missionaries had ever done to Christianity, and he stated that if their mission had had the resources to build more hospitals and employ more doctors, they would have been able to counter such appeals. 'What an opening for a real Surgeon, professing no magic save that of the Gospel!'[70] The ambiguity in this statement is telling. We may read Shaw in one way as saying that a 'real Surgeon' has 'no magic', only his skill as a surgeon. But also, he was implying that such a surgeon could, as a Christian missionary, bring into play the 'magic' of the Gospel. In this way his technical expertise would be supplemented by a higher, invisible power – that of faith.

Many missionaries believed that in certain cases the sick could be healed by trust in Christ and prayer alone. The CMS missionary Helen Bull thus reported a case from a village in which the missionaries had had little previous success in gaining a sympathetic hearing from the Bhils. A woman and her children had fallen ill during the monsoon of 1913 and she had put a charm of knotted hair string around her neck to ward off the evil eye. She had however once heard the missionaries preach, and had second thoughts. In Miss Bull's words:

> After a struggle she felt she must take it off, and she asked God to forgive her; and then said in her own simple way, 'since then day by day I have said, "O Lord, keep me, keep all my little ones, and my house and cattle, and take

> away all my superstition." And then triumphantly exclaimed, 'He has done it.'[71]

The cure for the Bhil woman and her children had in this case depended on faith, rather than in any medical intervention. On the whole, however, most missionaries recognised that in the majority of cases biomedical treatment would be required as well.

Although trust in Christ might bring a cure that could not be explained in scientific terms, faith in pagan deities and spirits was not considered to be able to bestow such benefits. In particular, the use of charms, exorcism and rituals to cast out evil spirits were seen to be profoundly anti-Christian. This was despite the fact that the Jesus of the New Testament had cured the afflicted by casting out malevolent spirits. The missionaries generally held that conditions had changed since the days of Christ, and that such methods were no longer appropriate to the times. In 1912, for example, 'C.F.H.' of the Church Missionary Society argued that Christians were now armed with the fruits of scientific knowledge, a knowledge provide by God through His Providence, and it was incumbent on Christians to apply it. Not to do so would be 'to despise God's wonderful gifts.' Changing tack somewhat, 'C.F.H.' also argued that miracle cures were associated in modern times 'with the grossest superstition' and that when applied by Christians they served only to discredit their religion:

> [M]any who have professed to hold what are usually known as 'Faith-Healing' views have gone abroad as missionaries and have brought grave dishonour on the name of Christ. Many have returned from abroad with wrecked constitutions, whilst others have died simply because they would not take quinine. Such cases stand self-condemned.[72]

The conclusion was not particularly logical – for, after all, many missionaries who did not believe exclusively in healing through faith also died in the field or had to retire home with shattered health. Also, it assumes that faith healing and Christian exorcism would be applied in isolation, rather than as one element in an all-round therapy. The real objection, it seems, was that miracle-cures were considered in the teleology of the post-Enlightenment age to be 'backward' and 'primitive', and it was feared that if modern Christians indulged in such practices they would bring ridicule on their religion. The mainstream attitude of missionaries towards exorcism and the casting out of evil spirits was therefore determined by a desire for their religion to appear in tune with the times. Moved by such concerns, the missionaries argued that God blessed the medical therapy that they applied, whereas that of folk healers and exorcists was 'Satanic', being likely to kill rather than cure.

The limits to Christian therapy

The blend of medical science, charitable sentiment and evangelical faith that was practiced by the mission healers was inevitably very alien to the adivasis' own structure of feeling. It was, moreover, by no means obvious to the latter that this form of therapy was superior to their own. The biomedicine applied by the missionaries was not the best that was available by any means, and they were not always successful in bringing about the desired cures. Very few of them were trained doctors. Few missionary organisations could afford to hire full-time medical workers, whether qualified foreign missionaries, local medical assistants, or trained nurses. Whole areas of biomedicine were beyond their financial reach. They could afford only the most basic drugs and medical equipment. Biomedicine often obtained its most dramatic results in surgery, but this was not possible in any major form without sterile and well-equipped operating theatres, and well-trained nurses for the necessary after-care. For many years, the only place with such a surgical facilities in the adivasi region of western India was Shepherd's Hospital in Udaipur, and even that was not located in an adivasi tract as such. Cases that came to Lusadiya requiring radical surgery had to be referred to Ahmedabad or the mission hospitals in Anand, both far to the south. Very few Bhils were prepared to subject themselves to the uncertainties of such a journey. When the need for surgery was drastic and urgent, the patient lacked even that choice, and most probably died in consequence.[73] In Lusadiya, adequate surgical facilities came only in the 1940s, along with a doctor, Margaret Johnson, who had the competence to perform more major operations.[74]

A failure in treatment could provide a setback to the work of the missionaries. In 1924 D.K. Salvi – an Indian Christian who was qualified as a hospital assistant – was running the Lusadiya hospital and dispensary in the absence of any fully-qualified medical missionary. The son of a former lay pastor fell ill with blood poisoning, and although Salvi worked hard to save him, he died after three days. The ex-pastor, who was a relatively wealthy and influential Bhil, immediately turned on the missionaries and accused Salvi of having killed his son. He also spread 'horrible lies' about the work of the hospital. There was an immediate falling-off in the numbers of patients. Only after working hard for several months to counter this malign influence did Salvi gradually – so it was reported – regain the confidence of the local people.[75]

Even if the best contemporary biomedical treatment had been available, it would in any case have been often inadequate to the task. This was particularly so during major epidemics. Although the major outbreak of plague of 1896–8 largely passed these tracts by, the cholera epidemic that accompanied the great famine of 1899–1900 caused massive mortality amongst adivasis. The little drinking water that was available in wells became infected, passing the disease to a people already malnourished and weak. The missionaries worked tirelessly trying to relieve the suffering, and several of them succumbed to the disease themselves. C.S. Thompson died under a tree on the road to Kherwara in May 1900, and R.B. Mawhinney and William Mulligan, both of the Irish Presbyterian Jungle Tribes Mission, followed him in July and August.[76] When the rains eventually came there was an epidemic of dysentery, and then a peculiarly severe outbreak of malaria. Many adivasis died besides the crops they had at last been able to raise.[77] During this crisis there was no indication that missionary medicine was in any way superior to the healing methods of the adivasis – many of whom resorted to cauterisation. Disease spared none, regardless of the treatment applied.

The charitable motives of the missionaries were also not necessarily appreciated in the spirit intended. The idea that white sahibs and memsahibs should devote their lives to the welfare of people like the Bhils was too unlikely to gain an easy acceptance. There was, rather, considerable suspicion of the motives of the missionary doctors, one of the least of which was a fear of conversion to Christianity. When C.S. Thompson offered medical help to the Bhils in 1880, their first reaction was that he was trying to harm them, or even lure them to their death. It was commonly believed that the British were in the habit of performing human sacrifices to ensure the success of their various projects,[78] and it was rumoured that this ritual was performed in secret in their hospitals and dispensaries. Fears of the malicious intent of the 'English doctors' continued. When Dr Jane Birkett upbraided a Bhil woman in 1906 for failing to seek treatment for her baby who was suffering from a bad case of ophthalmia, the reply was: 'I am told that if I take her to you and you put medicine in her eye the eye will burst!'[79] Such suspicions could only be broken down gradually. One of the best ways to do this was to take medicine to people in their own villages, where they could accept or reject treatment on their own terms. They were used to wandering Aryurvedic physicians coming to collect herbs and sometimes provide treatment, and could understand the itinerating medical missionary in such terms. Once they did allow themselves to receive the attentions of the missionary, their confidence then rested on the efficacy of the cure.

The greatest obstacle to mission medicine was however that they were fighting a whole culture of belief and practice that was not only deeply internalised amongst the adivasis, but also rigidly enforced by the patriarchs, elders and exorcists of the community. Although the adivasi elites tended to raise no objection to people of their village being treated by touring missionaries for a range of minor complaints, they were far less willing to allow them to go to the missionaries when a witch or evil spirit was believed to have caused an illness. Such attacks were seen to threaten the well-being and health of the community as a whole, and it was considered imperative that they be dealt with in the appropriate manner, though exorcism. Individuals were not considered to have a right of control over their own bodies in such matters; they were members of kin groups who had to conform to the wishes of the wider family or clan, so as not to offend and bring misfortune to either the living or the spirits of ancestors. We can see, furthermore, that refusal to accept such a therapy was also a challenge to the power and prestige of the elders and exorcists. This provided a further reason for their opposition. Treatment could thus become a battlefield between the adivasi elders and the missionaries. The missionaries understood this very well, seeing this as a struggle that was not so much over the technology of healing as a confrontation between two conflicting systems of belief. They tended to depict this as a battle against 'idolatory' and 'superstition', or between God and the Devil.

In such cases, those who persisted in taking treatment from the missionaries brought themselves into conflict with influential members of their own society, and even if the treatment succeeded and they developed a new faith in Christ, they often found it hard to become formal converts due to opposition from elders, exorcists, and relatives. To take one case, Jane Birkett's carriage-driver fell seriously ill in early 1919. His relatives brought in an exorcist to treat him, but his condition worsened. When he appeared to be at death's door, his brother went to see John Brand – Birkett was then on leave – and begged him to treat the case. Brand agreed. In Birkett's words: 'The prayer of faith, together with medicines and proper diet, won him back to life and health, and he promised the doctor that he would serve the Lord Jesus....'[80] Time went by, and he failed to come forward for baptism. The reason, according to Birkett, was that his relatives had put pressure on him not to do so. There were, she said, many similar cases.

The pressures continued, even on adivasis who had been converted and baptised. Converts were expected by the missionaries to accept only mission-based therapy for themselves and their close relatives. For example, in one case of 1906, Jane Birkett noticed on a visit to the house of a Christian convert that a 3-year-old girl had a knotted string around her neck. When she asked what it was, she was told it was a charm to cure her sore eyes. Birkett told them that the whole idea was absurd, and made them remove the string. Later in the day, the girl was brought to Birkett's tent for treatment.[81] Many converts continued, nevertheless, to believe in the power of charms and exorcism, and resorted to them at times of crisis. Even if their belief in this respect had become uncertain under missionary influence, there were always strong community pressures for them to take treatment from the exorcists. When, however, they did so they were likely to suffer a strong

Figure 5.3

'Christian congregation in Khetadra, 1904.'
From a photo album in the possession of Hilary Griffiths, a daughter of Paul and Margaret Johnson, who served in the Bhil Mission during the 1940s and 1950s.

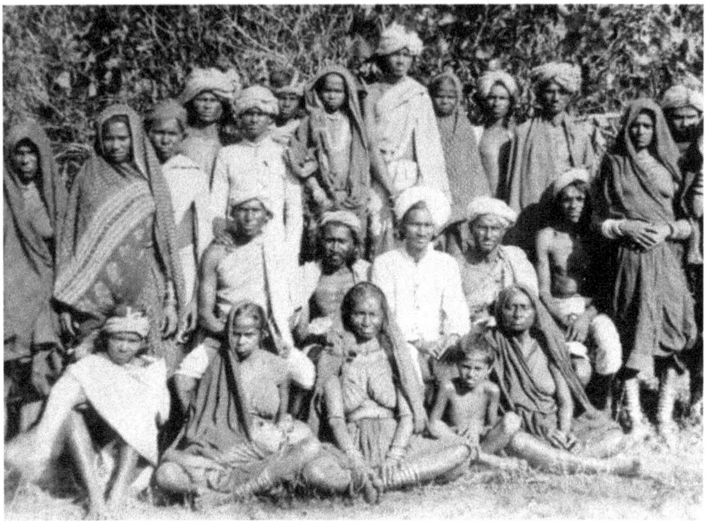

rebuke from the missionaries, and, if they persisted, even suffer excommunication. In 1914, for example, a Bhil woman who was married to a Christian convert fell ill. When her father-in-law proposed to take her to the mission hospital at Lusadiya, a local exorcist told him that if he did this his son – her husband – would fall ill and die. The woman's own father was eager to take her for treatment, but the will of the exorcist, as exercised over the father-in-law, prevailed. The woman died as a result. Arthur Birkett was so disgusted by this that he excommunicated the whole family.[82]

In the Bhil village of Khetadra, where there was a small community of converts, the Birketts had a long-running battle on this score that stretched over many years. They have provided a detailed account of one such encounter in November and December 1906, when they had set up camp in the village so as to preach, heal and minister to the Christians. Jane Birkett was called to see a convert, a woman who had given birth four months previously and since that time had been sick, growing ever weaker. On being questioned, she said that the illness was caused by 'Satan':

> [W]ho was trying to get her back to idolatry and spirit worship. Satan came in dreams to her in the night and threatened her because she had left off idolatry. Her first husband had practiced exorcism and had worshipped the exorcised spirits in his house, where he had a special alter to them, and she thought he now wanted her and her Christian husband to return to the old practices, and that because she had not complied Satan was tormenting her with this mysterious illness.[83]

The Christian couple had been told by an exorcist that for five rupees he would remove the spirits from both the woman and the house. So far they had resisted this solution. They had gone to live with a neighbour, and were considering abandoning the old house and building a new one elsewhere. Jane Birkett 'taught them and prayed earnestly with them for peaceful sleep for the woman.' The woman's husband also prayed with great zeal. In this case the couple appear to have internalised the vocabulary of the missionaries, though the haunting was understood in terms of the Bhils' own cosmos of belief.

A week later news was brought to the Birkett's tent at night that the Christian woman who was being haunted by Satan had 'yielded to her heathen instincts and practice and has had the exorcist in!' The two missionaries went straight over to reason with the woman and her husband. The husband and wife were however adamant that 'nothing but their old custom of exorcising evil spirits could avail in the present circumstances – medicines and prayer would never cure her.' Jane Birkett claimed that the woman had in fact been recovering her strength in the week since they had prayed together. Other villagers then intervened, abusing the missionaries, stating that if the woman followed their advice she would inevitably die and her blood would be on their heads. They threatened that if they did not leave, their tent would be burnt down next day. The missionaries retired to their tent 'very sore at heart'. Next morning they took comfort when they found the reading for the day was from Isaiah 53:

> Enlarge the place of thy tent, and let them stretch forth the curtains of thine habitations: spare not, lengthen thy cords, and strengthen thy stakes. Fear not; for thou shalt not be ashamed; neither be thou confounded; for thou shalt not be put to shame....

Heartened by God's Word, they resolved to stay put. News was brought to them that the exorcism had continued for the whole of that night, and that fifteen evil spirits had been captured by the exorcist and carried away in a sack. The missionaries camped there for another month, preaching and treating patients, without suffering the threatened fate. Jane Birkett commented at the end of their stay that:

> [T]he Bhils are very shy indeed; even when they seem to be very friendly on some lines they still cling to their own idea of treatment, so progress here will be very slow. We can only pray that as they grow in grace they may have grace to care properly for their own bodies.[84]

The Christian converts of Khetadra continued to cause problems for the Birketts. In 1915 they discovered that Waga Koya, a lay pastor who led the congregation there, had been taking part in 'superstitious practices' for many years previously. He had himself asked for help from a 'wizard', eg. an exorcist, on at least one occasion. Several converts had left the church, and the Birketts felt that Waga Koya's behaviour was to blame. This seems unlikely, as the pressure to use the exorcists was as likely to have come from the converts as from the lay pastor. Waga Koya was ordered to go to work in Kherwara, far away. He seems to have been genuinely baffled by this, stating that he had done no wrong and begged to be allowed to stay in Khetadra. As a result of this, fifty-one of the converts of that village were excommunicated.[85]

There were other, more gruesome cases involving converts. In 1915, a girl in a family of Bhil converts of Abapur village died of tetanus. The father, Makana, and his brother, Jalji, consulted an exorcist to discover the cause of her death. They were told that the wife of the headman had bewitched her. They two men went to her house at night with the intention of killing her while her husband was out guarding his crops in the field. They attacked her with an axe, cutting off one arm and slashing the other to the bone. They tried to cut her throat, but her screams brought her husband running and they fled.[86]

The missionaries found it particularly hard to fight the hold of such 'superstition' and they often saw it as posing the greatest obstacle to their evangelical and medical work. Arthur Birkett stated in December 1915 that his difficulty in this respect was weighing on him more and more, even to the extent of keeping him awake at night. During the hot weather that year he had almost suffered a breakdown in consequence.[87]

There were, nevertheless, the occasional victories to provide heart to the missionaries. Jane Birkett thus wrote of a young Christian couple whose only son had fallen gravely ill. Their elder relatives and even leading Christian converts told them that exorcism was the only remedy, but they insisted that they would place their faith in God and God alone. Birkett commented: 'God honoured their faithfulness and restored the child to them.'[88] John Brand told similarly of a great spiritual battle over the treatment of an Indian lay preacher who had fallen sick, Premji Hurji. Many of the local converts believed that Premji was a victim of sorcery, and they tried to persuade him to combat the evil power in the traditional way. Brand reassured him that he would recover through a combination of his treatment and the power of prayer. Premji remained steadfast to his Christian faith, and when he eventually recovered, Brand interpreted it as demonstrating 'the power of God to heal' – a revelation of the superior power of Christ compared to local 'wizards'.[89]

The results of these struggles were sometimes ambiguous. In 1918, for example, there was a battle between the missionaries and an exorcist in Lusadiya village itself. Jiva Dala, the oldest Christian of the place and the local postmaster, was suffering from what was described in the report as 'brain-softening'. He was treated by John Brand, but persuaded by his non-Christian relatives to also consult an exorcist. It seems that his wife also put pressure on him to do this. The exorcist used both 'mantras' – magical phrases that are recited during exorcism – and cauterisation. In the latter case, Jiva Dala was branded with a hot iron across the back of each hand, the instep of each foot, above his forehead, and just below his chest. This was all done at once by force, and he was left in agony. His brother, another leading Christian of the village, had approved of this treatment. He recovered eventually. The missionary W. Wyatt commented:

> [I]f he finally recovers, I expect the Bhagat will get the credit for the cure, while the fact that many Christians were praying for his recovery will be ignored. I have seen many bullocks cured of lameness and other ailments by branding, but it would seem a somewhat drastic remedy for a brain affection![90]

Rather than depicting this as a struggle between 'superstition' and scientific medicine, the missionary interpreted it as a battle between two systems of belief and practice. While the Christians provided medical treatment and prayer, the exorcist applied cauterisation and mantras. Both thus sought to cure through a combination of appeals to a higher force and physical treatment. Surprisingly, Wyatt even admitted that the Bhagat's chosen treatment in this latter respect could have been effective.

The mission hospital could provide a place of refuge for those who sought to escape the influence of community patriarchs and the exorcists. When a Christian woman of Biladia village fell ill in 1925, she feared that she would come under the influence of 'a heathen who deals in Black Magic, and who lives close to her house.' To resist this pressure, she went to Lusadiya for treatment as an inpatient.[91] It is not clear from the report as to her exact reasons for so doing. She might have had faith in Christian medicine as against exorcism, but it is more probable that she believed either that the exorcist and his henchmen would not pursue her so far or that the evil spirits which were haunting her lacked power within the confines of the hospital.

If the latter was the case, her faith was not so much in biomedicine as in the superior temporal and/or supernatural power of the missionaries.

Too often, however, the power of the missionaries was not only seen to fail, but to be inferior to that of more powerful forces. In 1929, a Bhil convert of a poor farming family brought his 7-year-old nephew to the mission school at Kotada. The boy quickly learnt the alphabet, gave intelligent answers to questions about the Bible, and sang hymns with zeal. One day he told his mother that he wanted to be 'a Jesus child'. Soon after this he suddenly dropped down dead. He had no history of illness, and the local missionary, Miss Carter, was baffled as to the cause. She suspected that 'an enemy hath done this', without stating exactly what she thought that this 'enemy' might have done. She noted that the non-Christian Bhils of the area had been plotting for some time to force the converts to renounce their Christianity. She could however see very clearly that the boy's sudden and inexplicable death was a grave setback to her work in the area.[92]

Conclusion

Despite all their efforts, the Christian missionaries won few adivasi converts during this period. There were no waves of mass conversion, as amongst the Vankars of central Gujarat – a community classed as 'untouchable' – in the period 1890–1910.[93] The mass movements amongst adivasis of those times were led by people such as Govind amongst the Bhils in 1913, and in South Gujarat, the Devi mediums of 1922–3.[94] Compared to these movements for self-assertion, the impact of the missionaries was very slight indeed. The opposition from the community elders increased, if anything over time. In 1926 the leading Bhils of the Lusadiya region even convened a meeting to discuss strategies for preventing the spread of Christianity in their community.[95] This is not to say that the missionaries failed entirely, for they did manage to establish a few Christian communities that have managed to survive and flourish.[96] There was something of a breakthrough in this respect during the great famine of 1899–1900, when they established orphanages for children whose parents had died. Most of these children subsequently became Christian, forming the nucleus for a number of Christian farming settlements.[97] There was also an unexpected wave of conversions in 1925–6 in a Bhil village of Mewar that had been visited by James Shepherd many years before, in which well over a hundred people expressed their faith in Christ.[98] As a result of all this, the numbers of adivasi Christians ministered to by each of the major mission denominations could be counted thereafter in hundreds, rather than in tens.

Little of this could be attributed primarily to medical work. As a vehicle for successful proselytism it proved – in this area at least – to be much overrated. In the late 1920s most adivasis were continuing to refuse to go to the mission stations for treatment, even when seriously ill, for fear of offending the community elders and the exorcists. A significant minority were, however, seeking out treatment. They would not have come if they had not had some sort of confidence, or perhaps hope, in the medical therapy available at these places. As indicated in the previous section, this confidence was not so much based on a belief in biomedicine as in an often-uncertain faith that the power of the missionaries might prevail against the counter-power of the elders and exorcists. Although this reveals that there were many subordinate adivasis – and particularly adivasi women – who wanted to escape the oppressive and often-exploitative controls exercised over them by their elders, it also meant that acceptance of the missionaries was in most cases an act of rebellion that would be limited to particular individuals and their families. This did not provide a strong base for the mass conversion of whole communities.

It might be argued that despite their lack of success in winning souls, the missionaries did at least help to inculcate alternative medical values through their work. We need to emphasise, however, that these were not those of a purely secular scientific medicine of the sort normally associated with post-Enlightenment modernity. The missionaries' own 'modernity' had developed alongside this and represented an alternative – that of an evangelical Christianity that was reinforced though not superseded by science.[99] In their healing mission, they believed that their superior medical knowledge was of only limited efficacy. As important was the power of Christ's love and compassion for the sick and injured that, working through them, brought relief from pain and suffering.

The supernatural was seen to not only endorse the rational and scientific, but also to bless the endeavours of Christians in ways that went beyond science. It is clear from the reports of the missionaries that their invocation of the supernatural brought their practice more in tune with popular local belief about disease causation than bureaucratic colonial medicine – which was rigidly secular in its application – had managed to do. However, in appealing to a deity that was very alien to the adivasis, it was hard to turn this to their advantage. Also, their abhorrence for the practice of exorcism – seen by them as a device of the Devil – prevented them from practising the sorts of ritual that most adivasis expected of their healers.

The chief impediments to Christian therapy were, however, that the majority of adivasis continued to be convinced of the efficacy of, and indeed, imperative need for exorcism, and that the majority of adivasi elders believed that the missionaries' strictures against indigenous form of therapy posed a major threat to their own political and moral hegemony. It was for these two reasons that the community leaders did all they could to undermine the often dedicated and selfless medical work of the missionaries amongst the adivasis, for the most part with considerable success.

Notes

1. In using the term 'adivasi' to describe these groups in the past I am aware that my usage is anachronistic. However, rather than deploy a series of evolving terms – such as 'early tribes', 'aboriginals', 'jungle tribes', 'scheduled tribes' and the like – I have used the term that these people commonly use to describe themselves in contemporary India. It will be clear from the text that other terms were used at different times. For a fuller justification of my usage in this respect see my book *The Coming of the Devi: Adivasi Assertion in Western India* (New Delhi: Oxford University Press, 1987), 11–16.
2. S. Muthiah (ed.), *A Social and Economic Atlas of India* (New Delhi: Oxford University Press, 1987), 27.
3. On this, see in particular D. Hardiman, 'Power in the Forest: the Dangs, 1820-1940', in D. Arnold and D. Hardiman (eds), *Subaltern Studies VIII* (New Delhi: Oxford University Press, 1994); A. Skaria, 'Timber Conservancy, Desiccationism and Scientific Forestry: The Dangs 1840s–1920s', in R. Grove, V. Damodaran, S. Sangwan (eds), *Nature and the Orient: The Environmental History of South and Southeast Asia* (New Delhi: Oxford University Press, 1998).
4. On usurers, see D. Hardiman, *Feeding the Baniya: Peasants and Usurers in Western India* (New Delhi: Oxford University Press, 1996); on liquor dealers see D. Hardiman, 'From Custom to Crime: The Politics of Drinking in Colonial South Gujarat', in R. Guha (ed.), *Subaltern Studies IV* (New Delhi: Oxford University Press, 1985).
5. [Anon.], *The Rajputana Gazetteer* (Calcutta: Superintendent of Government Printing, 1879), 76; R.S. Mann, 'Bhils of Rajasthan', in K.S. Singh (ed.), *Tribal Movements in India* (New Delhi: Manohar, 1983), 310; N.N. Vyas, *Bondage and Exploitation in Tribal India* (Jaipur: Rawat Publications, 1980), 19–20.
6. See P.C. Shah, *Tribal Life in Gujarat* (Bombay: Bharatiya Vidya Bhavan, 1964), 27–9.
7. D.P. Khanapurkar, 'The Aborigines of South Gujarat' (unpublished Ph.D. thesis: University of Bombay, 1944), 712.
8. Songs set out in *ibid.*, 936–7.
9. Report by G. Jervais, 9 September 1844, Maharashtra State Archives, Bombay, Revenue Department 81/10, 1844.
10. Recent investigations by the Gram Seva Samaj, Vyara, have revealed a high prevalence of sickle-cell anaemia amongst adivasis in South Gujarat. Although only recently discovered, it is unlikely that this is a new phenomenon. Interview with Jinabhai Darji, Vyara, 10 December 2000.

11. T.H. Hendley, 'An Account of the Maiwar Bhils', *Journal of the Asiatic Society of Bengal*, 44, pt 1, 4 (1875), 362–3.
12. Mrs A.I. Birkett, 'In the Bhil Country', *Mercy and Truth*, 5, 57 (September 1901), 207–8.
13. Mrs A.I. Birkett, 'Camping out in Khetadra', *Mercy and Truth*, 11, 124 (April 1907), 103–4.
14. [Anon.], 'Central Provinces and Rajputana Mission, Lusadia', *Mercy and Truth*, 11, 130 (October 1907), 319.
15. The twenty years were from 1877 to 1898 inclusive. T.H. Hendley, *General Medical History of Rajputana* (Calcutta: Government of India, 1900), 130–1.
16. Hendley, *op. cit.* (note 11), 362.
17. Hendley, *op. cit.* (note 15), 148.
18. H. Lambert, 'The Cultural Logic of Indian Medicine: Prognosis and Etiology in Rajasthan Popular Therapeutics', *Social Science and Medicine,* 34, 10 (1992), 1071. See also D. Arnold, *Colonizing the Body: State Medicine and Epidemic Disease in Nineteenth-Century India* (Berkeley: California University Press, 1993), 121–5. Arnold examines indigenous forms of inoculation on 125–33.
19. Hendley, *op. cit.* (note 11), 363.
20. D.C. Pal and S.K. Jain, *Tribal Medicine* (Calcutta: Naya Prokash, 1998).
21. Hendley, *op. cit.* (note 11), 363.
22. Birkett, *op. cit.* (note 12), 208.
23. Interview with Janubhai Thakre, a well-known Dangi healer, Dhavalidod, 11 December 2000. Thakre still uses this technique, along with herbal remedies and exorcism. It is possible that cauterisation operates by stimulating the immune system.
24. A. Skaria, *Hybrid Histories: Forests, Frontiers and Wildness in Western India*, (New Delhi: Oxford University Press, 1999), 57–8.
25. This was reported in 1878 for the Bhils of eastern Gujarat. District Deputy Collector's Report, Panchmahals District, 5 July 1878, Maharashtra State Archives, Bombay, Revenue Department, 1878, Vol. 15, Comp. 1024.
26. Collector's Report, Panchmahals District, 21 July 1876, Maharashtra State Archives, Bombay, Revenue Department, 1876, Vol. 10, part 2, Comp. 1518.
27. *Missionary Visitor*, 11, 7 (July 1909), 235.
28. J. Campbell, *Notes on the Spirit Basis of Belief and Custom* (Bombay: Government Central Press, 1885), 143. There were many variations on this ceremony that were informed by a similar intention. For example, the goddess might be induced to enter the body of a goat or buffalo, which was then driven beyond the boundary of the village. R.E. Enthoven, *Folklore Notes*, Vol.1, *Gujarat* (Bombay: British India Press, 1914), 88.
29. Skaria, *op. cit.* (note 24), 60.

30. Birkett, *op. cit.* (note 13), 103.
31. A.I. Birkett to E.H.M. Waller, 24 June 1914, Church Missionary Society records, University of Birmingham [hereafter CMS], G2 I 8/0, 1914, doc. 31.
32. A. Skaria, 'Women, Witchcraft and Gratuitous Violence in Colonial Western India', *Past and Present*, 155, (May 1997), 109–41.
33. For an analysis of how the British conceived of this 'civilising mission' with regard to the adivasis of western India, see Skaria, *op. cit.* (note 24), 154–5 and 192–200
34. Sir Lepal Griffen, 17 March 1883, National Archives of India, Foreign Department, Political-I, 212–58, June 1883.
35. C.S. Thompson to G.B. Durrant, Baulia 14 March 1893, CMS, G2 I 6/0, 1893.
36. Interview with Captain Stockley, Commander of the Mewar Bhil Corps, 20 May 1914, CMS, G2 I 8/0, 1914.
37. 'Annual Report of the Church of the Brethren for the Year Ending 31 March 1910', *The Missionary Visitor* (June 1910), 17.
38. Report from Valsad Mission for 1905, *The Missionary Visitor* (June 1906), 7.
39. G. Carstairs, *Shepherd of Udaipur and the Land he Loved* (London: Hodder and Stroughton, 1926), 80–1.
40. *Ibid.*, 161–2, 239–40.
41. R. Carter, *Battling and Building Among the Bhils* (London: Church Missionary Society, 1914), 15.
42. *Ibid.*, 17.
43. *Ibid.*, 17.
44. 'Bhil Mission', *Mercy and Truth*, 5, 50 (February 1901), 44.
45. J. Birkett to H. Moloney, Lusadia, 11 January 1905, CMS, M/FL I 5.
46. From a statistical table in *Mercy and Truth*, 12, 144 (December 1908), 410.
47. This Institute was established by the Scottish medical missionary, Dr Colin Valentine, in 1881. See J. Wilkinson, *The Coogate Doctors: The History of the Edinburgh Medical Missionary Society 1841 to 1991* (Edinburgh: The Edinburgh Medical Missionary Society, 1991), 30.
48. Mrs A.I. Birkett, 'Lusadia and the Present Opportunity', *The Mission Hospital*, 27, 305 (June 1923), 125.
49. These figures are all from annual reports in the CMS medical mission monthly *Mercy and Truth*, which was renamed *The Mission Hospital* in 1921.
50. 'Bhil Country: Lusadia', *The Mission Hospital*, 31, 355 (August 1927), 208.
51. 'Annual Report of the Church of the Brethren for the Year Ending 31 March 1907', *The Missionary Visitor* (1907), 20–1.
52. 'Annual Report of the Church of the Brethren for the Year Ending 31 March 1910', *The Missionary Visitor* (June 1910), 14.
53. C.F.H., 'Principles and Practice of Medical Missions', Chapter 9,

'Professional Work', *Mercy and Truth* 16, 190 (October 1912), 347.

54. Carstairs, *op. cit.* (note 39), 183.
55. A.I. Birkett to E.H.M. Waller, 24 June 1914, CMS, G2 I 8/0, 1914, doc. 31.
56. Mrs A.I. Birkett, 'Medical Work at Lusadia', *Mercy and Truth*, 11, 127 (July 1907), 205.
57. C.F.H., 'Principles and Practice of Medical Missions', Chapter 4, 'Itineration', *Mercy and Truth* 16, 186 (June 1912), 185.
58. 'Central Provinces and Rajputana Mission, Lusadia', *Mercy and Truth*, 11, 130 (October 1907), 319.
59. 'Report by Miss H. Bull, Kotra', *Church Missionary Society Report of the Mission to the Bhils for the Year 1914* (Surat: IP Mission Press, 1915), 16, CMS, G2 I 8/0, 1915, doc. 25.
60. G.W. Blair, *Station and Camp Life in the Bheel Country: A Brief History of the Origin, Aims, and Operations of the Irish Presbyterian Jungle Tribes Mission, with an Account of the Bheels: Their Manners, Customs, Religion, &c.* (Belfast: Jungle Tribes Mission, 1906), 85.
61. Carstairs, *op. cit.* (note 39), 141.
62. N. Quaiser, 'Politics, Culture and Colonialism: Unani's Debate with Doctory', in B. Pati and M. Harrison (eds), *Health, Medicine and Empire: Perspectives on Colonial India* (New Delhi: Orient Longman, 2001), 317
63. For a study of the place of 'English medicine' in contemporary Rajasthan, see H. Lambert, 'Plural Traditions? Folk Therapeutics and 'English' Medicine in Rajasthan', in A. Cunningham and B. Andrews (eds), *Western Medicine as Contested Knowledge* (Manchester: Manchester University Press, 1997), 193 and 196.
64. Wilkinson, *op. cit.* (note 47), 21–2.
65. For Jain traditions of medical charity see V. Sangave, *Jaina Community: A Social Survey* (Bombay: Popular Prakashan, 1980), 230 and 280. For nineteenth-century medical philanthropy see Arnold, *op. cit.* (note 18), 269–74.
66. R.E. Svoboda, *Ayurveda: Life, Health and Longevity* (New Delhi: Penguin, 1993), 20.
67. *Ibid.*, 30.
68. H. Lankester, 'Medical Missions in Theory', *Mercy and Truth*, 4, 38 (February 1900), 41.
69. A. Neve, 'Gifts of Healing', *Mercy and Truth*, 15, 176 (August 1911), 266. Neve worked in Srinagar, in Kashmir, for many years.
70. Report by C.L. Shaw, in *Church Missionary Society Report of the Mission to the Bhils for the Year 1913*, CMS, G2 I 8/0, 1914, doc. 27, 15–16
71. Report by A. Helen Bull, in *Church Missionary Society Report of the Mission to the Bhils for the Year 1913*, CMS, G2 I 8/0, 1914, doc. 27, 18.

72. C.F.H, 'Principles and Practice of Medical Missions', Chapter 1, 'Introductory', in *Mercy and Truth*, 16, 181 (January 1912), 23.
73. For one such case for 1925 – a time when there was no qualified doctor working in the Bhil mission – see report by F. Meigh, in *Church Missionary Society: Report of the Mission to the Bhils for the Year 1925*, G 2 I 3/0, 1926, doc. 50, 7.
74. R. Mash, 'Margaret Fitzhugh Johnson, Doctor and Missionary (1941–1963)', (unpublished BA dissertation, University of Brighton, 2001).
75. Report by Mrs C.L. Shaw, in *Church Missionary Society: Report of the Mission to the Bhils for the Year 1924*, CMS, G 2 I 3/0, 1925, doc. 52, 22.
76. Carter, *op. cit.* (note 41), 23; Blair, *op. cit.* (note 60), 103.
77. Carstairs, *op. cit.* (note 39), 217.
78. A.T. Shuttleworth, Conservator of Forests, Northern Division, to Chief Secretary to the Government of Bombay, Revenue Department, 6 April 1871, Maharashtra State Archives, Bombay, Revenue Department 1871, Vol. 18, comp. 552.
79. Birkett, *op. cit.* (note 13), 103.
80. 'Report by Mrs Birkett for 1919', *Church Missionary Society: Report of the Mission to the Bhils for the Year 1919*, CMS, G 2 I 3/0, 1920, doc. 73, 3.
81. Birkett, *op. cit.* (note 13), 103.
82. A.I. Birkett to E.H.M. Waller, 24 June 1914, CMS, G2 I 8/0, 1914, doc. 31.
83. Birkett, *op. cit.* (note 13), 102.
84. *Ibid.*, 104.
85. 'Bhil Mission', *Report of the CMS Western India Mission 1916*, CMS, G2 I 3/0, 1916, doc. 35, 75.
86. R. Carter, 'The Power of Darkness in the Bhil Mission', *The Bombay Church Missionary Gleaner*, November 1915, CMS, G2 I 3/0, 1915, doc. 107, 2–3.
87. A.I. Birkett to E.F.E. Wigram, Lusadia, 6 December 1915, CMS, G2 I 3/0, 1915, doc. 110.
88. J.L.J. Birkett, 'Lusadia Medical Work', in *Church Missionary Society Report of the Mission to the Bhils for the Year 1914*, CMS, G2 I8/0, 1915, doc. 25, 8.
89. Report by J. Brand, in *Church Missionary Society Report of the Mission to the Bhils for the Year 1913*, CMS, G2 I8/0, 1914, doc. 27, 8–10.
90. W. Wyatt, *Report of the CMS Western India Mission 1918*, CMS, G2 I 3/0, 1919, doc.109, 49.
91. Report by C.L. Shaw, *Church Missionary Society: Report of the Mission to the Bhils for the Year 1925*, CMS, G 2 I 3/0, 1926, doc. 50, 22.
92. Report by R. Carter, in *Church Missionary Society: Report of the Mission to the Bhils for the Year 1929*, CMS, G 2 I 3/0, 1930, doc. 56, 8–9.
93. This is described in J. Tremayne Copplestone, *History of Methodist Missions*, Vol. IV, *Twentieth-Century Perspectives (The Methodist Episcopal Church,*

1896-1939) (New York: The United Methodist Church, 1973), 790–98

94. For Govind see D. Hardiman, 'Assertion, Conversion and Indian Nationalism: Govind's Movement amongst the Bhils', in Rowena Robinson and Sathianathan Clarke (eds), *Religious Conversion in India: Modes, Motivations, and Meanings* (New Delhi, Oxford University Press, 2003). For the Devi movement see D. Hardiman, *op. cit.* (note 1), in particular 151–65.
95. Report by C.L. Shaw, in *Church Missionary Society: Report of the Mission to the Bhils for the Year 1926*, CMS, G2 I 3/0, 1927, doc. 22, 4.
96. Interview with Peter Galji Bhanat, Samaiya village, Vijaynagar Taluka, Sabarkantha District, 15 December 1997. Peter's father was converted by the CMS missionaries who were based in nearby Biladia.
97. Carter, *op. cit.* (note 41), 32–7
98. Carstairs, *op. cit.* (note 39), 290–1.
99. On this form of 'modernity' see 'Introduction' in P. van der Veer, *Conversion to Modernities: The Globalization of Christianity* (New York, Routledge, 1996), 8–20.

6

Colonialism, Cannabis and the Christians: Mission Medical Knowledge and the Indian Hemp Drugs Commission of 1893–4

James H. Mills

This chapter considers the ways in which missionaries in nineteenth-century India forced the issue of cannabis into the political arena of the House of Commons by the 1890s. By examining the links between Thomas Evans and his colleagues in south Asia, and temperance campaigners such as William Caine in Parliament, the chapter argues that ideas generated about medicines and drugs by missionaries could have impacts not simply on metropolitan discourses, but also on metropolitan politics and power relations.

Mission medical knowledge

The strength of most recent academic accounts of mission medicine lies in the way in which they have dealt with issues arising from the power of the medical missionaries and of the resistance to their designs. Megan Vaughan's work considers the setting up of hospital systems by churches, the success of surgery, the opportunities for evangelisation at the bedside, the struggle over maternity and the effects of African assistants.[1] Terence Ranger establishes the theoretical basis of mission medicine before examining the circumstances of the arrival of missionary medicine in Masasi, the campaigns against yaws and measles, the survival of the African lay therapy group and the issue of adaptation of Western techniques to local medical practices and models.[2] In a similar vein, the Comaroffs explore the possibility that medical missionaries were 'motors of history'[3] in southern Africa and discover that 'like all aspects of the civilising mission the healing ministry had unintended consequences'.[4] Rosemary Fitzgerald chooses to focus on the practical problems of the Protestant missionaries in India and is concerned to show that 'despite indications that missionary medicine had established itself among sections of the people, it touched only the fringes of India's vast population.'[5] Taken together, they offer a comprehensive analysis of the operations of mission medicine and its outcomes.

Less compelling, however, has been the way in which such studies have dealt with missionary knowledge. Megan Vaughan asserts that:

> [T]he image of the 'sick African' and of Africa as a 'sick continent' to be pitied and despised is one which, though not entirely of the missionary societies' making, was greatly influenced by the reports which they sent home, and one which retains a strong hold even now.[6]

Yet she produces little evidence to back up her point and is forced to admit that she found it 'hard to measure the precise impact of the medical missionary discourse on British perceptions of the "African".'[7]

The Comaroffs are similarly assertive of the impact of missionary knowledge on metropolitan ideas and on Western discourses. They start from the conclusion that:

> As comparative anatomy and physiology developed, and took hold of African bodies, two things followed. Both were deeply rooted in the signifying economy of colonialism. First, like much early travel writing, the new discourse eroticized the 'dark continent', often reducing it in the clinic to the ostensibly excessive reproductive organs of its women. And, second, as the medical gaze moved into the unknown interior, it treated the black female physique as a natural site for explorations in pathology. This was especially marked in researches on the relationship between disease and unruly fecundity, a relationship quintessentially associated with Africa.[8]

They then assert that 'influential in this respect, of course, were the writings of David Livingstone who, it will be recalled, continued to treat difficult obstetric cases even after he lost enthusiasm for healing.' The problem with this is that they simply describe Livingstone's writing on the African female in isolation and entirely fail to show that his work was quoted by other writers and at other times. In other words they fail to demonstrate where and when Livingstone's work was actually influential in the developments that they describe.

Even more ambitious is their claim that:

> [T]he enduring legacy of the medical mission lay, rather, in something more subtle: in its quiet impact on European consciousness during an age when parochial paradigms of knowledge and practice were undergoing reformation, an age when Europe was caught up in constructing the modernist self. This self, a biological individual/ist with an enclosed physique and discrete parts was knowable in the first instance by contrast with its sable opposite: the uncontained, unrestrained African female body.[9]

This is an important thesis and would place medical missionary knowledge at the heart of Western culture if it were not for the fact that the Comaroffs provide absolutely no evidence to show that the work of Christian doctors in Africa was disseminated, let alone read and quoted, in wider circles and networks. Indeed, the only convincing assertion that they make on the subject of medical missionary knowledge is a minor point about Livingstone, that 'he also published accounts of a range of African diseases; several were to be of lasting professional significance,'[10] as they at least provide references to show where this was the case.

This study will take a detailed look at the issue of missionary medical knowledge partly to provide proof that the assertions of Vaughan and the Comaroffs are broadly correct, that is that medical knowledge generated by colonial missions could have lasting impacts on metropolitan imaginations and on Western discourses. There are other reasons that such a study is important, however. The first is to consider whether missions acted as did prisons, hospitals and lunatic asylums in modern empires, as rare observatories at which the colonial doctor could bring samples drawn from the local population under the glare of Victorian science in order to gather knowledge about that population as a whole. It has been argued that colonial governments had little access to local society and therefore relied on the information supplied by their doctors at medical sites to draw a range of conclusions on issues ranging from typical diet to the dangers of drug use.[11] This study will see how far mission medicine was similarly an agent of colonial knowledge.

A second further reason for such a study is to build on existing research that has convincingly argued that missionary medical knowledge could have wider political impacts. Maina Chawla Singh has examined American missionary women in India and has concluded that a medical idiom was used by female medical missionaries to create an image of a moral universe where Indian women were trapped in a world of illness and decay. In providing examples such as that from an 1881 publication, *Women's Medical Work in Foreign Lands*, which portrays the zenana as 'dark, dirty, miserable dwellings, where fevers, ophthalmia and other ills breed unchecked,'[12] she argues that this was no idle Orientalist fancy. Rather, such ideas about disease were central to an important and strategic process of representing a gendered problem in India that demanded a gendered response in America. As Singh concludes:

> [T]hese missionary discourses of 'degradation in heathen lands' and more importantly of the 'plight of the heathen woman' as the passive, victim figure in the midst of this perceived degradation, were to become the building blocks for a domestic cult among women's missionary societies in North

> America. As a phenomenon that transformed women's modest prayer groups and 'cent societies' into institutionalized chartered women's missionary boards that grew large in size and budget, this movement touched the lives of thousands of North American women in Protestant denominations... the Gospel, aimed at 'saving' the 'heathen women', thus became a liberating force for missionary women themselves offering spaces for feminist articulation and legitimizing what were essentially radical moves in challenging established sex roles.[13]

Kathleen Lodwick's work has similarly shown how it is possible to trace the influence and impact of medical missionary ideas in wider circles. She has looked at the way in which medical missionary knowledge was mobilised in support of the anti-opium campaigns mounted against the drugs trade in Asia. In considering the impact of such publications as *Opinions of Over 100 Physicians on the use of opium in China,* she concludes that:

> Medical missionaries in China gathered the first scientific data on the nature of the drug, helping to convince even the most hardened sceptics that opium really was harmful. The missionary doctor's scientific evidence was used by the International Opium Conferences in 1909 and 1911–12 in their deliberations.[14]

Lodwick's case study also suggests a final reason why a detailed study of the impact and influence of mission medical knowledge is important. When considering the legacies of missionary medicine,[15] it is perhaps to knowledge rather than to institutions and processes that historians might turn in looking for lasting impacts. It can be argued that ideas about opium generated by colonial missionaries continue to shape moral agendas on drugs to this day, and this chapter will argue that ideas about cannabis similarly continue to bear the imprint of the missionaries.

In focusing on the case of cannabis drugs and missionaries at the end of the nineteenth century in India, this chapter will consider three ideas. The first is that the information produced by missionaries in south Asia on the subject of cannabis medicines and drugs was shaped by their own convictions about the virtues of temperance and also by the association of medicinal preparations of the plant with local, rival religious groups and practices. The second is that the place of these missionaries in wider information networks ensured that the representations of cannabis medicines and drugs that they constructed drove the Parliamentary campaign to force the Government of India to organise a Commission to enquire into the issue of cannabis use in India. Finally, the third idea is that the broader politics of cannabis and colonialism acted to prevent the views of the missionaries from becoming officially endorsed, as the Government of

India's revenues from the trade in cannabis drugs in Asia were too great to forego. Taken as a whole, the article demonstrates the cultural and political nature of the knowledge generated by missionaries about Indian medicines and the ways in which, despite the questionable nature of this information, it could in turn produce wider outcomes and become embroiled in broader debates. The article will consider the evidence of medical missionaries but also that of other evangelists without formal medical training where they paid particular attention to issues of medicine and drugs.

William Caine and his cannabis campaign

On 2 March 1893 the Secretary of State for India declared in the House of Commons that the Government of India would establish a Commission to examine the issue of cannabis use among the communities of south Asia. Although preparations of the cannabis sativa plant were largely unknown in Britain in the 1890s they became the subject of a sustained campaign by individual MPs in the Commons after 1891 when Mark Stewart MP stood up in the House of Commons on 16 July:

> [T]o ask the Under-Secretary of State for India whether his attention has been called to the statement in the *Allahabad Pioneer* of the 10th May last that ganja 'which is grown, sold and excised under much the same conditions as opium', is far more harmful than opium, and that 'the lunatic asylums of India are filled with ganja smokers'.

He pressed his point, asking further of the Under-Secretary:

> [W]hether he is aware that the possession and sale of ganja has been prohibited for many years past in Lower Burma and that the exclusion of the drug was stated in the Excise Report of that province for 1881–82 to have been 'of immense benefit to the people'.

The reason for his curiosity was that he wanted to know:

> [W]hether he [the Under-Secretary of State] will call the attention of the Government of India to the desirability of extending the same prohibition to the other Provinces of India?[16]

Mark Stewart was an experienced temperance campaigner by the 1890s and a member of the vociferous anti-opium campaign that finally cornered the Government on the issue in the last decade of the nineteenth century. He had been badgering the authorities about opium for almost twenty years. As early as 1875 he had urged the House of Commons to pass a motion that:

> [T]he Imperial policy regulating the opium traffic between India and China should be carefully considered by Her Majesty's Government with a view to

> gradual withdrawal of the Government of India from the cultivation and manufacture of Opium.[17]

This had failed, but the campaign continued, reaching a crescendo in 1891, when Sir Joseph Pease successfully brought forward the motion in the Commons that 'this House is of opinion that the system by which the Indian opium revenue is raised is morally indefensible, and would urge upon the Indian Government that it should cease to grant licences for the cultivation of the poppy.'[18] Stewart remained at the forefront of the campaign in this period, speaking alongside Pease in, for example, the debate on the subject of 3 May 1889 when, assuming a religious authority, he pronounced that 'the opinion of the Christian Churches in this country is that the Indian Government ought no longer to be the producers and manufacturers of this drug.'[19] This tone had been adopted by Pease who had argued that 'this trade, demoralizing to so large a portion of mankind, stands in the way of the spread of the Christian faith that we all desire.' Opium was not the only intoxicant to worry Stewart; since the 1870s he had also been a supporter of legislative measures against alcohol consumption. He had supported the Intoxicating Liquors (Scotland) Bill of 1875 and had announced in the following year that in the case of intemperate use of spirits in Ireland 'he would rather that moral suasion were used to remedy the evil complained of but that having failed it was high time to legislate on the subject.'[20]

Indeed, it seems that cannabis was of little real interest to Mark Stewart as an issue in itself and was rather seen as just another intoxicant and just another way of darkening the reputation of the Government of India in the House of Commons by emphasising its murky dealings in drugs. Stewart had raised the subject of ganja only once before in begging:

> [T]to ask the Under-Secretary of State if he can inform the House of the number of shops or houses in each province of British India licensed for the retail sale of opium, ganja and bhang respectively and in how many of these opium is allowed to be smoked or otherwise consumed on the premises.[21]

Evidently, the focus of this query was opium even though cannabis products were briefly mentioned. Indeed, he never bothered with the subject of cannabis preparations again after his question about the lunatic asylums of India in 1891 although he did continue to concentrate on the issue of opium, at one point confronting Gladstone on the subject and demanding to know 'if it is the intention of Her Majesty's Government to bring in a Bill, with a view to legislation, on the opium question this Session, in accordance with the Resolution passed by this House in 1891?'[22]

It was one of Stewart's colleagues in Parliament, William Sproston Caine, who instead took up the issue of cannabis use in India. On the face of it

Caine and Stewart were unlikely colleagues. The latter was a member of an old aristocratic family – the Stewart clan of Kircudbrightshire in the lowland borders.[23] The former, on the other hand, was from a family that had only relatively recently built its fortune from iron ore mining in Cheshire. What the two had in common was an interest in temperance reform. Caine was raised as a Baptist and he came to serve as president of institutions such as the Baptist Total Abstinence Society and the National Temperance Federation.[24] His commitment to issues of temperance was such that he resigned his seat in the House of Commons over the matter of compensation for public-house licence-holders and was appointed to the Royal Commission on liquor licensing laws that sat between 1896 and 1899.[25] It was this commitment that meant he was a also a determined member of the anti-opium campaign, writing at one point that:

> I have been in East-End gin palaces on Saturday nights, I have seen men in various stages of delirium tremens, I have visited many idiot and lunatic asylums but I have never seen such horrible destruction of God's image in the face of man as I saw in the Government opium dens of Lucknow.[26]

He stood up in the Commons on 14 February 1893 in order to:

> [B]eg to ask the Under-Secretary of State for India whether the Indian Government has yet forwarded to the India Office the further Despatch dealing with the case of ganja and other drugs, promised in paragraph 4 of its Despatch, dated 14th October 1891?[27]

He evidently suspected the Government of India of dragging its feet but instead learnt from George Russell, who was now the Under Secretary of State for India, that it had indeed arrived accompanied by a range of papers and that it would be 'laid upon the Table if my hon. Friend will move for them.' Caine did indeed apply to see the report and it was sent for printing on 8 March. Before even seeing this response from the Government of India to Mark Stewart's question he piped up again, this time to demand action:

> I beg to ask the Under-Secretary of State for India if the Secretary of State for India will instruct the Government of India to create a Commission of Experts to inquire into, and report upon, the cultivation of and trade in all preparations of hemp drugs in Bengal, the effect of their consumption upon the social and moral condition of the people, and the desirability of prohibiting its growth and sale.[28]

He also insisted that 'the Commission shall be partly composed of non-official natives of India'.

To what seems to have been his surprise, George Russell stood up and declared 'the Secretary of State proposes to request the Viceroy to appoint a Commission to inquire into the cultivation and trade in hemp drugs and he will be glad if the result of their inquiry is to show that further restrictions can be placed upon the sale and consumption of these drugs.' The Indian Hemp Drugs Commission (IHDC) had been established, although Caine seems not to have expected this as he had a Resolution on the subject lined up on the Order Book that he had to arrange to be withdrawn.[29] He was dogged in ensuring that the matter was seen to as a matter of urgency, asking questions throughout June about who was going to be on the Commission and finally receiving his answer on 7 July. Cannabis had become a matter of concern in the House of Commons for the first time and William Caine had secured the IHDC to examine the drugs and medicines prepared in India from the plant.[30] He had done this more or less single-handedly, as he had followed up Mark Stewart's original question of 1891 and had persisted in returning to the subject throughout the early months of 1893 despite the fact that no-one else spoke in his support or in condemnation of cannabis in the Commons. The question remains, therefore, of why Caine had mounted this successful campaign.[31]

William Caine, Thomas Evans and the missionaries of India

There is no published record that suggests that William Caine ever showed a knowledge of, or an interest in, cannabis products before his trip to India late in 1888 to promote the Anglo–Indian Temperance Association. He had formed this in that year with fellow temperance MP, Samuel Smith, with Caine taking the post of Honorary Secretary, a position he held until the end of his life. On 30 April 1889 they offered the following resolution which was put to the ballot in the House of Commons:

> In opinion of this House, the fiscal system of the GOI leads to the establishment of spirit distilleries, liquor and opium shops in large numbers of places, where, till recently, they never existed, in defiance of native opinion and the protests of inhabitants and that such increased facilities for drinking produce a steadily increased consumption, and spread misery and ruin among the industrial classes of India calling for immediate action on the part of the GOI with a view to their abatement.[32]

The resolution was carried, and the result was that the Government of India was contacted and asked to defend its position by the Secretary of State for India, which it did in 1890 through an attack on the alleged misrepresentations that Caine had relied upon.[33]

However, Caine's knowledge of temperance issues in India after his trip there in 1888/9 went beyond spirits and opium as he seems to have formed an opinion on all of the intoxicants used in the country. He was no simple across-the-board kill-joy and his biographer speaks of his approval of one beverage:

> Mr Caine frequently denounced the mistaken policy of taxing the toddy-palm. The toddy-palm yields a liquid which for ages has formed one of the staple articles of food of the poorer classes in India. Whilst fresh it is perfectly innocuous and wholesome. When fermentation takes place, the result is only a slightly intoxicating beverage.[34]

There was no such treatment for cannabis which Caine denounced in 1890 as 'the most horrible intoxicant the world has yet produced.'[35] In that year he published a guide book for those travelling to India in which he committed his first words on cannabis to paper. While describing things to do on a wander around Lucknow he inserted the following passage:

> Here and there throughout the bazar are little shops whose entire stock consists of a small lump of greenish pudding, which is being retailed out in tiny cubes. This is another 'Government monopoly' and is majoon, a preparation of the deadly bhang or Indian hemp known in Turkey and Egypt as Haseesh, the most horrible intoxicant the world has yet produced. In Egypt, its importation and sale is absolutely forbidden and a costly preventive service is maintained to suppress smuggling of it by Greek adventurers; but a Christian Government is wiser in its generation and gets a comfortable income out of its sale. When an Indian wants to commit some horrible crime, such as murder or wife mutilation, he prepares himself for it with two anna's worth of bhang from a government majoon shop. The little rooms, open to the street, of which the sole furniture is some matting and a few Hukas, are churras or Chandu shops, farmed out by the government of India to provide another form of Indian hemp intoxication which is smoked instead of eaten.

This description was, of course, closely followed by an account of drinking dens and opium parlours. Fast on the description of cannabis users, he creates the image of:

> [T]he groups of noisy men seated on the floor [who] are drinking ardent spirits of the worst description, absolutely forbidden to the British soldier, but sold retail to natives at three farthings a gill, of which two farthings go to the exchequer [who were sat nearby the] large native house... through a door of which streams in and out a swarm of customers. It is perhaps three o'clock in the afternoon. Entering with them, you will find yourself in a spacious but very dirty courtyard, round which are ranged fifteen or twenty small rooms. The stench is sickening, the swarm of flies intolerable, and there

is something strange and weird in the faces of those coming in from the street. This is the establishment of another Government contractor, the opium farmer.

Caine's ideas about cannabis were closely bound together with his fears about alcohol and opium in India and were caught up in his political opposition to the colonial government there.

If the date of these pronouncements on cannabis suggests that the trip to India in 1888/9 was significant in the formulation of his thinking on cannabis then it is the company that Caine shared while there that explains how he came to develop his opinions. Attention focuses here on the Reverend Thomas Evans, a man of whom it was said that Caine 'always spoke in the highest terms'.[36] Evans had served as a Baptist missionary in India since 1855. Born in Trefdraeth, Newport, in Wales in 1826 he had been a lifelong opponent of intoxication as a result of his childhood experiences of his father's drunken rages. He had become concerned about the Government of India's income from taxes on alcohol in 1874 during a residence at Monghyr and later wrote that:

> [I]n India, the manufacture and sale of liquor is under Government control and as a loyal Briton, as well as a friend of the people of India and a Christian missionary, I could not support a policy which secured extra revenue at the cost of impoverishing and demoralising the people.[37]

By the 1880s he had taken to sending letters to the British newspapers and these drew him to the attention of MPs in the House of Commons for whom the issues of temperance, the opium trade, and the Government of India were all entwined. William Caine contacted Evans in the summer of 1888 and proposed that they travel together across India to stir up interest in temperance issues on a speaking tour.

Caine's choice of Evans was a practical one. The latter had been in India for over thirty years and had extensive contacts across south Asia. Sent there as a member of the Baptist Missionary Society, he travelled widely and had at various times been based in Agra, Mathura, Delhi, Calcutta, Allahabad, Monghyr, Ootacamund, and Rangoon. In his memoirs he detailed friendships and professional contacts with a host of British and American missionaries, evangelical laymen and chaplains of the cantonment churches. In other words, Evans would have seemed to be the ideal man to lead Caine and his Anglo–Indian Temperance Association to those likely to be attracted to its agenda.

The speaking tour with Caine began on 11 November 1888 in Bombay and by 1 January 1889 Caine and Evans had appeared in cities across Gujarat, the Punjab, the United Provinces, Bihar and Bengal. After a week in Calcutta the tour moved to the south and, by 8 March, Caine and Evans could boast that they had:

> [S]ucceeded in addressing nearly one hundred public meetings and visiting almost every large centre of population throughout British India. Upwards of forty temperance societies were formed in consequence of these meetings and were affiliated to the Anglo–Indian Temperance Association. Many others were subsequently established and there were soon seventy affiliated branches.[38]

The biography of William Caine provides a similarly hectic version of the trip, 'the second visit Mr Caine paid to India was as the representative of this Association. During his tour he addressed nearly one hundred public meetings, many of them of enormous proportions. He was accompanied throughout his journey by the Reverend Thomas Evans.'[39]

Evans' views on cannabis are made clear in his written response to the IHDC. Evans wrote:

> It appears to me a superfluous labour to make an enquiry whether the use of hemp drugs are or are not deleterious in their effects upon those who indulge in them. That they are so is a fact well known throughout the world.[40]

He reported that 'I have myself seen idiots wandering about in large towns in the North-West, especially in Patna, who had become so by indulgence in charas and ganja,'[41] and he quoted lunatic asylum statistics from Lower Bengal to make his point about the relationship between mental health problems and use of cannabis, arguing that 53% of cases in the government's hospitals were due to consumption of the plant's preparations.[42] Evans was also concerned to place cannabis in a comparative context and he argued that 'the indulgence in opium is bad enough, but not half as injurious as that of ganja, and about four times more ganja is consumed in Bengal than opium.'[43] All of this was a preamble to an attack on the Government where he applied his broader arguments on all intoxicants in India to the specific issue of cannabis.

> What I and others charge the Government with is the sad fact that by the cultivation of hemp drugs in Lower Bengal under Government sanction and control, and by the incentives given by the State to increase the production and the sales for revenue purposes, the Government itself becomes the producer and the monopolised merchant of the vile traffic through which thousands of its own subjects are ruined. This is a serious charge, but it is as true as it is regrettable, and it applies to opium and liquor as well as to hemp drugs.

In accordance with this attack he called for a radical change of policy on the part of the Government:

> Let the Government wash its guilty hands clean of the traffic as far as its own dealings with it are concerned… to my mind by far the best measure is prohibition.[44]

Evans' views of cannabis were evidently severe and elsewhere in the IHDC testimony suggests that these were convictions that had been held for some time. The Reverend Prem Chand reported that:

> I am a Baptist Missionary. I was once under Mr Evans and worked with him for 7 or 8 years in Monghyr. Thence I went to Calcutta for 4 years and from Calcutta I was transferred to Gaya. Mr Evans knew my views. I saw him in December last but we did not then talk over the hemp drugs. When Mr Evans and I worked together in Monghyr we often conversed about them, and had common experience about them. We worked together in the cause of temperance.[45]

It would appear therefore that William Caine had travelled across India with a man whose experience of the country spanned four decades and had allowed him to form damning opinions about cannabis based on his lifelong conviction about the evils of intoxicants. It is also clear that in Evans, Caine had found a companion who was given to discussing cannabis drugs and their evils.

Indeed, Evans would not simply have appeared as an isolated voice to Caine. Evans' account of the speaking tour is interesting when cross-referenced with the witness lists of the IHDC. While travelling with Caine, Evans recounted visiting the Reverend S.J. Long in Coimbatore. When confronted by the IHDC Long had reported that 'I also think that ganja calls for more restriction than alcohol at the hands of the Government' despite the fact that he readily confessed that he had no experience of the deleterious effects of cannabis.[46] Evans also recalled encountering W.H. Campbell while speaking in Cuddapah.[47] Campbell presented the IHDC with the unappetising information that cannabis:

> [I]s put into curry, especially brain curry. This is common at funeral ceremonies amongst various sudra castes. It is pounded or pressed into meat, especially such pieces as the heart or liver, and the whole is roasted and eaten.[48]

Indeed, Evans also noted that while with Caine he had met with the Reverend Prem Chand, mentioned above, who happily admitted to the IHDC that he was a long-time supporter of Evans' stance on the drugs.[49]

Prem Chand's evidence is particularly important as he confessed in his report to the IHDC that 'Mr Evans sent me the paper of questions and I despatched my answers through him'.[50] In other words, a glimpse is caught here of Evans actively contacting missionaries that he knew to have negative views of cannabis in order to orchestrate responses to the IHDC's inquiries. Evans appears here not simply as someone with a dim view of cannabis products and not simply as someone known to discuss these views and to know others with similarly critical opinions. He appears to be a man ready to rally others to the cause of publicly damning cannabis intoxicants.

It is little wonder then that William Caine, after a tour of India in the company of Evans, went on to write such lurid and damning accounts of cannabis drugs. Indeed, having established the Anglo–Indian Temperance Association, Caine also founded its journal with the ironic title *Abkari*, after the local name for the excise system in India. This was used as a mouthpiece so that Evans could reach a wider audience still, and he wrote in 1892 for example to condemn 'the State traffic in the noxious ganja poison'.[51]

It is tempting to wonder what Caine might have thought of cannabis had he not been accompanied by Thomas Evans. After all, even within the missionary presence in India there was no clear or unanimous view on cannabis. Indeed, the returns of the IHDC show that few missionaries had an opinion of any sort on the issue of cannabis drugs in India. The IHDC complained that:

> [E]very effort was put forth by the Commission to obtain missionary opinion on the subject of their inquiries and it is a matter of some regret to them that their efforts have met with but little success.

Apparently it found that there was a dearth of knowledge of the issue of cannabis among Christian churches in India:

> Not only was it announced through Local Governments that the Commission desired to receive communications from religious bodies of all denominations but the Commission themselves also communicated freely with persons of this class. But the large majority of them declined to come forward as witnesses and many, including Churchmen, Dissenters and Roman Catholics communicated letters either to Government or direct to the Commission excusing themselves on the ground of want of knowledge. As an example of the want of knowledge of the subject or lack of interest evinced by missionaries, it may be observed that in one instance (in the Madras Presidency) the Commission made over 70 copies of their questions to two sects of missionaries professing to represent one-fifth of the whole missionary enterprise of the Madras Presideny. Yet the total number of

missionaries in this Presidency who sent in answers or statements to the Commission was only 15.[52]

Among those that did reply there were those that had obviously done so out of a sense of duty and who knew little. The Reverend Thomas of the London Missionary Society was perhaps the most honest in admitting that 'I have given the matter of hemp drugs very little attention until I was asked the other day.'[53] Reverend I.C. Archibald in Chicacole in the Madras Presidency stated baldly that 'although I have had some nine years of residence in this country, the bulk of the questions I am unable to answer,'[54] and the Reverend G.A. Lefroy of the Cambridge Mission in Delhi confessed that 'I know scarcely anything about the matters with which this commission deals'.[55]

Others had evidently gone to the effort of hastily gathering some information in order to provide some evidence to the IHDC. George Pittendrigh, a Free Church of Scotland missionary in Madras, candidly made it clear that 'it was not till after I heard of the Commission that I made any special enquiry into the matter... no-one seemed to know anything about it.'[56] The Reverend Ball of the Church Missionary Society in Karachi qualified his statements with an introduction that stated:

> I have completed thirteen years of service in Sind, but till within the past few weeks I have not taken advantage of any opportunities I might have had to inform myself regarding matters connected with hemp drugs, and the information I now give, such as it is, has been gathered by personal enquiry from natives.[57]

John Kerry, a missionary in Dacca, readily confessed that:

> [M]y attention was not drawn to the use until I was asked in connection with this Commission... generally I have seen nothing of the effects of ganja or its use until I searched for them.[58]

Some of those who had stories to tell and opinions to offer were positive in their assessment of cannabis drugs. Reverend Dutt, a missionary in Khulna in the Bengal Presidency related the remarkable tale of a former colleague. He described him as:

> [O]ne man who had derived benefit from using ganja in moderation. He was a preacher of the Baptist Mission and lived to nearly 100 years old. He used to take one chillum daily before going to bed... this man was my friend for 14 or 15 years but I never knew that he smoked.[59]

J.P. Jones, stationed up in Assam, offered the observation that 'men often work well when taking ganja,'[60] and A.E. Ball serving in Sind noted the medical uses of cannabis preparations:

> I gather that Bhang is recommended in cases of venereal disease and that ground into powder it is useful for external application to piles. For the same disease a pinch of powdered bhang with an equal quantity of sugar is eaten by some in the morning. Tincture of charas and charas pills are said to be good for cough and asthma. When cattle refuse their food, bhang is often given to them to produce appetite. When a calf dies and the cow refuses to give milk when another calf is brought, bhang is given and the cow under the intoxicating influence of the drug gives milk and never refuses to do so afterwards. Bhang creates appetite, helps digestion and used moderately, may be beneficial.[61]

The Catholic missionary, the Very Reverend A. Chelvum in Vizagapatam, stated clearly that 'the moderate use is beneficial.' He went on to confirm that he thought that:

> [A]lcohol in moderation contributes to health by refreshing and relieving the mind and body… I should receive either a spirit drinker or ganja smoker into my congregation. If he were given to excess, I should inculcate moderation.[62]

Others were more negative. Dr H.M. Clark was a medical missionary at Amritsar who stated that he had qualified as 'a Doctor of Medicine and Master of Surgery of the University of Edinburgh'. He reported on his experiences of the Punjab and in particular of preparations of charas, the pure resin exuded by the female plant. From the outset he was keen to make clear that 'I can find no other word to describe the effects of charas other than they are frightful,' and his overall conclusion was that 'as far as my experience goes the effects of hemp are always and altogether bad.'[63] A fellow medical missionary, the Reverend D. Morison who was working in Bengal, was broadly in agreement with these assessments although his particular study was of ganja, the dried flowering tops of cultivated female hemp plants which have become coated with resin. He noted that:

> [I]t over stimulates the appetite, causing the smoker to gorge himself with food which he cannot digest, and thus leading to indigestion; it does not give staying power, but the reaction is severe. It demands the stimulant again or the smoker is quite helpless and useless; it is never used as a febrifuge, indeed if a ganja smoker has an attack of fever, he dare not indulge in his usual pipe as it aggravates his condition. The ganja-smoker is as liable to fever as others. It has no prophylactic power in malarious districts.

Taken as a whole he was convinced that:

> [I]t impairs the physical organism, saps the muscular energy by over-stimulation and leads to loss of muscular vigour, producing emaciation.[64]

Missionaries who lacked a medical training did not feel, however, that assessments of the health impact of cannabis drugs were beyond them. Reverend Phillips of the London Missionary Society, who served in Calcutta, was particularly interested in the psychological implications of use of the preparations. He stated that:

> I believe that this question of insanity from the use of ganja is a very serious one.... It creates such horrible visions, intensifies so unnaturally all the powers of mind and body, exhausts physical and mental energy, and places its victim in the direct line for the mad house.[65]

Others preferred to venture their opinions on the moral and social effects of these drugs. Reverend Heinrichs, who worked in the Krishna District of the Madras Presidency, wrote:

> I may say that their use generally induces laziness on the part of the consumers. People who indulge in ganja smoking never like to work hard and appear to be physically weak in constitution. These drugs are never used as an aphrodisiac but on the other hand it is said that the use of the drug tends to produce impotence.[66]

From Karachi, the Reverend Ball contented himself with passing on the report that:

> [T]he sweetmeat majum in which bhang is mixed is eaten by some as an aphrodisiac.... I gather that prostitutes use it for this purpose [and] I should say that a large proportion of bad characters are excessive consumers of these drugs.[67]

Prejudice, pride and missionary information

William Caine became a champion of the anti-cannabis cause in Parliament – leading to the establishment of the Indian Hemp Drugs Commission – because he had happened to fall in with a missionary, Thomas Evans, who was at that time probably the most powerful critic of the drug within the evangelical community in India. It is not at all clear, however, that Evans was representative of missionary opinion in India in general on the topic.[68] Neither is it clear that Caine was well-informed. A survey of the opinions expressed by those opposed to cannabis suggests that a number of prejudices shaped their position and that little by way of scientific or sociological rigour had troubled their thinking.

The most obvious of the prejudices was the abhorrence of intoxication typical of those committed to the temperance movement.[69] In some of the responses the temperance agenda of the missionary is implied rather than stated, so that Reverend Phillips in Calcutta, whose concern about the mental health implications of the drug was mentioned above, admitted that 'I hardly care to distinguish between opium, alcohol and ganja. I regard them all as bad.... I am prepared to prohibit all three intoxicants on account of the evil which I see done by them all.'[70] The Reverend Long of Coimbatore, whom Thomas Evans encountered on his tour with William Caine, also acknowledged that he was 'Secretary of a Temperance Association which takes note of intoxicating drugs as well as liquor'. Long confessed that he viewed intoxication in a negative manner as he reported that 'I may say I have never seen a member of the Native church drunk, but I know some take liquor and we disapprove of this, whether in moderation or excess.' His recommendation was that 'because I think the hemp drug more dangerous, the physical effects so injurious, and the habit so difficult to leave off, I also think that ganja calls for more restriction than alcohol at the hands of the Government.' This, however, was his conviction rather than his experience talking, as he also admitted that before the inquiry 'I had no experience of the drugs or their effects. I had come on no cases of ill effects from the use of the drugs.'[71] Writing in a similar vein, the Reverend Thomas, a member of the London Mission working in Vizagapatam, stated:

> I am myself a total abstainer; but the London Mission does not make a point of total abstinence. Most of our Native Christians are total abstainers; but this is not made compulsory. I should myself not permit a member of the church to use hemp drugs. I should strictly forbid it. If he did not obey I should not permit him to remain a member. I should not take the same course in regard to alcohol (spirit) provided that no effect came to my notice, and that the use was not a confirmed habit but only occasional. I should treat the use of opium precisely as I should treat the use of ganja. The reason of the difference in my attitude towards alcohol is that I think the drugs seem to affect the man more directly.[72]

All this despite the fact that he admitted that 'I have given the matter of hemp drugs very little attention until I was asked the other day.'

Another apparent reason for the antipathy of the missionaries towards cannabis preparations was that they were frequently associated with their rivals, the Hindu holymen. Their use of such substances was taken as an index of their degeneration. In Bengal, Reverend Dutt pointed out that:

> [W]henever Fakirs and Kartabhajas assemble together for religious purposes they, as a rule, take ganja. The taking of ganja is considered by them essential, and it generally becomes excessive and consequently injurous to health.[73]

The Canadian Baptist, Reverend H.F. Laflamme, argued that:

> [T]he mats or peculiar home of the religious mendicants, sanyasis or, as they are termed in these parts, bairagalu, have usually quite a garden plot attached in which the hemp plant is cultivated, but only to supply the need of the monks and their disciples. Such monasteries exist, I am informed, at large places like Samalkota, Chicacole, Berhampur, etc.[74]

He also stated that 'I had frequently met bairagis in the course of my evening preaching at the temples in the villages... there would be many disciples and poor people smoking with the bairagis on these occasions.'[75] In his report to the Commission, the Reverend Goffin of the Madras Presidency fulminated that:

> [T]he religious mendicants who use it largely do so probably 1. because they are a lazy, bad class of men; 2. because it helps them to bear the hardships of their peculiar kind of life; 3. because the half-crazy, imbecile demeanour it produces is not unfavourably regarded by the people.[76]

The Christian missionaries' views of their competitors in India's religious market and the orientalising impulses of those convinced of the inferiority of Asian cultural systems, were combined here to condemn cannabis use.[77]

Other prejudices are evident. The Reverend Morison, a Medical Missionary in Rampur Boalia, was concerned about sex and the use of cannabis substances and feared that it:

> [U]tterly demoralises a young lad. The sexual desires are so stimulated that, if he can afford it, he will spend his days and nights with prostitutes. Laziness follows the over-stimulation of muscular and sexual functions.[78]

This narrative is a disapproval of promiscuity and prostitution rather than an assessment of a plant substance.[79] However, the broader conclusion is clear. The missionaries who took a dim view of cannabis did so because it fell foul of their own convictions and prejudices and not because any of them had conducted extensive or informed study of the plant, its products and their uses. In falling in with those who held such negative opinions on cannabis, William Caine found himself influenced by facts and information that had rather shaky foundations.

Conclusions

The story of Caine, Evans and the IHDC offers a number of perspectives on the issues raised in the opening of this chapter. First of all, the story shows how the ideas generated about medicines and drugs by these missionaries and medical missionaries in India were able to enter wider information networks and to impact upon metropolitan discourses. Disseminated through such sources as the publications of William Caine and the pages of *Abkari*, the judgements of cannabis made by Christians in South Asia came to dominate thinking on the subject in political circles in London to the extent that the Government of India was forced to establish the IHDC in order to investigate and respond to the claims that originated in India. This, despite the fact that these claims originated not in medical or scientific observations, but in the imaginations of a group, the Christian evangelists, who had professional and moral objections to the uses made of cannabis medicines and drugs in South Asian culture. Here then is evidence that backs up the assertions of writers like Vaughan and the Comaroffs that medical ideas and images generated by missionaries in colonial contexts had impacts on metropolitan discourses.

That these ideas could occasion a parliamentary campaign on the issue of cannabis, a drug that was after all largely unknown in Britain at the end of the nineteenth century,[80] and the fact that these images could force the Government of India to order the IHDC seems to corroborate the process identified by Singh and Lodwick in which ideas and strategies generated by missionaries in colonial contexts impacted not simply on metropolitan discourse but also on metropolitan politics and power relations. Singh demonstrated how this operated in remaking gender relations within American evangelical organisations, while Lodwick showed how missionary beliefs became powerful weapons in the hands of anti-opium campaigners. This chapter has highlighted how the issue of cannabis drugs and medicines as constructed by missionaries in India became another stick with which the coalition of temperance campaigners, imperial critics, and anti-opium activists in the House of Commons attempted to beat the British Government over its administration of India and its revenue from opium sales in Asia.

That the IHDC rejected the ideas and opinions on cannabis medicines and drugs that had their origins in India with the missionaries is discussed more fully elsewhere.[81] However, the fact that they were rejected provides an interesting source of reflection on the third issue raised in the opening of this chapter. It may well have been the case that the British authorities had very limited access to Indian society and as such privileged information coming from the few sites that they had for gathering data, such as the prisons, the army barracks, and the hospitals. The rejection of missionary information on cannabis drugs and medicines shows, however, that not all European observers and not all European observatories were automatically given credence by the Government of India. It seems that, in the production of official, colonial knowledge, the authorities were careful to privilege only those sites that were producing data that was acceptable in the wider political economy of British imperialism.

The cannabis sativa plant is a complex organism that can yield a variety of substances available for use as medicines and intoxicants, which can have a range of physical and psychological impacts on users that are complicated by a number of variables that include diet, emotional state, circumstances of consumption, and so on. It has had its advocates and its opponents throughout history and across societies and cultures. There was, however, no significant debate on the topic in British political circles until the missionaries forced it onto the agenda in the 1890s. Much has happened since the end of the nineteenth century to shape the ongoing relationship between the British people and cannabis, but it remains the case that the overtly negative judgement of cannabis drugs and medicines that was first established in the country's politics in 1893 remains dominant in government discourse over a century after it was first planted there by the missionaries of India. This is despite the fact that alternative judgements have been offered on cannabis, by administrators, by scientists and doctors, and by consumers and users. In sifting the archaeology of negative ideas about cannabis at the start of the twenty-first century, it is perhaps possible to agree with the Comaroffs that:

> [T]he enduring legacy of the medical mission lay, rather, in something more subtle: in its quiet impact on European consciousness during an age when parochial paradigms of knowledge and practice were undergoing reformation.[82]

Notes

1. M. Vaughan, *Curing Their Ills: Colonial Power and African Illness* (London: Polity Press, 1991), 55–76.
2. T. Ranger, 'Godly Medicine: The Ambiguities of Medical Mission in Southeastern Tanzania' in S. Feierman and J. Janzen (eds), *The Social Basis of Health and Healing in Africa* (Berkeley: University of California Press, 1992), 256– 84.
3. J. Comaroff and J. Comaroff, *Of Revelation and Revolution: Christianity, Colonialism and Consciousness in South Africa* (London: University of Chicago Press, 1991), 7.

4. J. Comaroff and J. Comaroff, *Of Revelation and Revolution: The Dialectics of Modernity on a South African Frontier* (London: University of Chicago Press, 1997), 358.
5. R. Fitzgerald, '"Clinical Christianity": The Emergence of Medical Work as a Missionary Strategy in Colonial India, 1800–1914' in B. Pati and M. Harrison (eds), *Health, Medicine and Empire: Perspectives on Colonial India* (Hyderabad: Orient Longman, 2001), 131.
6. Vaughan, *op. cit.* (note 1), 74.
7. *Ibid.*
8. Comaroff, *op. cit.* (note 4), 354.
9. *Ibid.*, 357–8.
10. *Ibid.*, 356.
11. See D. Arnold, *Colonizing the Body: State Medicine and Epidemic Disease in Nineteenth Century India* (Berkeley: University of California Press, 1993), 113–15; J. Mills, *Madness, Cannabis and Colonialism: The 'Native-Only' Lunatic Asylums of British India, 1857–1900* (Basingstoke: Palgrave, 2000), 63–5.
12. M. Chawla Singh, *Gender, Religion and 'Heathen Lands': American Missionary Women in South Asia, 1860s–1940s* (New York: Garland, 2000), 121.
13. *Ibid.*, 130.
14. K. Lodwick, *Crusaders Against Opium: Protestant Missionaries in China 1874–1917* (Lexington: University Press of Kentucky, 1996), 3.
15. Comaroff, *op. cit.* (note 4), 358–62; Vaughan, *op. cit.* (note 1), 74.
16. 'Papers Relating to the Consumption of Ganja and Other Drugs in India' in *British Parliamentary Papers*, Vol. 66 (London: Hansard, 1891), 3.
17. *Hansard*, 225 (3rd Series), 571, 25 June 1875.
18. J. Rowntree, *The Opium Habit in the East: A Study of the Evidence Given to the Royal Commission on Opium 1893/4*, (London: King, 1895), 4.
19. *Hansard*, 335 (3rd Series), 1174, 3 May 1889.
20. *Hansard*, 230 (3rd Series), 1351, 12 July 1876.
21. *Hansard*, 342 (3rd Series), 713, 13 March 1890.
22. *Hansard*, 9 (4th Series), 1454, 9 March 1893.
23. M. Stenton and S. Lees, *Who's Who of British Members of Parliament*, Vol. 2 (Brighton: Harvester, 1978), 237.
24. See D. Fahey, 'Caine, William Sproston' in J.S. Blocker, D.M. Fahey, and I. R. Tyrrell (eds), *Alcohol and Temperance in Modern History: An International Encyclopedia*, Vol. 1 (Santa Barbara: ABC-Clio, 2003), 128.
25. G.S. Woods, 'Caine, William Sproston (1842–1903)', rev. H.C.G. Matthew, *Oxford Dictionary of National Biography* (Oxford: Oxford University Press, 2004): accessed 29 Oct 2004: www.oxforddnb.com/view/article/32238.
26. *Hansard*, 335 (3rd Series), 1160, 3 May 1889. For more on Caine and his anti-opium activities see J. Mills, *Cannabis Britannica: Empire, Trade and*

Prohibition, 1800–1928 (Oxford: Oxford University Press, 2003), 99–105.

27. *Hansard*, 8 (4th Series), 1360, 14 February 1893. The accompanying papers included Hem Chunder Kerr's report on the manufacture of cannabis substances for the Indian market. This is discussed in more detail in J. Mills, 'Cannabis in Colonial India: Production, State Intervention and Resistance in the Late Nineteenth-Century Bengali Landscape' in M. Steinberg, J. Hobbs and K. Mathewson (eds), *Dangerous Harvest: Drug Plants and the Transformation of Indigenous Landscapes* (New York: Oxford University Press, 2004), 221–31.
28. *Hansard*, 9 (4th Series), 822, 2 March 1893. The following two quotations also originate from this article.
29. This motion moved that 'In the opinion of this House the growth, cultivation and sale of bhang, ganja, charas and other preparations of hemp by the Provincial Governments of India produce much misery, poverty, insanity and moral deterioration among the people of India; and whereas similar results in Turkey, Egypt and Greece have led to the absolute prohibition in those countries of the manufacture and common sale of hemp drugs, it is desirable that the Secretary of State for India should order a commission of experts to enquire into and report upon the cultivation of and trade in all preparations of hemp drugs in Bengal, the effect of their consumption upon the people of that presidency and the desirability of the prohibition of their sale; not less than one half of such commission to be composed of non-official natives of India' in *Abkari* (14 July 1893), 111.
30. This was not the first time that Caine had forced the Government of India to conduct a survey of its policy on intoxicants. As a result of his endeavours in 1889 it conducted a 'ponderous inquiry' into liquor that resulted in it raising taxes in order to reduce consumption. See I. Tyrrell, 'India' in Blocker *et al., op. cit.* (note 24), 309. For a detailed study of relations between various British and local groups in India on the issue of 'liquor' see D. Hardiman, 'From Custom to Crime: The Politics of Drinking in Colonial South Gujarat' in R. Guha (ed.), *Subaltern Studies IV* (Delhi: Oxford University Press, 1985), 165–228.
31. Caine was so successful despite being an isolated voice on cannabis as the Government of India and the British Government were seeking to obfuscate the opium issue. For more on the reasons that Gladstone's administration had for its approach to cannabis and opium see Mills, *op. cit.* (note 26), 100–105.
32. J. Newton, *WS Caine MP: A Biography*, (London: Nisbet, 1907), 237.
33. Tyrrell, *op. cit.* (note 30), 309.
34. Newton, *op. cit.* (note 32), 241.
35. W.S. Caine, *Picturesque India: A Handbook for European Travellers* (London: Routledge, 1890), 292. The following two quotations originate from this

source.

36. Newton, *op. cit.* (note 32), 236. The details of Caine's career are all taken from this volume.
37. T. Evans (edited by D. Hooper), *A Welshman in India* (London: James Clarke, 1908), 172. All details of Evans' life and career are taken from this volume. He is not mentioned in Blocker *et al., op. cit.* (note 24), or in B. Harrison, *Dictionary of British Temperance Biography* (Sheffield: Society for the Study of Labour History, 1973).
38. *Ibid.*, 176.
39. Newton, *op. cit.* (note 32), 236. For more on this speaking tour and its outcomes see L. Carroll, 'The Temperance Movement in India: Politics and Social Reform', *Modern Asian Studies*, 10, 3 (1976), 417–47.
40. *Report of the Indian Hemp Drugs Commission 1893/4* (Simla, 1894), v. 5, 304. Hereafter IHDC.
41. *Ibid.*
42. For an analysis of asylum statistics and colonial knowledge about cannabis see Mills, *op. cit.* (note 11), 43–65.
43. IHDC, v. 5, 304.
44. IHDC, v. 5, 305.
45. IHDC, v. 4, 436.
46. Evans, *op. cit.* (note 37), 204.
47. *Ibid.*, 200.
48. IHDC, v. 6. 361.
49. Evans, *op. cit.* (note 37), 209.
50. IHDC, v. 4, 436.
51. T. Evans, 'The Cultivation of "Ganga" by the Indian Government' in *Abkari*, 3 (1892), 14–17.
52. IHDC, v. 1, 5.
53. IHDC, v. 6, 385.
54. IHDC, v. 6. 383.
55. IHDC, v. 5. 487.
56. IHDC, v. 6, 385.
57. IHDC, v. 7, 294.
58. IHDC, v. 4, 445.
59. IHDC, v. 4, 444.
60. IHDC, v. 4, 583.
61. IHDC, v. 7, 295.
62. IHDC, v. 6, 387.
63. IHDC, v. 5, 452.
64. IHDC, v. 4, 336.
65. IHDC, v. 4, 438.
66. IHDC, v. 6, 382.

67. IHDC, v. 7, 296.
68. Indeed, the conflicting positions of the missionaries reflect the wider division of opinion on cannabis among the British in India, and also among scientists and doctors back in the UK, throughout the nineteenth century. See Mills, *op. cit.* (note 26), 34–46, 69–92.
69. There is a wealth of studies on the temperance movement in the UK in the nineteenth century. The best place to start for understanding the relationship between religious groups and temperance is M. McKean and G.W. Olsen, 'Evangelical Temperance (United Kingdom)', in Blocker *et al., op. cit.* (note 24), 225–7. The broader context for understanding Christian campaigns can be found in L.L. Shiman, *Crusade Against Drink in Victorian England* (Basingstoke: Macmillan, 1988), and a useful introduction to the relationship between temperance movements and imperialism is R. Room, 'Drink, Popular Protest and Government Regulation in Colonial Empires', *The Drinking and Drug Practices Survey*, 23 (1990), 3–6.
70. IHDC, v. 4, 440.
71. IDHC, v. 6, 368-369.
72. IHDC, v. 6, 385.
73. IHDC, v. 4, 443.
74. IHDC, v. 6, 372.
75. IHDC, v. 6, 378.
76. IHDC, v. 6, 356.
77. See E. Said, *Orientalism* (London: Routledge and Kegan, 1978) and J. MacKenzie, *Orientalism: History, Theory and the Arts* (Manchester: Manchester University Press, 1995).
78. IHDC, v. 4, 336.
79. See R. Pearsall, *The Worm in the Bud: The World of Victorian Sexuality* (Stroud: Sutton Publishing, 2003) for a broad survey of attitudes in this period; for an amusing taste of Victorian sexual conservatism see G. MacDonald, *Once a Week Is Ample: Or, the Moderately Sensual Victorian's Guide to Restraint of the Passions* (London: HarperCollins, 1997).
80. Mills, *op. cit.* (note 26), 140–50.
81. *Ibid.*, 121–3.
82. Comaroff, *op. cit.* (note 4), 357.

7

African Medical Personnel of the Universities' Mission to Central Africa in Northern Rhodesia[1]

Linda Beer Kumwenda

The medical work of the Northern Rhodesian diocese of the UMCA was consistently marginalised by the male-dominated missionary hierarchy due to its status as 'women's work'. Understaffed and under-funded, it relied heavily on its small team of male medical orderlies. Whilst the scarcity of such orderlies often placed them in a position of power, they were under-represented in publications intended for missionary supporters. An examination of the records of the UMCA enables us to identify individuals and demonstrate how the orderly became an integral part of the medical work. By the presentation of selected brief 'biographies', it is shown why the colonial government's appeal to missions to set up training schemes for female nurses from the late-1940s was such an attractive proposition for the UMCA.

In October 1976 orderly Jonathan Mutakasha received a letter from the Anglican bishop of Northern Rhodesia. 'Your record of forty-seven years of unbroken service at Fiwila' he wrote, 'is... unsurpassed by any other person in the Anglican Church in Zambia. It is that fact that you have remained at one place that distinguishes you from other people.'[2] Mutakasha's record was not unique, however. Many mission stations had such men in their employ. The Universities' Mission to Central Africa (UMCA), an Anglican body that forms the subject of this paper, employed a number of such orderlies, sometimes for long periods. For example, Philemon Chupa, an orderly at both Msoro and St Francis, began his career in 1949, and was still working in 1998.[3] Francis Kweche, also of Msoro and St Francis, began his career in 1951, and was also still employed in 1998.[4] For the London Missionary Society, Philip Shilengwe at Mbereshi, who began his employment in 1943, was still the '"backbone" of the hospital' in 1963.[5] He was reinstated some years after his retirement, during the 1970s.[6] The Brethren, known as

Christian Missions in Many Lands, also had their long-standing employees, such as Basoni Samulozela from 1940 to 1968, and Gibeon Chipishi from 1948 to 1987, both employed at Kalene in Northwestern Province.[7]

The purpose of this paper is, firstly, to recover a little of the experience of those like Jonathan Mutakasha, upon whom the medical services of the UMCA depended. Their experience was both created by, and significant in the creation of the power struggles that existed between the clerical, pedagogic and medical spheres of the mission. These circumstances in part underlie the abandonment of training of male orderlies by the UMCA and its involvement in the early stages of training for females. This shift in focus will be dealt with in the latter sections.

African medical personnel[8]

Patterson and Hartwig were among the first historians to acknowledge the need to examine the various issues surrounding African medical personnel when they included 'nursing' and 'the use of paramedical personnel' as two items in a long list of health-related concerns requiring investigation.[9] They did not suggest how these topics should be approached or what issues might be illuminated. Ten years later, Arnold noted the possible role played by African staff in the increasing acceptance of Western medicine by Africans.[10] Vaughan has also made suggestions regarding the utility of such a study. Concerned with the false dichotomies which she perceived in some of the literature, she proposed that the study of 'African practitioners of scientific medicine might prevent this tendency, whilst not obscuring the differences that are present'.[11] Elsewhere she has asserted that research into the role of African medical personnel – in particular their practice and representation of biomedicine, and how they have been perceived within their own communities – is required for an analysis of the possible uses made of colonial public-health intervention as 'hegemonic practices contributing to the maintenance of colonial order'.[12]

Despite these calls for research, the subject has until now only been treated within wider studies. Ranger raises the matter in his analysis of the UMCA in Masasi when he demonstrates that missionary medics saw the training of local staff as a necessary part of their drive for modernisation, in this being opposed by the clerical staff who believed more in 'adaptation'. Much hope was placed in African medical assistants as providing a means to eradicate 'superstition'.[13] Vaughan also makes this point.[14] Iliffe has provided us with 'a collective biography of East African Doctors' that explores 'what Africans of great skill and responsibility have tried to do with political freedom.'[15] Sayenda argues that the increase of trained assistants – who in effect became 'semi-relatives' – lessened the authority of the 'lay therapy group'[16] within the mission hospital, and also of the missionary staff.[17]

Zvogbo's study of medical missions in Southern Rhodesia gives details of when and where formal training began, viewing it merely as 'progress', with no analysis of how this fitted into the wider missionary strategy.[18]

The Northern Rhodesian government employed African medical personnel from an early stage.[19] They were also found working on the Copperbelt in mine hospitals from the late-1920s. Government reports, however, are far less informative about these people than the mission records. The letters and journals of the missionaries inform us of the qualities that were considered to make an orderly either 'good' or 'difficult'. They believed that the actions of the medical workers illustrated what they perceived to be the character deficiencies of 'the African'. They saw this as a process of development, and that in time the orderly might attain Western standards of behaviour. Through anecdotes about these workers they reinforced racial stereotypes for a Western audience.[20]

Missionary records also highlight ways in which training empowered Africans, with many using their qualifications to escape the confines imposed by the missionary milieu. They reveal the grievances held by Africans against their employers, especially regarding working conditions, and show some of the steps they took to ameliorate their situation. There is evidence that African medical staff had the upper hand at times and that they were able to bargain successfully with their employers. The missionaries were also concerned about the prevalence of male nurses at a time when few women had received education. In common with government officials, they were concerned about the 'proper' roles of male and female medical staff. Africans were themselves just as concerned about this issue, though for different reasons.

The Universities' Mission to Central Africa in Northern Rhodesia

The UMCA was formed in 1858 as a direct result of Livingstone's famous appeal on 4 December 1857 at the Senate House at Cambridge. The Northern Rhodesia Diocese was formed on 4 December 1907 in celebration of the fiftieth anniversary of this address.[21] Unlike other mission societies working in Northern Rhodesia, the UMCA did not select a 'sphere of influence', but set up stations in various places that were not occupied by the others, such as Mapanza (Southern Province), Msoro (Eastern Province), Chipili (Luapula Province), and Fiwila (Central Province). Bishop May described Northern Rhodesia in graphic terms as 'a sea of long established missions, dotted with islands… of unoccupied territory; and our extension can only be by way of occupying the islands – and occupying them quickly before they are covered by the sea.'[22] The UMCA missionaries lived very isolated lives as a result, particularly as they were required to take a vow of celibacy, which meant that they had no family for company.

From the outset, the mission was dogged with financial and staffing problems. Medical work was sidelined for many years as a result. High Anglican doctrine stressed community rather than personal salvation. Priests were central to this endeavour. Schools were considered to provide a better means than hospitals to underpin the church. Unable to obtain or finance a doctor, medicine became 'women's work' by default and was thus the most precariously situated when financial cutbacks were necessary. By 1918 with only a 'skeleton crew' of nine priests the bishop reported that 'I feel myself bound to say that till the stations are manned, the women's work must wait.... We must have more men.'[23]

The absence of women within the mission did not mean that medical work was entirely neglected. Both bishop and priests provided basic medical ministrations to converts and others whom they met on their travels. Some, such as Padre Ruck, even established dispensaries for basic medical treatment. Yet in the late-1920s, when medical work began to take a firmer shape – largely because of a more consistent presence of nurses – even Ruck appeared to show signs of hostility to this development. In Ruck's case, and perhaps in others, the fear was that their vow of celibacy might be put under strain by the presence of nurses. This created tensions within the mission station that at times presented itself as an antagonism toward medical work.

The rule of celibacy did not come into existence until at least twenty-five years after the UMCA was founded. According to one account, it was initiated by Smythies, the Bishop of Zanzibar from 1883 to 1894, as he believed that it allowed the priests to move more easily from one mission station to another as required by the diocese. Also, it was thought that 'climate and conditions of life were... unsuitable for married people and children.' In addition, wives and children were considered to place an unnecessary financial burden on the mission. Whatever the practical reasons for the rule, it was justified by the argument 'that the acceptance of it for the sake of God's work was pleasing to Him and should be regarded as a vocation'.[24] Those who later decided to marry were required to resign, although the bishop could invite them to rejoin the mission as a married couple. Their position within the mission was however seen as anomalous, and their missionary colleagues often resented their presence.

While for some the vow of celibacy was central to their missionary calling, and a 'tradition... at the very heart of the UMCA',[25] for others it was merely something they had to take as a condition of their membership of the mission. Tensions were created when missionaries with these differing understandings lived together in close proximity on the same mission station. The vow required missionaries to live a religious life, in the monastic sense, but did not give the protection of a single-sexed community of celibates. Ruck was one of those priests for whom celibacy was an ideal, and he found that the hybrid system of the UMCA was in this respect riddled with 'inherent defects' and that there were 'inevitable difficulties and dangers… in dealing with members of the other sex'.[26] Some priests, Ruck included, 'begged' the Bishop 'not to reintroduce ladies'.[27]

This issue posed problems for medical work from the start. For example, Gladys Salisbury set up a practice at Mapanza in 1915 that was counted as being very popular with the local people. Very soon, however, she and the local UMCA padre, Moffat, decided to get married. Although they wanted to continue to work at Mapanza, they were compelled to leave. The medical work thus came to a premature end. Following further such 'incidents' the bishop drew up some regulations that were designed to prevent priests and women workers from being alone together. Even so, by 1936 there had been 'numerous matrimonial alliances'.[28]

The presence of white female nurses created other frictions. There were clashes of authority, and disputes over the demarcation of different disciplinary skills. These problems were compounded for the nurses by the fact that they were isolated on the scattered mission stations, and thus unable to put up a united front to fight for their interests in an effective manner. As medical work increased in importance, the conflicts intensified. It was rare for such disputes to come out into the open. As one of the religious sisters at Mapanza complained in writing to one of her nursing colleagues in 1938: 'Magazines so often give the bright side alone.'[29] The records reveal, however, that disputes between the male priests and the white female nurses could at times become extremely acrimonious. The complexities of such disputes may be appreciated through an examination of one case, that of Msoro, where Padre Goodall was priest in charge.

A conflict at Msoro

Victoria Watson was stationed at Msoro as 'nurse-in-charge' of St Luke's Mission Hospital from 1939 to 1944. She interpreted her title to mean that she had ultimate control in all medical matters at the station.[30] Padre Goodall held a different opinion. Writing to his bishop, he asked:

> Who is in charge of the Hospital work? Has the priest in charge the right should he wish to do so to forbid the nurse to go unattended except for a native orderly and at her own will and discretion stay out all night or parts of the night sleeping any how in native huts without reference to the priest without his express permission or even without his knowledge?[31]

He enumerated an assortment of grievances regarding the unwarranted authority that Watson had taken upon herself, including the 'indiscriminate' admission of patients and the engaging of African medical staff.[32] In his response, the bishop said that the control of medical *policy* was in the hands of the priest in charge, although he should try to accept advice from those with technical expertise. He also stated that he himself had overall authority.[33]

Watson felt that Goodall's criticism went further: 'without the co-operation of the Priest in Charge of what use is the Hospital?' she enquired of the Bishop.[34] Her words were to be echoed only a year later by her successor from 1944 to 1949, Mary Young. The latter's criticisms were even more far-reaching. In a memo to the bishop of 1945 she stated that Goodall appeared to be hostile to mission medical work in general, openly stating that such work should be the responsibility of the government. His attitude, she said, led him to be antagonistic towards the medical staff as a whole, including the African orderlies. She accused him of instilling his personal views amongst the catechists under his training, and alleged that he discouraged them from making use of the medical facilities at Msoro. As the catechists were particularly important in encouraging people on their tours of the villages to seek medical help from the mission, this affected the general use of the hospital. Under Goodall's influence, Young argued, the catechists continued in 'their old superstitions and [use of] native medicines.'[35]

There were other elements that contributed to the antipathy between Goodall and Young. Soon after her arrival at the mission she discovered a number of cases of bilharzia and/or hookworm during the course of a routine health inspection of boys at its boarding school. Many of the boys refused to be treated; whereupon Young attempted to force them, arguing that it was a waste of time educating children who were not fully fit. She also felt the inspections served no purpose if they were not followed up by appropriate treatment that eliminated the source of infection. She saw the boys' refusal as a breach of mission discipline. Her attitude led the boys to eventually stage a strike, in which the girl pupils joined them. Padre Rogers and Misses Field and Trentham (both teachers) allowed the boys to remain without treatment if they so wished, and 'begged' Young to be more lenient in her attitudes. Bishop Selby Taylor concurred with their decision, arguing that there were various risks inherent in compulsory treatment and that the time for it had not yet arrived.[36] In common with his predecessor, Bishop May, Selby Taylor believed that at the present 'state of development' they had no choice but to tolerate the indigenous *mchape* medicine. In commenting on why he allowed so many of their converts, including catechumens, to resort to such treatment, May had stated: 'I cannot regard the acceptance of Muchape medicine as a grave offence on the part of our untutored Christians... friendly ridicule effects more in such cases than ecclesiastical censure.' The best course of action was to 'be just a little blind'.[37]

A further incident brought matters to a head between Goodall and Young. In July 1945, Nebat, a catechist, was bitten by a mamba. Goodall –

the first missionary on the scene – discouraged the use of indigenous medicines and sent for Young. Nebat was taken to the hospital and treated. As a precaution, Goodall took along Holy Oils and the Sacrament, but was told by Young that Nebat was recovering; indeed, he had not been bitten at all, but was merely in a state of panic due to having been refused indigenous medicines. Young continued to insist that Nebat was merely feigning his symptoms, even as his condition deteriorated. Although it was against his better judgement, Goodall agreed to send away those who had gathered around the hospital awaiting Nebat's death. Within minutes of their departure Nebat died. At the funeral, Young was accused in public both at the church and by the graveside by Nebat's brother-in-law Joseph – also a catechist – of causing the death by denying Nebat the use of indigenous medicine. Young called for Joseph's dismissal, an action that Goodall refused to comply with.

Each had their own interpretation of the root of the events surrounding Nebat's death. Young felt the whole incident to be the direct result of Goodall's alleged instilling of a negative attitude towards the medical work amongst the catechists. For his part, Goodall believed that Young had alienated the local people by applying compulsion and showing contempt for local remedies. He felt that she had been wrong to deny Nebat the treatment that he wanted. Indigenous medicine would have done him no harm and the time was not yet ripe to launch an attack on it. He argued that 'the best way of getting the confidence of the people [is] by pandering to their foibles.' He believed, furthermore, that it was wrong to be harsh on Joseph, since his actions were dictated by the fear of repercussions from the village if he made no protest.[38] He denied that he was hostile to medical work. The Bishop believed the impasse to be so serious that either Goodall or Young would have to be moved.[39] In the event, Goodall was transferred to Chipili and the Bishop informed Young that he did not wish her to return after her home leave. As she herself put it, 'you do not consider me an asset to the Mission.'[40] Goodall appears to have exhibited a more positive attitude to the medical work at Chipili, where he worked hard to help Nurse Rowley set up an outstation dispensary at Mulipula.[41] Goodall's apparent change of attitude is perhaps explained by the following log book entry of 1948: 'Fr Goodall writes to announce engagement to Miss Rowley.'[42]

Goodall was not the only one to criticise Young, for the bishop received several letters of complaint against her from his parishioners. Fanuel Mwanga, for example, listed a number of specific complaints against her, relating mainly to her treatment of his child who died under her care. He stated that: 'We do not like the work that Dona Young does at this hospital,' and he asked that she be replaced.[43]

African orderlies at Msoro

The hostility to the European nurses, coupled with a general lack of funds for medical work, led to a greater emphasis being placed on male African medical orderlies. At Msoro, both Victoria Watson and Mary Young had made a systematic attempt to train such orderlies. Junior and senior exams were set, and some were then sent for a short course of about three months to the African Medical Training School in Lusaka, after which they took another exam. This training did not, however, qualify them to work in a government hospital. These orderlies came to be regarded as an essential component of the medical work of the missions; 'for just as the catechist must always be the backbone of our evangelistic work so medical work can never expand as we should like it to grow without trained orderlies.'[44] In their own way, nevertheless, these orderlies were just as problematic for the mission as the white female nurses.

As with the problems over the nurses, the missions did not generally air these difficulties in public. Blood, in his history of the work of the UMCA, made few references to the work of the African medical staff, but when he did mention them he merely stated in a bland way that: 'The work of these African orderlies reflects the greatest credit not only upon themselves but also on the nurses, who undertook their training.'[45] In reality, the relationship between the white missionaries and these orderlies was fraught with tension. There were numerous problems, some moral, some relating to the ambiguities of authority within the mission, and others concerning the difficulties caused by the highly gendered division of duties. Indeed, the African medical staff largely becomes visible in the mission records because they were in conflict with the European staff. Among other things, these accounts reveal how closely their medical careers were bound up in the life of the Church and how their behaviour helped determine the acceptance of mission medicine within their communities.

Records of the UMCA both in England and Zambia allow for the construction of about twenty brief biographies. The five biographies presented are of orderlies who worked at Msoro. These biographies must be seen and understood in the light of the prevailing circumstances at Msoro, where modernising nurses worked in opposition to adaptive clerical and teaching staff – both male and female.

One of the earliest of the trainees was William Katumbi. He began working at Msoro in July 1940, but does not appear in the documents until the end of 1943. He enters the records because he had, according to the nurse-in-charge, become very lazy and was not accepting responsibility. Although she did not wish him to leave she informed him that he would not be allowed to sit his final examination or stay on at Msoro unless he

Figure 7.1

'Orderly from Chipili.'

Central Africa, volume 55, number 665, May 1938.

Courtesy Rhodes House Archives, Oxford.

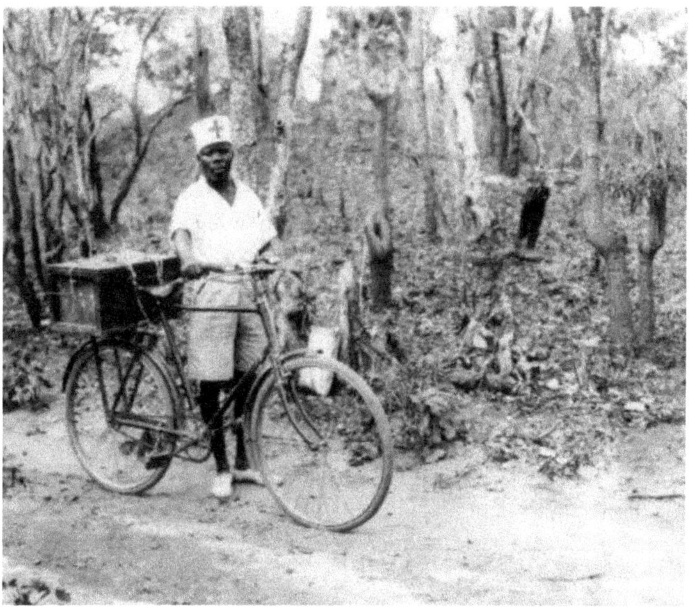

improved. William began to take his medical work more seriously from this time, and worked alongside his colleague Eliam, giving injections, dispensing medicines and doing some microscopic work. However, in the December of the following year a more serious shortcoming came to light. William was accused of adultery with the wife of a trainee catechist, and possible rape. The woman, Cecilya, said that she had been seduced by William the previous year when she had taken her child to the hospital with measles, and that now the catechists would not allow their children to be taken to the hospital because they did not trust William. Although William vehemently denied the charges against him the priest felt that the evidence was such that he would have been convicted in a local court. He gave him a month's notice and penance. Cecilya was suspended from Communion until the Bishop made a judgement on whether or not she was also guilty, as the European nurse believed.

The Bishop was concerned that this case might have implications for the acceptance of Western medical care by African women. 'I hope that William understands that so long as hospital orderlies behave in the way that he behaved, women will not be prepared to come to the hospital, and that is a very serious matter.'[46] The Bishop's judgement was that William should serve penance of two months, and Cecilya one month. However, he also felt that he should be allowed to return to work, in order that he might be able to go to Lusaka for a short course and examination as some of his colleagues had done. If he completed the short course at Lusaka successfully he should then be placed elsewhere.

The new nurse, Young, was on William's side, even though she had earlier been censorious when another orderly had committed misdemeanours. She blamed the incident on William's unhappy marriage and the deliberate behaviour of Cecilya. She believed William to be a keen orderly with potential, and she was eager that his career should not be ruined. Even if he was not able to work at Msoro again, she felt that a career in a government hospital might be open to him.

Cecilya's husband, Justin Mpanga, made his side of the story known, and his situation is evidence of a further strand of tension existing on UMCA mission stations. The divide that was often evident between the missionaries working in the different spheres of education, medicine and evangelism was often reflected in the attitudes of the Africans who worked in these respective arenas. As a rule, trainee catechumens were of a lower educational standard than both teachers and orderlies, and as such were looked down on by the latter. Joseph wrote:

> I was strongly to take the case to... Government, but being of the Kristianity [*sic*] I have obey the Priest in charge to hear what the Lord will say to his servant. ...I surprised to [*sic*] much with this man. Is it a law or not that we had come here to offer our wifes [sic] to the medical orderly? So in this way they have to make us discourage even to carry on our business. Because when we are leaving the Compound such people... talk to our wifes and dispiese [sic] us to much that we are good for nothing we are uneducated men. So soon every one has to call us only rough names.[47]

William left Msoro that month, and did not go to Lusaka for additional training.

Eliam Zilinde was from Nyasaland, but began his medical career at Msoro in 1941. It was intended that he should be trained for about three years at Msoro and for a further three-to-four months at Lusaka, after which he would take an examination at the African Medical Training School. Watson, who trained him at Msoro, felt however that his progress was being hampered by the fact that she did not have enough time to give adequate theoretical training. The teaching he received enabled him to give injections and dispense medicines. He was reported as having 'made great strides with the microscope.'[48] In spite of his progress and commitment to his work, Eliam dreaded the prospect of taking an examination in Lusaka as he lacked confidence in his academic ability. He was, however, better in practical work than his colleague William Katumbi. Both were scheduled to go to Lusaka, and were encouraged by the exam success in 1944 of orderly Wallace Apuleni, who was trained at Mapanza.

Eliam eventually went to Lusaka at the end of 1945. He returned to Msoro in April 1946, much improved as an orderly, and with a good report from the Superintendent, Dr Purnell. However, he had failed his Medical Assistant examination. Eliam was particularly distraught about this as he had come to appreciate the value of an official certificate, and he requested that he be allowed to take the UMCA's own examination in Nyasaland. He had passed the UMCA's internal Northern Rhodesia exams, but these had little value at a wider level.

Having failed his exam, Eliam was placed on probation for six months. During this period he was involved in a controversial case that led to questions being raised about his competence. The missionary nurse Mary Young had instructed Eliam to give assistance to the wife of Francis Mngawa, a teacher, during childbirth. It is not clear whether Eliam willingly took on the duty, or was coerced by Young, who had a reputation for being 'fierce'. The baby died the following day. Receiving no adequate explanation for Eliam's actions from the missionaries at Msoro, Mngawa wrote to the Bishop. His main anger was directed at Young and his wife rather than Eliam:

> I have no power and I do not know what shall I do. I told Miss Young that Evelina will not be my wife. She will devoced [*sic*] because of you. This matter was taken to the Padre and Dona Treatham. It was long talk tried to make my heart cool. Although I believe to keep my wife, but I shall not join her or to help her, because she is not a woman now is a dog.
>
> For this reason I wish very much to devoce her because of Miss Young. I do not want her to join me. I want to take a second wife. I am still waiting for you. Dona has spoilt all this Area now she is very great enemy.[49]

In his reply, the Bishop assured Mngawa that in his view the fault lay with Young and not Eliam.

Eliam's downfall came in the end, however, not because of any medical incompetence. In August 1947 it was discovered that a great deal of soap was missing from the hospital drug store. The staff houses were searched, in the course of which drugs were discovered in Eliam's house. He was put under penance, with further punishment awaiting the judgement of the Bishop. Before this judgement could be passed the stolen soap was discovered. It had been hidden away by Eliam's wife before their house was searched. During the preceding five years Eliam had been using the drugs, soap, money, and other goods to bribe Headman Kasezya, the father of a woman who was soon to give birth to Eliam's child. It also transpired that Eliam had taken a second wife, the niece of a church elder. The deception of the mission had involved many lies and bribes, and several church members, including elders, were implicated. It thus became a community matter that, in the words of the priest in charge, required 'corporate penitence... if the Body of Christ is to be healed in this place'.[50]

Eliam, Kasezya and a third man were taken to Fort Jameson in handcuffs. Eliam was sentenced to one year's hard labour. On his release he was not invited to return to Msoro hospital. While he was still in prison, the Bishop had written to the provincial medical officers at Fort Jameson as well as in Nyasaland to try to find employment for him on his release. Whether through the auspices of the Bishop or not, Eliam eventually found employment at Riscorn Hospital in Southern Rhodesia, where he worked using a microscope. From there he wrote to the Bishop, quoting liberally from Psalm 51, in which David prays to God for mercy following his adultery with Bathsheba. He thanked the Bishop for the training he had received and requested that he be provided with a written statement of what he had been taught. The Bishop obliged with a copy of a Junior Medical Orderly Certificate.

Nicholas Jim began his first period of work as a medical orderly at Msoro in 1935, and left after almost three years to work in a non-medical job in Southern Rhodesia. During this time he was, the bishop noted, 'a terrible nuisance'. He was a 'careless worker', and indulged in 'indiscreet behaviour' when visiting villages as an itinerant orderly, although there had been no specific case against him.[51] In 1943, he went to Mapanza in order to complete Standard Six, after which he was keen to return to Msoro to work in the hospital. He had asked to return there two years previously, but the nurse-in-charge, Victoria Watson, had at that time told the priest not to consider it.

This second application was looked upon more favourably, even though Watson was still in charge. Whilst there had been 'strong suspicions of women and excessive beer drinking', the priest admitted that he had 'always liked him' and would welcome his return.[52] The Bishop wrote to Watson to win her over, arguing that Nicholas was older, and she should not make his return difficult, as working at Msoro would entail financial sacrifice for him. This time she was willing to receive him, partly because she was experiencing problems with William Katumbi, but also because she hoped that as an older man he would be a good example to the three junior orderlies who had just been suspended temporarily for staying out of the hospital compound the whole of Christmas night.

Nicholas began working at Msoro in July 1945. By September he had already fallen foul of the strict new European nurse, Mary Young. 'His chief trouble', she said, 'is constant disobedience and unwillingness to correct his mistakes. He will not accept hospital discipline.'[53] The Bishop felt that Nicholas should be given the benefit of the doubt. He had gone to Msoro at 'considerable personal sacrifice,' and they could not expect too much of him so soon after restarting his medical career. Young asserted that he was 'corrupting' the juniors, and suggested that he go away to think things over. News of Nicholas's treatment reached Festo Michael in Nairobi, and gave him reason to be 'afraid to do work with Dona Young'.[54] Nicholas disappeared from the records at this point.

It is unclear when Festo Michael began his career with the UMCA. He had, however, at least two years' experience before the start of the second world war. During the war he joined the 7th Northern Rhodesia Field Ambulance corps and was stationed in both British Somaliland and Nairobi. On his discharge he stated that he intended to return to medical work for the UMCA. This was a source of cheer for the priest in charge at a time when he found much to discourage him. There was, he felt, great indifference amongst the African Christians, caused by the 'materialistic spirit' engendered by war conditions.[55]

Festo nevertheless had some misgivings about returning to Msoro, for he had heard about some of the problems surrounding the medical work there. The Bishop attempted to allay his fears.

> It might be that Miss Young is fierce, I do not know... but I see no reason why you should find that difficult because, as you say, you have been in the army all these years and there you have army discipline which is probably more strict than hospital discipline.
>
> Miss Young is only newly out in this country and she requires all the help that we can give her: I know that you would be able to give her a great deal of help and if she is fierce, we will have to try and explain to her that such methods are not suitable in a mission hospital.[56]

Although Festo still declared that he was 'afraid to work with her', he returned to Msoro hospital in May 1946. Young reported almost immediately that she found him 'just a little superior with his army experience.'[57] The correspondence does not reveal how Festo adjusted to missionary medical work over the next one and a half years, as he was not mentioned in the records. As was often the case, he became visible again because of a sexual offence. In October 1947, he was found guilty of adultery at Chief Msoro's court. The court fined him £12; the priest-in-charge gave him one month's penance and a month's suspension from the hospital, after which he would be allowed to resume his duties again.

The priest was, however, puzzled by the extent of Msoro's fine, and on questioning Festo eventually discovered that the offence was not just adultery, but incest. The priest was still willing to allow Festo to return, but requested guidance on the case from the Bishop, as he was unsure whether this would be insensitive to the mores of the local community whom – he believed – thought the offence to be particularly heinous. Indeed they had already shown their displeasure by confiscating his 'not inconsiderable possessions'.[58] The Bishop's judgement on the case was that the penance should be increased to three months, but that the suspension from hospital duties should remain the same. Whether he ever worked at the hospital again was up to Festo. 'I doubt whether he will be prepared to face the shame', opined the Bishop, 'but if he is I think that we should try to help him to do so.... If he is not willing to work at Msoro we might be willing to consider employing him elsewhere.'[59]

Festo evidently did not wish to continue to work at Msoro hospital, or elsewhere in the UMCA Diocese. Local rather than mission judgement deprived Msoro of a trained orderly at the same time as they lost the services of their only other experienced medical worker, Eliam Zilinde.

During the early 1950s there was no European nurse at Msoro, but the tradition of training at that station was to some extent continued by Valentino Mtaja. He was one of at least two orderlies who worked for the UMCA in Northern Rhodesia who were trained at the UMCA hospital at Likoma, Nyasaland, by Dr Wigan. He began his training there in the late 1920s, and was transferred to Northern Rhodesia in 1939.

Valentino's first appointment in Northern Rhodesia was at a small outstation seventy miles west of Fiwila; Kakwe Lesa, or God's Little Place. This had been set up as a theological school, and the dispensary was a new venture on the station. During his first full year at Kakwe Lesa he treated thirteen inpatients and 929 outpatient cases. In the following year the figures increased to fifteen outpatients, and 2,232 outpatients. In 1942, the Annual Report noted that he had done very good work, and that 'the Territory could do with more like him'.[60] Yet by 1943 he had been transferred to the main station at Fiwila, and it was there that the particular personality traits that affected the rest of his career with the UMCA began to reveal themselves.

The situation at Kakwe Lesa had suited him well. He had been in charge and had had a certain amount of autonomy. At Fiwila his work was supervised, and he became discontented with his job, which affected his attitude to both the missionaries and local people. The Bishop wrote to him early in 1944, and remarked that he was not 'the same happy Valentino I used to know at Kakwe Lesa'.[61]

His response to the new situation was of some concern both to the priest-in-charge, Munday, and the Bishop, for Valentino was a valuable worker whom they could ill afford to lose. 'I think we should try to satisfy Valentino's demand as much as possible', the Bishop instructed Munday.[62] It was decided to send him to another UMCA outstation – Cibondo, thirty-five miles from Chipili – where he would again be responsible for setting up a new dispensary. 'It is a great responsibility', the Bishop wrote to Valentino, 'I am anxious that the people of the district should have a very good picture of the kind of treatment they receive in a UMCA dispensary.'[63]

This, for reasons that are not clear, was not the solution that Valentino had wanted. He was 'extremely angry', and was not placated by Mrs Munday's patronising attempts to soothe him by telling him 'how lucky he was to have such a "call", about the need for an experienced man to start the new dispensary in a crowded area.' Whatever Valentino's thoughts on the move, it was proclaimed by the missionary to be 'a relief to be quit' of him.[64]

In spite of his misgivings, Valentino moved to Cibondo in early 1944. Within just three weeks he had treated over two hundred and fifty cases. This demand for medical services goes some way to explain why the bishop had been so keen to keep hold of him. He was constantly being asked to open new dispensaries, but he lacked orderlies to staff them. During his first full year at Cibondo, Valentino dealt with seventy-eight inpatients, and 3,665 outpatients. The dispensary was, noted DC Thomson, 'especially being run well.'[65]

In 1948, Valentino treated 187 inpatients and 5,628 outpatients, an 'almost embarrassing' situation.[66] The dispensary needed another orderly to cope with the large volume of work, but neither the money nor the staff were available. Even so, the following year the Bishop felt that it was time for Valentino and his 'charming and very devout wife,' Agnes, to move on to yet another station: Msoro.[67]

Msoro's medical work was in crisis. Over the preceding five years the station had had three different missionary nurses, with no more than two at any one time. These nurses had been unable to work together, or with their African staff and the other missionaries on the station. One left to work in Nyasaland, the other two were asked not to return. Neither were there any African orderlies any more, as those who had been there had moved away, probably because of the difficulties they had encountered working with the European staff. In 1949 Miss Mounsey arrived, a new missionary nurse with 'a natural grace' making her 'most successful in dealing with the Africans'.[68]

She began to train another orderly, Elasto, but not only was he 'more or less illiterate', but he was found guilty of stealing the medicinal brandy.[69]

Prior to Elasto's misdemeanours the Bishop had suggested to the nurse that what was needed was a competent orderly to set the medical work back on its feet again. Valentino was seen to fit the bill. The Bishop was aware of the characteristics that could make such a move disastrous. 'He is a man who works very much better by himself,' he explained to Mounsey, and 'unfortunately he has a habit of showing some of his less pleasant traits to the Europeans.' However, he had done 'splendid work' at Cibondo, and he was well liked by the Africans there.[70] Understandably, Mounsey proclaimed herself to be 'rather dubious', not wanting to be prevented from giving her personal supervision to the patients. Yet, even while the Bishop tried to convince her of Valentino's fitness for the job – 'he has a real sense of vocation, he works extremely hard and the patients all seem to like him' – he again left her in no doubt as to the kind of man Valentino was. He 'tends to become morose and moody', he added to the list of positive qualities.[71]

The Bishop discussed the matter fully with Valentino and tried to organise matters in such a way that he would find work at Msoro congenial. Despite this, he continued to be disenchanted after his arrival there. In a letter of March 1950 he wrote to the Bishop:

> Please my Lord you may understand my words, what I am thinking is to leave the work on Sept this year; because you don't trusted [*sic*] my complaining.
>
> I am not an animal that can not fill [*sic*] bad. You may be thanking [sic] that I have worked in your Diocess [*sic*] for ten years with many complain, but you do not help. And now I am tired with your work. I may go back home. I am not pleasing with with [*sic*] your treatment.
>
> I wished to work in your Diocess, but now I am unable to work more years because I am not an animal.[72]

A few months later, and fortunately for Valentino, Mounsey was stricken by the Northern Rhodesia UMCA 'epidemic', for she had left Msoro in order to marry Padre Robertson, whom she had met there and who had subsequently been stationed at Mapanza. Thus, the UMCA's hybrid system worked in favour of Valentino, for not only did Mounsey leave, but the priest-in-charge was one who had a deep commitment to celibacy, and so opposed the Bishop's plan to send a married couple to Msoro as a means for providing a replacement European nurse at the station. The priest urged the Bishop to allow Valentino to continue alone in the hospital, and even to supervise the new young orderlies. The Bishop agreed to this 'temporarily', but the extreme difficulty in recruiting European nurses experienced both by the Mission and the Government, together with the setting up of the training hospital at nearby Katete, ensured that Msoro hospital remained under Valentino's charge until he left the UMCA in 1956.

Valentino showed his commitment to the UMCA in a letter to the Bishop shortly after Mounsey's departure.

> I hope to carry on the work for a little while as you have asked me. I am pleasing with your kind as always you done your kindness to me. I am only not please with this district of Msoro through unkindness people; and because you are shortage of nurses I will help you for little moment.[73]

The Bishop continued to bombard the Women's Secretary in England with requests for a nurse for Msoro, even though Valentino had threatened to leave if one came. The Bishop's opinion was that however good Valentino was, 'it is not the same as having a nurse' – a euphemism for the lack of maternity services.[74] No nurse was forthcoming, and Valentino continued his work faithfully, with the help of three or four orderlies and dressers that he had largely been responsible for training. The Bishop's opinion remained positive towards him, and he also won the respect of the Government Provincial Medical Officer who consistently reported very favourably on the medical work at Msoro during Valentino's tenure. The PMO increased the normal government grant of £50 for a dispensary run by an African orderly to £150, being so impressed by Valentino's work and 'outstanding personality'.[75]

In spite of this there was some underlying discontent. The reason was never overtly stated, but there were hints that Valentino was dissatisfied with his salary. This was a common theme amongst mission orderlies, who were well aware that they could command higher salaries in government institutions or at the mines. He eventually left in 1956 to take up government service at Kalindalwalo Dispensary in Petauke. He had nonetheless begun something of a family tradition of medical work both for the UMCA and the government. In August 1958, his daughter Prisca began the Medical Assistant course at St Francis', Katete, and passed her final examination in March 1962. Following in her father's footsteps, she was said to be 'thoroughly competent and responsible', but 'can be temperamental.' Ten years later she was still working as a nurse, at Chingola Mine hospital.[76]

These examples of moral lapses and increasing demands for salaries in line with those of government institutions and mines were replicated on all the UMCA mission stations. For the Bishop, such incidents were 'one of the bitterest disappointment of workers in Africa,'[77] and no doubt contributed to his readiness to co-operate when the Government indicated that it was prepared to fund the development of nursing training for African girls at mission hospitals.

The genesis of the Zambian female nurse

By the 1940s the Colonial Office was stressing that if medical services were to be improved in Africa, the priority was to build up a solid body of African 'subordinate' medical staff rather than construct new institutions.

> If any real and permanent advance in health conditions is to be made and if general Colonial policy is to be implemented, peoples of the Colonies, not only men, but women also, must be encouraged to interest themselves and be trained to participate fully in all health services. This is being put in the forefront of medical progress.[78]

The African female nurse was seen as the key figure for the 'civilisation' of the female 'masses.' After training, such a nurse was expected to become:

> [A] leader in the village community – to visit patients in their own homes, and advise women about household problems, hygiene of the home, the care of children and infants; conducting propaganda among village people, inculcate better use of food... and better cooking methods, visit schools, inspect children, carry out health education in schools... and generally be an exponent of better health for all in the community.[79]

It was believed that employing female nurses would lead to 'improved standards of nursing and greater quietness' within the hospital environment.[80] In some colonial territories this shift had been considered in the late-1930s, and had been hastened by the exigencies of the war, with male orderlies being required in military hospitals. However, a complete switch to a female nursing staff was not envisaged. The male nurse was still required – not as a nurse in his own right, but to save the female nurse from the indignity and impropriety of caring for male patients who suffered from either mental illness or venereal disease.[81]

It took some time for Northern Rhodesia to catch up with this wider colonial programme. This was partly due to the very slow development of girls' education. Even in 1950, the majority of girls who entered Western-style schools only completed up to Standard II. Those who did go further 'had the advantage of being able to profit from the... mistakes made in... boys' education;' such as an 'over-emphasis on the merits of academic learning.' Thus there was 'very little chance of an African girl becoming a "blue-stocking".'[82] Another reason for the paucity of female nurses was that there was a long-standing prejudice amongst colonial medical officers against the use of African women. 'The native female of this territory is at present inherently unsuited to such work,' wrote the Principal Medical Officer in

1926, 'and I hold the opinion that she should be at present altogether disregarded in this connection.'[83]

This attitude continued over the next decade, though there were two isolated 'experiments', neither of which became the basis for future training schemes.[84] Although it was evident to the Medical Department that there was 'considerable opportunity and indeed need for the employment of native girls,' not only were they not sufficiently educated, but, in words that resonated with UMCA thinking during the early years of its Northern Rhodesian presence, it was considered that: 'The most pressing need is still for trained native boys.'[85]

Opinions were, however, beginning to shift. The medical system was expanding, with more and bigger hospitals, leading to an increasing recruitment of European nurses.[86] With the increase in their numbers, and the presence of a matron-in-chief, nurses gained a stronger voice in decision-making. Also, as treatments became more technical, the care that had until then been largely provided by the relatives of patients came to be seen as inadequate. New standards in infrastructure meant that relatives were not so easily accommodated. Gradually, they were eliminated from the caring process.

In 1941, Selby Taylor – a strong supporter of medical mission work since his arrival in Northern Rhodesia as a padre in 1935 – was enthroned as Bishop of that Diocese.[87] He was eager to take up the challenge of training nurses as he believed that it would put the mission in the vanguard of 'Africa's medical progress'.[88] His original plan was to secure the services of a doctor to work at Msoro who would train male orderlies as a part of his duties. This would have entailed major reconstruction work at that mission.[89] However, this provided a problem for the Bishop, as Chipili hospital also needed to be rebuilt, and there was insufficient financing for both projects.[90] At this point Dr Trefusis came forward. He had originally joined the UMCA as a priest in 1914. During his early work with the UMCA he developed the view that health care was an essential part of the gospel, and in 1924 he returned home to study medicine, obtaining BM and BCh degrees in 1930. He returned to Northern Rhodesia in 1946, having previously been employed in the Dioceses of Nyasaland and Zanzibar. His particular vision was for the training of medical orderly evangelists, and thus, initially at least, he seemed well suited for the new project in Northern Rhodesia. His plan to build a new training school at Liulu having been thwarted in the previous year, he was eager to take up the challenge in Northern Rhodesia.[91] He was appointed to work at Msoro, and this station was then chosen by Selby Taylor to receive the limited funding available.

It was soon realised that Msoro was not a suitable place for such a project. The road from there to Fort Jameson had to cross seven rivers and was impassable during the wet season. Dr Trefusis was in favour of selecting a site in the Eastern Province, and since he was essential to the project the search for a new site began. Selby Taylor had further reason for preferring a completely independent medically-centred mission. The interdisciplinary strife that had been so prevalent on the other stations would thus be obviated, since Trefusis would be in complete control of the work. This, remarked the Bishop, would be 'the only satisfactory position'.[92] Yet, paradoxically, this position led to a far greater threat to the medical work than any interdisciplinary strife that had occurred heretofore.

The Government was also in favour of finding a site in Eastern Province. In the past – under the directorship of Dr Haslam – the Health Department had found little space for the missions in its development plans. This began to change in the late-1940s. It was now considered that missions had a greater understanding of 'the African woman', who, perceived as morally vulnerable, could be better kept in hand in the mission environment.[93] The Government had launched its Community Development programme at the beginning of 1947, and the sub-boma was to be at Katete. It suited their plans if there was to be a new mission hospital there. Indeed, the PMO invited Trefusis to begin his work there, and took him on a tour of inspection to assist him in his search, the venture also being supported by local chiefs.[94] A site was found along the Great East Road, about thirty-five miles from Msoro. This site was outside of the UMCA area, and was in fact already occupied by the Dutch Reformed Church and the Roman Catholics.[95] This was not a problem initially, as an amicable agreement was reached between all the parties. It became a source of friction only later when the whole project appeared to be on the verge of collapse.

St Francis, Katete

The seeds of the crisis were sown even as the foundations of the St Francis Hospital at Katete were being laid. Trefusis was resolute in his intention to train male orderlies; orderlies who would 'follow in the footsteps of St Francis... infused... with his spirit'. These men, having undergone a training in a mission hospital 'saturated' with St Francis, would then go out into the villages, and as medical evangelists, run dispensaries.[96] There was no place for female, hospital-based nurses in his vision. Yet even as he rejoiced over his chance to fulfil his dream, Selby Taylor was forming a very different plan in league with the Health Department.

The UMCA – in common with other mission societies – was approached by the Health Department with regard to the training of female medical staff. Selby Taylor agreed with these officials that missions were better equipped to train girls, and he made it publicly known that 'at Katete we are hoping to do our share in training women.'[97] In contrast to the earlier emphasis on educating women so that they would make good wives and mothers, there was now a serious desire to train women to work as female staff in mission hospitals.[98] The Bishop had other, pragmatic, reasons for going along with the Health Department initiative. As always, the UMCA was in financial difficulties, which were only exacerbated by the building of a completely new mission, rather than the upgrading of an existing one. If the Mission fell in with the scheme for training girls they would receive a pound for pound grant, up to a limit of £2,500.[99] This was an important consideration for a diocese that had been informed by the Home Board that medical expenditure should not exceed government grants.[100] A further indication of the Bishop's determination in this respect was that he planned to transfer the girls' school at Msoro to St Francis, in order that the Upper School might be a recruiting ground. This objective received the full support of the DMS.[101]

Trefusis appeared oblivious of the Bishop's strategy and he quickly set about alienating the health authorities. Since the latter were to make a substantial contribution to the work they felt it their right to impose certain criteria upon the building of the hospital. When Trefusis refused to comply with their demands, the grant failed to materialise. Trefusis proclaimed himself 'free but poor! – and happy', having gained greater 'bargaining powers', by disentangling himself from the demands of the Health Department.[102] He did this without consulting the Bishop, appearing to believe that he had full authority over the new venture.

Trefusis' highhanded manner with the Health Department was not, however, unduly detrimental at this juncture. Whilst funding from overseas supporters was declining, the mission was able to obtain monies from other sources. It had already been reckoned that even with government support additional finances would be required, and a successful application had been made to the Beit Railway Trustees.[103] The UMCA itself had also set up its own Development Fund, and allocated £1,000 to St Francis. Part of this sum was obtained from a source new to missions: a BBC wireless appeal for medical work in Africa. The Home Board also acknowledged that Northern Rhodesia had never received funding commensurate with that of the other dioceses, and could no longer be denied equal treatment.[104] Trefusis' dealings in other matters, however, led to a situation where the Bishop, other diocesan missionaries and the Home Board were led to wonder if 'the whole thing was a mistake.'[105]

In the meantime, the Mission had, in May 1949, acquired the services of two more doctors – Nichol and Kingdon. Both were better qualified than Trefusis, and it was intended that they would focus on the medical work while Trefusis applied his energies to building the new hospital and training school. He was unwilling to accept this and he thwarted the new arrivals at every turn. Kingdon left in September, ostensibly because of his wife's ill health, but he made his misgivings about Trefusis known. There was, he said, 'no future whatever for Katete as long as Trefusis remains there.'[106] Nichol left early in the following year, stating that Trefusis was out of touch with modern drugs, and 'old-fashioned' in his medical outlook. With his advanced medical qualifications, (MRCS, LRCP, MRCOG) Nichol felt unable to remain in a situation where his work was hampered by a man he considered to be incompetent. Trefusis' attitude and methods also alienated the Mission nurses, and the acting DMS and PMO were concerned that the 'efficient nursing team' that had developed at St Francis would disintegrate under his domineering presence.[107]

By 1951, the Mission had run out of money, and the theatre, sterilising room and anaesthetic room had yet to be completed. An appeal to the Government failed, as the Health Department was not prepared to provide funds so long as Trefusis was still in place.[108] The DMS had even criticised him personally at the Advisory Committee on Medical Missions in front of committee members from other societies.[109]

Both the Bishop and the Home Board were convinced that Trefusis should leave. Unable to detach himself from the medical work, the building project had come almost to a standstill. 'What I feel I should like to say to Trefusis' wrote the Secretary, is that:

> [W]hat was tolerable twenty or thirty years ago, because nothing better was then possible, is now quite intolerable. The days for amateurish makeshifts are past and unless this is realised it will be quite impossible to get medical staff for Katete. Nor do I think Government will continue to make grants.[110]

Whilst he remained at St Francis there was every possibility that the entire venture would have to be handed over to the Government. This would have wider ramifications for medical missionaries in Northern Rhodesia in general, as many in 'government circles' were opposed to mission–government co-operation, and a failure at Katete would become 'one more nail in the coffin of co-operation.'[111]

Removing Trefusis was not a simple task. He declared on a number of occasions that he had no intention of retiring nor leaving under any other pretext. However, leave he did. Early in 1952 he was transferred to Southern Rhodesia, to take charge of the station in Mashonaland.[112] The first step in St Francis' struggle for survival had been taken, and the Government funding that had been promised on condition that 'there will be no formal training of males…[and that] Dr Trefusis will be replaced' was received.[113]

The Mission had to be practically built up from scratch. With only a few buildings completed, and no doctor and only one nursing sister, very little

Figure 7.2

Images from St Francis School of Nursing, Katete, early-1950s.

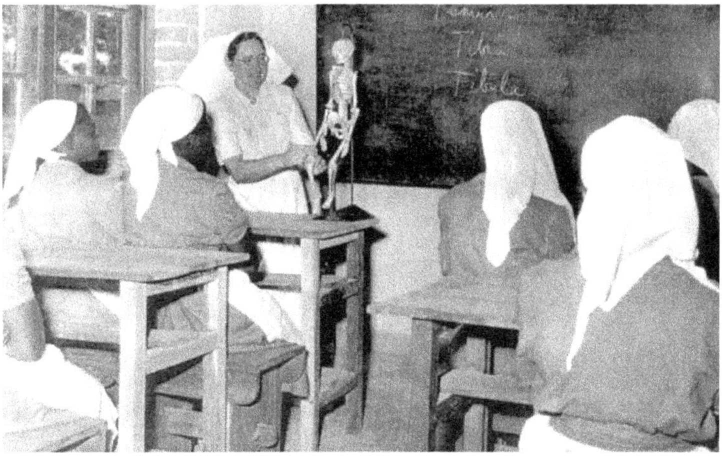

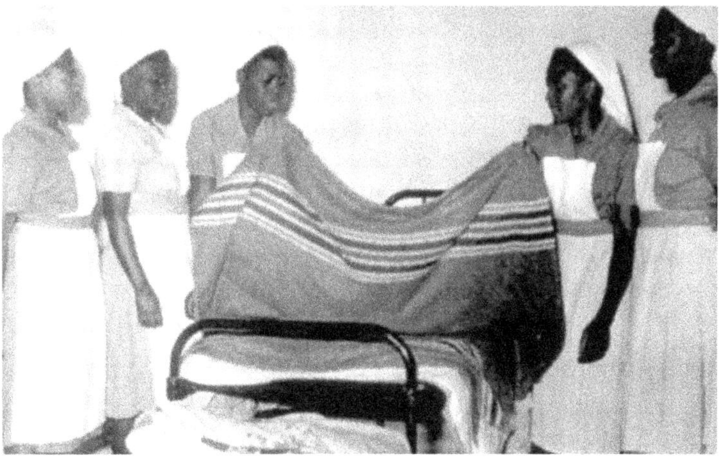

Images of female nurses differed greatly from those of medical orderlies. Whilst the latter were often depicted examining specimens intensely under a microscope or wielding a syringe, the former were shown, as here, making beds or sitting diligently at their desks.

progress had been made. The whole future of the venture depended on the acquisition of a doctor, since the training school would not be recognised by the Health Department without one.[114] At the same time the Mission was experiencing great difficulty in finding nurses suitable for educating trainee nurses.[115] Dr Eileen Welcher's arrival in late-1952 did little to relieve the problem since she was only a temporary appointee. It was not until the following year, when she said that she would stay until 1955, that the school gained official recognition.[116]

Although the UMCA had faced enormous difficulties in establishing the training school at St Francis, it was only the second to be officially recognised in the whole territory, the first being the Salvation Army mission at Chikankata in 1947.[117] Yet, in spite of the colonial rhetoric about nurses, who would 'really care for patients', the training provided by both these establishments was on the same lines as the course in Lusaka for men. It focused on preventive and curative medicine rather than nursing, with the girls receiving Medical Assistant certificates after three years of training. The first course for Enrolled Nurses did not begin until 1964.[118]

This failure to live up to the original intentions of the Health Department was in part due to a lack of commitment. A special course in nursing required a new syllabus. The Medical Missionary Advisory Committee had its first meeting in October 1949, and it was determined at the outset that it should discuss nursing and training issues. The training of nurses in particular required 'urgent attention,' and the Bishop specifically requested that the 'vocational' rather than the 'technical' side be prioritised.[119] In other words, at this stage the Bishop favoured the British Enrolled Nurse model, rather than the Northern Rhodesian Medical Assistant model. At the next meeting a Nurses Training Sub-Committee was set up specifically to discuss a syllabus and textbook.[120] In the following year this became a committee in its own right, being known as the Nursing Committee.[121] This was controlled predominantly by the Health Department rather than the missionary bodies, with the matron-in-chief, Miss Houlding, being firmly in control of it. It is hard to trace what happened to this Committee, but it is evident that no nursing syllabus was agreed upon, although the training was modified.[122] As yet, nurses had little power within the medical profession. Even after independence, all matters pertaining to nursing and midwifery – including the training, registration and enrolment of nurses and midwives – were dealt with by the Medical Council of Zambia, established in 1965. The General Nursing Council of Zambia was formed only in 1970.[123]

The training that began in 1952 did, however, prove liberating for many young African women. Although they were closely supervised in their working and free time while in training, their horizons broadened once they had gained their qualification. Eleven girls arrived at Katete in August 1952, although the records of only two of these girls survive.[124] Possibly they were the only girls to complete the course. As they were only educated to Standard

IV, they were only permitted to do the two-year course. The more advanced three-year course was only for girls with Standard VI education. Constance Bwanga completed her course in 1954, and was still practising in 1971. Rhoda Shilen completed in 1955, later trained as a midwife and in 1968 was working at the Wusakile Hospital, Kitwe.

Whilst nursing opened up new possibilities for young women; it also provided fathers with new choices and methods of control. Mathilda Chitelela, a 16-year-old girl educated to Standard VI level at Chipili, needed 'a strict eye keeping on her' as she had been receiving and sending letters to boys – a matter deemed not 'proper.' Rather than let her continue her education at secondary school her father decided in consultation with the Chipili missionaries that a 'safer' option for her would be a nursing education, with the discipline and supervision that went with it.[125] She qualified in 1957, with no untoward reports regarding her behaviour.

Anna Kawambwa, who had achieved a Standard VI education at Msoro, was twenty-one years old when she qualified in 1957. Normally, she would have been married well before this age, and it had been agreed that she would marry on qualification. When the time came, however, neither she nor her father wanted the marriage to go ahead. The reasons for this change of mind are not stated in the records. Her father, in particular, was adamant: 'I do not want Anah to be marred [*sic*] soon; also I have written to the man that there is no more marriage with Anah. I want Anah to do midwife course or to come here and work... I want Anna to go for this course very much.'[126] She started her midwifery training in 1960 and qualified the following year.

Another father who decided on a career in nursing for his daughter was Emilius Nalumpa. He was one of the first teachers to graduate from St Mark's Teacher Training School at Mapanza. He became an evangelist and later he trained as a priest in Lusaka, returning to work at Mapanza. His wife had been one of the first pupils at St Anne's School for Girls. The family was thus steeped in the ways of the UMCA mission. The couple had ten children; the first being Lucy, who was born in 1940. All ten children received a mission education, and by the age of sixteen Lucy had achieved Standard VI. Soon after she had finished school her father took her on a trip without telling her where they were going or why. The trip ended at St Francis. Lucy recalled:

> [My father told me] 'You're going to be a nurse'. So I didn't decide to become a nurse. Nor did I think what I was going to be because I still wanted to go further education, but those days the secondary schools were few. So, it was you go to Standard six, so what? For me, I didn't think of doing anything. I don't think I fancied being a teacher either, but, I think when I got to the hospital I didn't mind, because I found myself, I was doing *something*.[127]

Nalumpa intended that his daughter should return to Mapanza after her training and follow in his footsteps by working as a nurse–evangelist. Although she did return there when she had obtained her qualifications as nurse and midwife in 1960, she had other plans. As she said: 'I wanted to see other places.' Her father was powerless to stop her. When she went to Ndola to visit her brother she decided that she would not return, and she found a job at the mine hospital there. Whilst there, she heard from the British nurses who worked there how she might get to England to further her training, and in 1967 she travelled to England and became a State Certified Midwife. Although she returned to Zambia in order to upgrade her nursing qualification to Zambian Registered Nurse, she continued to work in England.

Conclusion

This paper has sought to shed light on the largely forgotten figure of the African medical orderly. Such people were crucial for the medical work of both the colonial medical service and medical missions. The study of the UCMA records shows that their position was often a difficult one, as their work was affected by disputes within the mission between the evangelists and the professional educationalists and medical specialists, as well as between male and female employees of the mission. There were also sharp and unresolved racial tensions. With the mission hospitals closely bound to the life of the church, they found that they were judged on their morals as well as on their professional skills. They resented the fact that their pay compared poorly with that of their counterparts in government service. However, in contrast to other missions – such as Christian Missions in Many Lands – where each station was autonomous, the UMCA had a process of appeal to the Bishop in Northern Rhodesia. This was utilised to good effect by the orderlies. As medical services began to modernise, the focus shifted towards female trainees, leading to an increasing pressure to co-operate with Government initiatives. The new female medical workers soon found that the qualifications they had gained with the help of the missions provided an avenue of escape from the confines of both the missions and their own communities.

Notes

1. This research was made possible through the funding of the Carl Schlettwein Stiftung, Basel.
2. Records held at St Francis' Hospital, Katete. Miscellaneous box one. Fiwila – details of hand over and staff. In other records he is named Jonathan Mutakasya.

3. Interview with Philemon Chupa, 4 August 1998 at St Francis' Hospital, Katete.
4. Interview with Philemon Chupa, 4 August 1998 at St Francis' Hospital, Katete. National Archives of Zambia (NAZ), Zambian Anglican Council (ZAC), Box 28571, Mapanza Medical 1949–64. Dr James Wright to Mapanza, 2 September 1955.
5. School of Oriental and African Studies (SOAS), Council for World Mission (CWM), Africa 1941–50, AF/43 Reports A–F, MEA Cole 1945–50, 1948 Report; SOAS CWM, Africa 1941–50, AF/44 Reports G–O, M. Morton 1938–44, 1943 Report; SOAS CWM, Africa 1961–70, AF/31 Reports I–R, J. Parry, 1963 Report.
6. Interview with Enoch Kapusa, 2 August 1998, Lusaka.
7. Interviews at Kalene, January 1998.
8. It should be made clear precisely what category of medical personnel will be dealt with in this discussion. It is not possible to do this by merely listing the titles attached to various workers. However, it is possible to do this in the negative sense. This discussion will not include sleeping sickness guards, sanitary overseers or malaria control boys. It will be concerned solely with those staff employed either in dispensaries or hospitals.
9. K. Patterson and G.W. Hartwig, 'The Disease Factor: An Introductory Overview' in Patterson and Hartwig (eds), *Disease in African History: An Introductory Survey and Case Studies* (Durham, NC: Duke University Press, 1978), 19.
10. D. Arnold, 'Disease, Medicine and Empire' in D. Arnold, (ed), *Imperial Medicine and Indigenous Societies* (Manchester: Manchester University Press, 1988), 2.
11. M. Vaughan, 'Healing and Curing: Issues in the Social History and Anthropology of Medicine in Africa', *Social History of Medicine*, 7, 2 (August 1994), 283–96.
12. M. Vaughan, 'Health and Hegemony: Representations of Disease and the Creation of the Colonial Subject in Nyasaland' in D. Engels and S. Marks, (eds), *Contesting Colonial Hegemony: State and Society in Africa and India* (London: British Academic Press, 1994), 195–6.
13. T. Ranger, 'Godly Medicine: The Ambiguities of Medical Mission in Southeast Tanzania, 1900–1945', *Social Science and Medicine*, 15B (1981), 271–2.
14. M. Vaughan, 'The Great Dispensary in the Sky', in M. Vaughan, *Curing Their Ills: Colonial Power and African Illness* (Cambridge: Polity Press, 1991), 65.
15. J. Iliffe, *East African Doctors: A History of a Modern Profession* (Cambridge: Cambridge University Press, 1998), 1.
16. For an explanation of the functioning of the 'lay therapy group' see J. Janzen,

The Quest for Therapy in Lower Zaire (Los Angeles: University of California Press, 1978); also S. Feierman, 'Struggles for Control: The Social Roots of Health and Healing in Modern Africa', *African Studies Review*, 28, 2/3 (1985), 80–1, for cautionary remarks.

17. S. Sayenda, 'Missionaries and Health: The Case of Malamulo Mission Hospital, 1907–1964', University of Malawi History Seminar, 1989/90, 5, 8–9.
18. C. Zvogbo, 'Medical Missions: A Neglected Theme in Zimbabwe's History 1893–1957', *Zambezia*, 13 (1986), 111–13.
19. M. Gelfand, *Northern Rhodesia in the Days of the Charter: A Medical and Social Study 1878–1924* (Oxford: Blackwell, 1961), 160. This page contains a photo of African medical personnel at Livingstone, dated 1911.
20. For the 'creation' of the African patient see M. Vaughan, 'Without the Camp: Institutions and Identities in the Colonial History of Leprosy', in Vaughan, *op. cit.* (note 14), 83.
21. The first Dioceses were Zanzibar, Nyasaland and Southern Tanganyika.
22. Rhodes House, Oxford (RHO), UMCA Annual Report 1918, xix.
23. RHO, UMCA Annual Report 1918, xix.
24. RHO, USPG/UMCA, SF 63A Conditions of Service. 'Marriage in the Mission.' A Memorandum written by the Secretary in 1944 and revised in 1952 by the then Secretary G.W. Broomfield.
25. NAZ ZAC, Box 28562, Bishop's Correspondence 1949–51, Msoro. Mudford to Bishop, 23 July 1950.
26. RHO, USPG/UMCA, SF 73, Vol. V, Letters from Bishop of Northern Rhodesia 1933–5, Spanton to Bishop, 11 September 1934.
27. NAZ ZAC, Box 28559, Staff Regulations 1928–36, European Staff (Conditions of Station life), Bishop Alston May, 12 September 1936, Bishop to Rogers, 24 October 1936.
28. NAZ ZAC, Box 28559, Staff Regulations 1928–36, Bishop to Rogers, 24 October 1936.
29. NAZ ZAC, Box 28559, Various Correspondence 1929–40, C.R. Evelyn to Hawkes, 8 September 1938.
30. NAZ ZAC, Box 28562, Bishop's Correspondence 1942–44 Msoro, Watson to Bishop, 11 May 1944.
31. NAZ ZAC, Box 28562, Bishop's Correspondence 1942–44 Msoro, Private Memo by Goodall to the Bishop, March 1944.
32. NAZ ZAC, Box 28562, Bishop's Correspondence 1942–44 Msoro, Private Memo by Goodall to the Bishop, March 1944.
33. NAZ ZAC, Box 28562, Bishop's Correspondence 1942–44 Msoro, Bishop to Goodall, 12 May 1944.
34. NAZ ZAC, Box 28562, Bishop's Correspondence 1942–44 Msoro, Watson to Bishop, 11 May 1944.

35. NAZ ZAC, Box 28562, Bishop's Correspondence 1945–46 Msoro, Memo from Young to Bishop, undated, but attached to letter from the Bishop to Goodall, dated 26 July 1945.
36. Details of this incident are found in several letters contained in NAZ ZAC, Box 28562, Bishop's Correspondence 1942–44 Msoro.
37. Bishop of Northern Rhodesia Annual Report 1934 in *Central Africa*, 630 (June 1935), 126, 128. For a brief explanation of *mchape* see W.M.J. Van Binsbergen, *Religious Change in Zambia* (London: Kegan Paul International, 1981), 165.
38. The events surrounding the death of Nebat are related in a number of letters and memos in NAZ ZAC, Box 28562, Bishop's Correspondence 1945–6, Msoro.
39. NAZ ZAC, Box 28562, Bishop's Correspondence 1945–46, Msoro, Bishop to Goodall, 29 July 1945.
40. NAZ ZAC, Box 28562, Bishop's Correspondence 1945–46 Msoro, Young to Bishop, 4 December 1946.
41. NAZ ZAC, Box 28556, Chipili Log Book 1943–9, eg. 24 May 1946, 23 October 1947.
42. NAZ ZAC, Box 28556, Chipili Log Book 1943–9, 6 March 1948.
43. NAZ ZAC, Box 28562, Bishop's Correspondence 1945–46 Msoro, Fanuel Mwanga to Bishop, 17 May 1946.
44. RHO, USPG/UMCA, SF 73, Vol. VIII, Letters from Bishop of Northern Rhodesia 1941–44, The Bishop's Annual Report for 1941.
45. A.G. Blood, *The History of the UMCA,* Vol. III, 1933–1957 (London: UMCA, 1962), 168.
46. NAZ ZAC, Box 28562, Bishop's Correspondence 1945–6 Msoro, Bishop to Rogers, 16 January 1945.
47. NAZ ZAC, Box 28562, Bishop's Correspondence 1942–44 Msoro, Justin Mapanga to Bishop, 31 December 1944.
48. NAZ ZAC, Box 28562, Bishop's Correspondence 1942–44 Msoro, Watson to Bishop, April 1 1944.
49. NAZ ZAC, Box 28562, Bishop's Correspondence 1945–46 Msoro, Francis Mngawa to Bishop, 23 July 1946.
50. NAZ ZAC, Box 28562, Bishop's Correspondence 1947–48 Msoro, Robertson to Bishop, 28 August 1947.
51. NAZ ZAC, Box 28562, Bishop's Correspondence 1942–44 Msoro, Bishop to Rogers, 10 December 1943; Watson to Bishop, 17 December 1943.
52. NAZ ZAC, Box 28562, Bishop's Correspondence 1942–44 Msoro, Rogers to Bishop, 16 December 1943.
53. NAZ ZAC, Box 28652, Bishop's Correspondence 1945–46 Msoro, Young to Bishop, 24 September 1945.
54. NAZ ZAC, Box 28562, Bishop's Correspondence 1945–46 Msoro, Bishop

to Young, October 1 1945; Young to Bishop, October 15 1945; Festo Michael to Bishop, 19 October 1945.

55. NAZ ZAC, Box 28559, Annual Reports 1939–43, Msoro Annual Report, 1943, A.G. Rogers.
56. NAZ ZAC, Box 28562, Bishop's Correspondence 1945–46 Msoro, Bishop to Festo, 30 October 1945.
57. NAZ ZAC, Box 28562, Bishop's Correspondence 1945–46 Msoro, Young to Bishop, 25 May 1946.
58. NAZ ZAC, Box 28562, Bishop's Correspondence 1947–48 Msoro, James Robertson to Bishop, 29 October 1947.
59. NAZ ZAC, Box 28562, Bishop's Correspondence 1947–48 Msoro, Bishop to Robertson, 29 November 1947.
60. NAZ ZAC, Box 28559, Annual Reports 1939–43. Fiwila Medical Report 1941.
61. NAZ ZAC, Box 28554, Bishop's Correspondence with Fiwila. Bishop to Mtaja, 28 January 1944.
62. NAZ ZAC, Box 28554, Bishop's Correspondence with Fiwila. Bishop to Munday, 28 January 1944.
63. NAZ ZAC, Box 28554, Bishop's Correspondence with Fiwila. Bishop to Mtaja, 28 January 1944.
64. NAZ ZAC, Box 28554, Bishop's Correspondence with Fiwila. Muriel Munday to Bishop, 9 February 1944.
65. NAZ SEC2/874, Kawambwa Tour Reports 1940–8, Tour Report 3, 1947 by Thomson, DC, 16–30 September, Annexure 3 health.
66. UMCA, 1948 Review, *The King's Business*, 27.
67. NAZ ZAC, Box 28562, Bishop's Correspondence 1949–51 Msoro, Bishop to Mudford, 10 October 1949.
68. NAZ ZAC, Box 28562, Bishop's Correspondence 1949–51 Msoro, Mudford to Bishop, 13 September 1949.
69. NAZ ZAC, Box 28562, Bishop's Correspondence 1949–51 Msoro, Mudford to Bishop, 11 November 1949.
70. NAZ ZAC, Box 28562, Bishop's Correspondence 1949–51 Msoro, Bishop to Mudford, 10 October 1949.
71. NAZ ZAC, Box 28562, Bishop's Correspondence 1949–51 Msoro, Bishop to Mounsey, 16 November 1949.
72. NAZ ZAC, Box 28562, Bishop's Correspondence 1949–51 Msoro, Mtaja to Bishop, 26 March 1950.
73. NAZ ZAC, Box 28562, Bishop's Correspondence 1949–51 Msoro, Mtaja to Bishop, 19 September 1950.
74. RHO, USPG/UMCA, SF 73 IA Letters from Bishop of Northern Rhodesia re Women's Work. 1945–51. Bishop to Baber, 16 December 1950.

75. NAZ MH2/75 UMCA, Msoro, Vol. II, 1950–61. PMO to DMS, 25 March 1952.
76. Trainee records, held at St Francis', Katete.
77. RHO, USPG/UMCA, SF 73, Vol. IX Letters from Bishop of Northern Rhodesia 1945–47. Bishop's circular letter No. 16, 15 September 1947.
78. The National Archives (TNA), CO859/219/1 Nurses Reciprocity with the UK. *Colonial Nursing Service General Conditions of Service and Terms of Appointment* 1949, para. 3.
79. TNA CO 850/252/7, Training of Nurses in the Colonies. *Report of Committee on Training of Nurses for the Colonies* 1945 para. 13.
80. TNA CO 850/252/7, Training of Nurses in the Colonies. *Report of Committee on Training of Nurses for the Colonies* 1945 para. 17.
81. TNA CO 850/252/7, Training of Nurses in the Colonies. *Report of Committee on Training of Nurses for the Colonies* 1945 para. 17
82. E.R.G. King, 'On Educating African Girls in Northern Rhodesia', *The Rhodes–Livingstone Institution Journal*, 10 (1950), 65:71.
83. NAZ RC 343, Report on Work of the Medical Department, August 1925 – July 1926, 10–11.
84. These were the 'House of Life' at Mbereshi, and the government training that was established at Kasama during the late-1920s. The latter disappeared from the records after a couple of years. From the government's point of view, it was hoped that these two experiments would be important in contributing towards the provision of assistants to work on the female wards of European hospitals. (e.g. NAZ ZA1/9 28/7 1 Medical Orderlies, training of. April 1930–December 1931. Scheme for training medical orderlies.)
85. TNA CO799 16 Northern Rhodesia Administration Reports 1937. Medical Report on Health and Sanitary Conditions 1937, 13.
86. For example, in 1930 there were two matrons and twenty-four European Nursing Sisters. (TNA CO799 7 Northern Rhodesia Administration Reports 1930, Medical Report on Health and Sanitary Conditions for 1930, section 1). By 1948 there was one matron–in–chief, five matrons, eight senior nursing sisters, and sixty-two nursing sisters. (TNA CO799 26 NR, Administration Reports 1948, 9). In Sr Isabelle CSP *More Precious than Rubies* UMCA, No. 10, *Think it Over* Series, (undated, but post 1948, since there is a 1948 quotation), the urgency for female nurses due to increasing surgical intervention is highlighted.
87. NAZ ZAC, Box 28553 Msoro Log Book 1933–39.
88. The Bishop expressed this view in the UMCA, 1943 Review, *Spearhead of Africa's Advance*, 26.
89. RHO, USPG/UMCA, SF 73, Vol. IX Letters from Bishop of Northern Rhodesia 1945–47. Note dated 1 April, 1946.
90. RHO, USPG/UMCA, SF 73, Vol. IX Letters from Bishop of Northern

Rhodesia 1945–47. Bishop to Broomfield, 16 October 1946. For funding of different stations see RHO, USPG/UMCA, SF 70 Northern Rhodesia Finance, *inter alia.*

91. Details of Trefusis from Blood, *op. cit.* (note 45), 321; St Francis Katete prospectus, 1996, and from an interview with Dr Cairns, 3 September 1999, Poole. Dr Cairns was the MO at St Francis from 1958–95.
92. NAZ ZAC, Box 28562 Bishop's Correspondence 1947–48 Msoro, Bishop to Williams, 26 February 1947.
93. NAZ HM 4 CC /1/1/31 Christian Council 1949. Acting Director of Medical Services to George Hewitt, 23 June 1949, quoting letter from Chief Secretary to Bishop of Northern Rhodesia 3 July 1946, re. Statement of Government policy with regard to the relationship between Government and the mission societies, in connection with Mission medical work.
94. RHO, USPG/UMCA, SF 70 Northern Rhodesia Finance. Bishop's notes on Schedule 'A', dated January 1947.
95. Interview with Canon James Robertson, 28 August 1997, London. (Canon Robertson began working as a priest at Msoro in 1945). For a history of the DRC in Northern Rhodesia see G. Vestraelen-Gilhuis, *From Dutch Mission Church to Reformed Church in Zambia* (Netherlands: Wever, 1982).
96. Blood, *op.cit.* (note 45), 172.
97. *Testing Time* UMCA, Annual Review 1947, 24.
98. RHO, USPG/UMCA, SF 73, Vol. IX Letters from Bishop of Northern Rhodesia 1945–47. Bishop to Broomfield, 25 February 1947.
99. RHO, USPG/UMCA, SF 73, Vol. IX Letters from Bishop of Northern Rhodesia 1945–47. Bishop to Broomfield, 16 October 1946. RHO, USPG/UMCA, SF 73, Vol. X Letters from Bishop of Northern Rhodesia 1948–51. Robert to Broomfield, 5 February 1948.
100. RHO, USPG/UMCA, SF 70 Northern Rhodesia Finance. Mission Finance Committee. 20 February 1947.
101. NAZ ED/1/5/60 UMCA, Msoro, 1937–54. Bishop to Education Officer, Ft Jameson, 2 April 1948.
102. RHO, UMCA, SF 115A Northern Rhodesia Katete Hospital. Trefusis to Nugee (Lay Secretary UMCA), 3 June 1949. The records are unclear as to whether the Government withdrew the funding, or whether Trefusis rejected the offer.
103. RHO, USPG/UMCA, SF 73, Vol. X Letters from Bishop of Northern Rhodesia 1948–51. Robert to Broomfield, 5 February 1948.
104. RHO, UMCA, SF 115A Northern Rhodesia Katete Hospital. Robert Howard to Jameson, 9 March 1947.
105. RHO, USPG/UMCA, SF 73, Vol. XI Letters from Bishop of Northern Rhodesia 1952–54. Broomfield to Bishop, 1 April 1953. Bishop to Broomfield, 11 April 1953.

106. RHO, USPG/UMCA, SF 73, Vol. X Letters from Bishop of Northern Rhodesia 1948–51. Broomfield to Bishop, 8 September 1949.
107. NAZ MH3/17 E Province Tours Medical Reports 1945–52. One of two tours by PMO McGregor in 1951.
108. NAZ MH3/17 E Province Tours Medical Reports 1945–52. One of two tours by PMO McGregor in 1951.
109. RHO, USPG/UMCA, SF 73, Vol. X Letters from Bishop of Northern Rhodesia 1948–51. Bishop to Broomfield, 26 January 1951.
110. RHO, USPG/UMCA, SF 73, Vol. X Letters from Bishop of Northern Rhodesia 1948–51. Broomfield to Bishop, 4 October 1949.
111. RHO, USPG/UMCA, SF 73, Vol. X Letters from Bishop of Northern Rhodesia 1948–51. Bishop to Broomfield, 25 September 1949.
112. NAZ ZAC, Box 28552, *Church News* 1944–1952. April 1952. The exact circumstances of his removal are not made clear either in the *Church News* magazine, nor other records.
113. NAZ MH/3/56, tours by ADMS Thomas Evans, 1951–4. Tour of E Province, July 1951. Information regarding the difficulties surrounding the setting up of St Francis taken from several letters in RHO, USPG/UMCA, SF 73, Vol. X, Letters from Bishop of Northern Rhodesia 1948–51.
114. RHO, USPG/UMCA, SF 73, Vol. XI. Letters from Bishop of Northern Rhodesia 1952–54, Bishop to Broomfield, 26 March 1953.
115. RHO, USPG/UMCA, SF 73 IIA Letters from Bishop of Northern Rhodesia re. Women's Work. 1952–61. Oliver to White Cooper, 7 November 1952.
116. RHO, USPG/UMCA, SF 73, Vol. XI Letters from Bishop of Northern Rhodesia 1952–54. Bishop to Broomfield, 29 July 1953.
117. NAZ Health Department Annual Report for 1947, 7.
118. St Francis Katete prospectus, 1996, and interview with Dr Cairns, 3 September 1999, Poole.
119. Medical Missionary Advisory Committee report from meeting held 12 October 1949. Report filed at St Francis, Katete.
120. Medical Missionary Advisory Committee report from meeting held 26 January 1950. Report filed at St Francis, Katete.
121. NAZ MH9/5 Advisory Committee. Volume I. Record of meetings held 13 July 1950 and 5 December 1950.
122. There were originally three volumes in section MH9 Advisory Committee. Extant now are MH9/5 Medical Missionary Work, Vol. I (1950–51); and MH9/9 Medical Missionary Work, Vol. III (1956–61), Vol. II was destroyed when the section was re-catalogued. It is likely that serious understaffing contributed to the inactivity. For example, the approved establishment of European nursing sisters in 1950 was ninety-nine. There were in fact only seventy-eight actually employed. TNA CO 799 28, NR Administration

Reports 1950, 18.

123. The General Nursing Council of Zambia, Prospectus for Schools of Nursing and Midwifery, 1997. For the struggle for professional autonomy in South Africa see S. Marks, *Divided Sisterhood: Race, Class and Gender in the South African Nursing Profession* (London: The Macmillan Press, 1994), especially Chapter 5. See also S. Marks, 'The Legacy of the History of Nursing for Post-Apartheid South Africa', in A.M. Rafferty, J. Robinson and R. Elkan (eds), *Nursing History: Politics of Welfare* (London: Routledge, 1997). For the case of the British nurse see R. Dingwall, A.M. Rafferty and C. Webster, 'The Search for Unity', in *An Introduction to the Social History of Nursing* (London: Routledge, 1988), 77–97.
124. RHO, USPG/UMCA, SF 73, Vol. XI, Letters from Bishop of Northern Rhodesia 1952–54. Bishop to Broomfield, 3 September 1952.
125. Report from school principal, undated, in Trainee Records kept at St Francis, Katete.
126. Letters from father to Anna Kawambwa, held in Trainee Records kept at St Francis, Katete, 10 July 1957 and 8 August 1957.
127. Interview with Lucy Tandoh Nalumpa at Northolt, 3 January 1999.

8

'A Matter of Vital Importance': The Place of the Medical Mission in Maternal and Child Healthcare in Tanganyika, 1919–39[1]

Michael Jennings

This chapter considers the evolution of Maternal and Child Welfare (MCW) services in colonial Tanganyika. It argues that the creation and extension of mission MCW services in the 1920s and 1930s provided a major contribution to colonial provision of western biomedicine, and belies traditional depictions of missionary medicine as solely curative and qualitatively inferior to its secular counterpart. The work of missions in this area was a critical factor in forcing the colonial state to re-evaluate its relationship with the mission sector and shift to the funding of such services.

The place of the medical mission has suffered in the historiography from a series of broad generalisations and misconceptions, through artificial divisions created by both the historical literature and contemporary accounts, in which the place of the mission medical services in contributing to the evolution of national health systems in British colonial Africa has been downplayed and marginalised. Two themes from the historiographical literature and contemporary accounts have a particular relevance for this chapter. Firstly, there is the perception of missionary medicine as overwhelmingly curative. Missionary medicine has traditionally been defined in terms of its 'curative' focus, as opposed to the 'preventive' approach of colonial state medicine. In reality, this divide has been fluid at best. There were very good structural reasons why missionary medicine was perhaps more curative in its emphasis. However, it never worked solely in this field, and indeed played a considerable role in Tanganyika – as elsewhere – in the public health policies of the colonial state. From vaccination campaigns, to surveying and research on sleeping sickness, missions played a much fuller role in the medical sphere than a concentration on clinics and hospitals alone suggests. Moreover, the medical work of the mission was never confined to the sphere of the medical professional alone: education in medical and hygiene matters was an important element in the mission schools, for example. During the colonial period, one of the most significant contributions of medical missions in the public-health arena, alongside participation in national vaccination campaigns, was in maternal and child welfare.

The depiction of missionary medicine as a curative – and hence inferior – service, owes much to the self-interest of the colonial state in promoting such a view. During the pre-war period, the British colonial states were unsure of how to treat the mission medical services functioning in their territories. Without the presence of such services, the overwhelming majority of Africans would have little or no access to western biomedical health care. Yet, whilst the colonial state was unwilling to commit resources to expanding a network of colonial state health services and facilities, it refused to commit itself to supporting financially those operated by the missions. Depicting missionary medicine as somehow inferior, in promoting the notion that the key difference between mission and state services divided along the lines of curative versus preventive, the government sought to justify its unwillingness to commit resources to health care designed to meet the needs of rural Tanganyikans. In 1937 a secretariat minute to the Deputy Director of Medical Services declared:

> I think it is desirable at this stage to make very clear to the Missions the somewhat different outlook of the Government [medical practitioners] and the Missions, the former being concerned with the mass of the people and particularly with the prevention of the spread of disease; and the latter more particularly with the individual and with, so far, the curative aspect.[2]

The colonial state, in depicting missionary medicine in this manner, thus provided for itself an excuse for refusing regular and systematic grants-in-aid.

During the 1920s and 1930s, however, this position became increasingly untenable, and the issue of maternal and child health care was central to these shifting positions and contradictions within the colonial state. For these services fell easily into the preventive medicine arena; moreover, they tied up with colonial administrative fears over the low population and high death rates of infants. From the mid-1920s, despite considerable reluctance to establish any pattern of formal grants to missions for medical work, the maternal and child health services of these agencies were increasingly subsidised and supported by the colonial state. The administration could not afford not to support this sector. Maternal and child welfare was considered essential for the workings of the Empire, and it was the missions who actually undertook the work.

A second major theme amongst the historical literature has sought to define 'missionary medicine' as something peculiar to the Christian mission, stressing its evangelical and Christian theological underpinnings. In the rhetoric of Christianity, and the imagery of the missionary endeavour, the child has always held a special place. The symbol of innocence afflicted with the depredations of disease, suffering, and a most likely early death was used to promote the work of missions. The pictures now most strongly associated with modern day requests for donations for famine and other disaster – the small child with large eyes, looking directly into the camera and pleading for assistance; and the counterpart 'after' depiction of a child happy and playing – are echoes of missionary propaganda. Missions used the symbol of the child, that most pervasive image of Christian iconography, in order to mobilise support back home. The child was the means, to put it crudely, to open wallets and purses – as it is so often today. But behind the imagery, behind the use of the child as a symbol of all that the missionary movement was attempting to achieve, there was a real commitment to promoting the welfare of the child, and of its mother. Convert the mother, convert the child, and the entire community could thus be brought into Christianity.

This central place of the child and mother in Christian rhetoric, the targeting of these two groups for the purposes of evangelisation, has tended to colour the impression of maternal and child health services undertaken by medical missions. Indeed, the association of the Church with these two groups might suggest that medical missions were inevitably drawn to the provision of such services. The question might well be asked, what else would Christian doctors and nurses focus upon? In mothers and children, surely the Church and its medical mission had found its primary constituency? Akerele, *et al*, for example, assert that the pre-occupation of mission doctors with winning souls created a form of medicine that was targeted primarily towards these ends. They argue that the Christian discourse within which medical missionaries functioned led such services to focus upon particular medico-social 'tasks' such as relief for the leprous, the blind, and the handicapped.[3] In other words, biblical manifestations of disease and misery were more attractive to the missionary than the more mundane task of vaccination, for example. According to this perception, the welfare of children, expectant and new mothers, fell within a particular Christian vision of protecting the innocent.

However, the story of maternal and child welfare services is inevitably more complex. The clear shift to a systematic and structured response to the needs of women and children was not something inherent to missions alone. Medical missionaries were not in a realm of their own, cut-off from broader international trends in medicine. They had the same training that all doctors underwent, read articles in medical journals, were kept informed of latest developments, and participated in research trials of new drugs. In the 1920s, as the attention of medical authorities in the Empire and elsewhere turned to issues of nutrition, public-health education, maternal and child health, medical missionaries too responded to these new ideas and notions.

The shift towards medical care for children and mothers, for educating new mothers in hygiene, cleanliness, and care of babies and infants, occurred at all levels in colonial society – it was the exclusive preserve of neither the state nor the voluntary sector. Whilst the mission sector came to dominate maternal and child welfare services in Tanganyika – as in much of the British Empire – this reflected not so much a particular 'mission perception' of what medical tasks were most appropriate for a service firmly situated within a Christian context, but from the desire of the colonial medical department to minimise the costs of its own services by relying on the voluntary sector where possible. The evolution of maternal and child welfare emerged from this blend of Christian rhetoric, colonial state pragmatism, and international trends in public health.

Nevertheless, by the early-1930s the missions had stamped their claim to be the dominant provider of such services. It was the missions who became the driving force of maternal and child welfare work in the Territory, set the examples to be used by the colonial medical administration, and allowed the colonial state to claim it was fulfiling its mandate. A survey of Tanganyikan medical services on the eve of Independence found that the maternal and child welfare services of the Territory were overwhelmingly provided by the mission sector. It had almost double the number of antenatal clinics operated by central government, with twenty percent more attendances; missions ran more than double the number of child health service clinics than central government, with just under twice the amount of attendees.[4] This dominance reflected the important position of the mission medical sector in the health services offered in Tanganyika. Mission medical services were not simply one option for treatment along western bio-medical lines. For many Africans in the remote rural areas of Tanganyika, they were the only option.

Maternal and child health in Tanganyika: evolution of a policy

The late-1910s and early-1920s saw the emergence of maternal and child welfare services as a major concern across both Empire and Metropole. The first Midwives' Act of 1902 introduced regulation for the training and practice of midwives in Britain, but it was not until the 1920s that maternal welfare clinics and antenatal care were introduced in any widespread form across the country. Even in the 1930s, few English counties had a sufficient number of maternity beds: Gloucestershire, for example, had no obstetrician and very few maternity beds. Maternal mortality in England and Wales in

1934 mirrored that of the 1860s, and only thereafter began to decline.[5] In 1938, seventy-five per cent of all deliveries were still performed at home.[6]

The 1920s saw a similar flourishing of services targeting maternal and child health in other parts of the Empire. Concern for mothers and children began relatively early in British India, and largely within the voluntary sector – not just medical missionaries, but also committees and groups formed by concerned non-missionary women. Voluntary committees were established in some towns from the last quarter of the nineteenth century to promote western notions of maternal and child health. Funds were established to train indigenous midwives (*dais*). The first such scheme was established in Amritsar in 1866 under the charge of Miss Hewlett of the Church of England Zenana Missionary Society. Miss Hewlett established a training and certification programme in western midwifery for *dais*. In order to ensure regulation of practice following completion of the course, *dais* were encouraged to report each birth they attended with the promise of one rupee for each report. Miss Hewlett or her assistant would visit the new mother to ensure all was well following the report. The Victoria Memorial Scholarships Fund was established in 1903 to provide funds for extending training for indigenous midwives, but such efforts – as with provision of maternal and child health care – were confined largely to large towns.[7]

By the end of the First World War, efforts to promote maternal and child health became increasingly structured and widespread, albeit still largely sited in the voluntary sector. In 1918, the first institution to train health visitors was established. The Lady Chelmsford League, an organisation concerned with child health and well-being, was established in 1919, and its inauguration announced at the Child Welfare Exhibition in Delhi the following year. In 1924, the 'baby week' movement was started by Lady Reading, designed to promote better care of babies and promotion of child health throughout British India – giving rise to baby shows throughout the Empire. The rise of maternal and child health services in Tanganyika, therefore, occurred alongside its gradual evolution both in the Metropole and the wider Empire.

The colonial occupation of Tanganyika occurred during a period of turmoil, conflict, and ecological crisis in the region. Wars, natural disasters such as drought, and disease, took a heavy toll upon the population. The violence associated with the imposition of German rule further destabilised communities and led to large-scale death and a declining population trend. Up to the end of its period of rule, the German colonial administration remained concerned with population numbers. The British administration, although perhaps to a lesser degree, was similarly concerned with the state of the population in Tanganyika.[8] In particular, surveys pointed to the high infant and child mortality rates that existed across the Territory. In 1921, three surveys in northern and western Tanganyika painted an alarming picture. Charles Dundas, District Officer in Moshi, surveyed thirty-four WaChagga chiefs in 1921: the thirty-four chiefs had 285 wives between them, and 707 children had been born to these women. Only 405 survived to weaning (eighteen months /two years). In Ufipa district it was estimated that only 48.2% of children reached adulthood. In Kirando, near Lake Tanganyika, approximately 40% died before the age of two, and a further 13% before the age of ten.[9] Surveys in Tabora District in 1922 concluded that death rates of children varied between a minimum of 41%, and a maximum of 66% – with 295 of 447 children born in South Ugunda and Ngulu dying.[10]

The cause of these high death rates was ascribed to three main factors: the prevalence of disease – in particular syphilis, believed to be endemic in much of the population, and smallpox; cultural practices which harmed children – the practice of clitorodectomy was held responsible for many deaths in child-birth; and finally – and perhaps most importantly – poor care of children after birth. Infants were thought to be subjected to poor feeding practices, were left vulnerable to chills and pneumonia when taken out to the *shambas* and placed on the cold ground as their mothers worked, and a general carelessness by new mothers about disease.[11] The problem was defined as a failure of education: mortality rates could best be reduced through an effective preventive medicine and an education campaign that targeted new and expectant mothers. In addition, clinics targeted at the particular needs of child health, would assist in the reduction of disease, infant and child mortality, and hence a declining trend in the population of Tanganyika. The Chief Medical Officer declared:

> A campaign against venereal disease would probably result in a marked increase in the number of births, but the percentage of deaths can only be reduced by the spread of education, especially in the female population. Suitable diet, clothing and in the case of serious illness a visit to a Government or Missionary Hospital before the resources of the local witch-doctor have been exhausted, would have the greatest influence in reducing the present high infant mortality rate throughout the Territory.[12]

The task lay, medical authorities believed, under the remit of the Education Department. By 1921, the Tanganyikan colonial administration was seemingly ready to place resources into maternal and child health, albeit under the care of the Education Department rather than medical, in an effort to 'enable child welfare and maternity work to be taken up extensively in the future.'[13]

The rise of maternal and child welfare as a new focus of colonial concern reflected a gradual broadening in definitions and understandings of the key social determinants of health and well-being during the 1920s. The 1927 Orr–Gilkes Report identified the problem of malnutrition for the first time in British colonial Africa, and led to a series of colonial and international surveys on health and nutrition. The League of Nations 1933 *Report on Nutrition and Public Health* called for nutrition to be made an integral aspect of public health policy. The realm of what constituted public health during this period was widening rapidly. The needs of African society as well as colonial objectives came increasingly to encompass issues of general living standards, health, and social welfare, rather than the simple narrow economic concerns that dominated early colonial thinking. Concern for the health of African colonial subjects – and for the maintenance of a healthy labour pool – emerged as a critical element of public health policy in this period, dominated in large part by concerns for maternal and child welfare.

Whilst mothers and children had always received medical attention in government and mission hospitals and clinics, the first specialised medical service dedicated to maternal and child health in Tanganyika was established in 1924. A former missionary nurse, Miss B.G. Allardes, now employed by the colonial administration, was appointed as Sister-in-Charge of a new clinic for ante and post-natal care in Dar es Salaam. Her duties included daily visits to the Infectious Diseases Hospital and Government School, fortnightly visits to the wives and children based in the Kings African Rifles Camp, and to the police compound. Allardes supervised vaccinations of women and children, and conducted home visits of maternity cases where necessary. A 'model native house' was erected to function as both clinic, and example of European notions of cleanliness and good living. It consisted of two small wards, an office for Nurse Allardes, and a large out-patient room.[14] During 1925, further clinics were constructed or planned in various regions across the Territory: in Kahama and Mabama in Tabora Province; and in Tanga, Lindi, and Mwanza. In 1925, the clinic in Tabora inspected some 1,527 children, clinic staff attended thirty-seven births in the town, treated 617 children for 'minor ailments' and vaccinated 377 children.[15] It was proposed that a special medical officer permanently in charge of maternity and child welfare should be appointed to oversee the work and propaganda of these new clinics.[16]

The clinics were not to act in isolation: African District Sanitary Inspectors were expected to promote the new ideals of maternal care on their rounds, in a form of outreach programme. In particular, they were expected to promote the idea that babies should be breast-fed entirely for their first year. Colonial medical authorities believed that one major cause of infant death was feeding of solids to babies far too early:

> Whereas the African mother breast-feeds her child, as a rule, for a full year and sometimes longer, the beneficial results which would otherwise accrue are destroyed in the belief that the colostrum bearing milk is harmful, and that the mothers milk of itself is insufficient nourishment. The result is that from birth extraneous matter in the form of coarse indigestible carbohydrates is forced upon the child which naturally proves disastrous.[17]

Both African and European staff were requested in the Rules of 1925 to encourage African expectant mothers to attend clinics rather than relying on the 'harmful' unskilled care of traditional healers. Complications and problems should be reported as soon as possible, along with any illnesses of the new mother and child. The clinic was to be the centre of a propaganda effort to inculcate a new culture of child-care amongst African communities, with other health workers contributing as and when they could to promote the ideals of European maternal and child health.

Other propaganda efforts were introduced in order to spread this knowledge further. At Kahama, a baby show was organised in 1925 under the supervision of a nurse, the local Sub-Assistant Surgeon, and Senior Sub-Assistant Surgeon. It was designed to 'promote Maternity and Child Welfare'; to 'bring home to the Natives the importance of the care of the Infants and thus assist towards the increase of population;' and to 'contribute to Educational Propaganda and the spread of knowledge regarding Public Health and Hygienic Measures'.[18] Of the 3,500 babies inspected, only 30% were apparently in good health (28% had enlarged spleens, 20% with hereditary syphilis, 8% with yaws and other skin lesions, and 14% with anaemia, worms, or malnourishment). Prizes were distributed, and the afternoon ended with an address from the Administrative Officer urging mothers to take their children to the hospital and clinics to ensure their children remained – or became – healthy.[19] Such baby shows became annual events, organised throughout Tanganyika, and linked into the Empire-wide National Baby Week Council activities that promoted the use of such events as a propaganda tool.

Between 1921 and 1928 then, the colonial state initiated a drive towards maternal and child health care. It was driven by a perception that the Tanganyikan population was at a dangerously low level, or at least was in danger of becoming so. The needs of labour, economic planning orthodoxy, and the colonial political economy, demanded a large enough workforce to ensure development. Maternal and child welfare was one tool that might promote this. By the 1930s, it appeared that the tide in population trends had been turned, and the birth rate started to rise, as death rates dropped. Maternal and child welfare seemed to have been a successful public health policy that was paying dividends.[20] During the 1930s, maternal and child

Table 8.1
Confinements and attendances at MCW clinics, 1935–39:

	No. of Confinements	New Patients Mothers	New Patients Children	Total Attendances Mothers	Total Attendances Children
1927	**507**	**10,736**	**16,519**	**27,745**	**36,725**
1928	**1,645**	**16,686**	**24,870**	**74,349**	**90,747**
1929	**2,521**	**28,858**	**38,682**	**148,006**	**197,021**
1930	**2,399**	**24,569**	**31,553**	**164,833**	**219,133**
1931	**2,170**	**30,558**	**45,418**	**251,704**	**352,155**
1932	**2,344**	**35,283**	**46,806**	**273,763**	**454,401**
1933	**2,673**	**25,485**	**42,932**	**292,916**	**485,798**
1934	**3,809**	**28,554**	**41,163**	**269,254**	**395,648**
1935	**3,396**	**27,365**	**40,820**	**204,008**	**306,537**
1936	**3,614**	**30,689**	**48,648**	**177,432**	**294,174**
1937	**3,800**	**28,813**	**49,138**	**201,136**	**296,815**
1938	**4,927**	**28,525**	**43,432**	**201,136**	**264,281**
1939	**3,532**	**30,235**	**35,885**	**195,629**	**241,299**

[Source: Tanganyika *Annual Medical Reports* (*AMR*), 1927–38; *Report to the League of Nations on Tanganyika Territory*, 1939, 176, TNA 967.822. Note that where exact numbers do not tally between the two reports for years 1935–8, I have used the statistics in the *AMR*.]

welfare services expanded rapidly and provided care to large numbers of mothers and children (see Table 8.1).

However, this success in the creation and rapid expansion of such services hid an apparent withdrawal of the colonial state from its recent publicly stated commitment to provision of maternal and child health welfare. The Chief Secretary commented to the Director of Medical Services (DMS) as early as 1929:

> The expansion of Maternity and Child Welfare is a matter of vital importance… There are other missions also doing Welfare work.… This, however, to my mind, is not a disadvantage, for we could curtail our own expansion, except in selected areas, by letting the Missions do the work, under supervision and guidance, as at present, at a very small cost to [Government].[21]

In the mid-1930s, following the collapse of government MCW services in Kahama, this policy was made more explicit:

> I am aware that a start has been made to train native midwives at Kahama, but it is very late in the day now to make a beginning, and I personally would prefer to see maternity work outside the big towns left to the Missions, seeing that religious influence has considerable learning on the success of these operations.[22]

The provision of medical care to women and children was henceforth the sphere of the voluntary agency.

Even as late as 1943, the commitment of the British administration in Tanganyika to the development of adequate midwifery training, ante and post-natal facilities, and child health care, was ambiguous. The DMS declared: 'The social conscience of the local population has not yet reached the stage when the needs for improving the conditions for normal childbirth have wide recognition.'[23] Such problems, he continued, could only be challenged through development of organised Infant and Maternity Welfare Centres. A 'start', he wrote, had been made in Tabora, Tanga, and Dar es Salaam. As for midwives: 'I feel it is a mistake to train midwives who are spread abroad outside the controlling influence of supervised centres.'[24] The DMS failed, almost entirely, to acknowledge almost two decades of mission activity in this sector. More than just a 'start' had been made: but it was the missions who had taken on the burden of this work.

Why was the colonial state seemingly willing – if not keen – to disengage from active provision of maternal and child welfare services so soon after stating its commitment to this field of public health? Global depression from 1929 undermined the commitments to increased social welfare spending that the colonial government had indicated in the late-1920s. The state withdrew into provision of only those public health commitments it considered absolutely necessary for the continued development of the Territory. It was able to do this, however, only because there existed a sector that could undertake the social obligations inferred by the colonial enterprise. The key factor that allowed the state to divest itself of direct responsibility for this sector was the burgeoning interest of missions in this field of work. The rapid rise of mission activity in maternal and child welfare, the relative success of the missions in attracting ever more numbers of women to the clinics, and the cheapness that this option offered the colonial state, allowed the administration to draw back. Yet it was not until the post-war period that any real financial commitment to missionary medical work was made. During the 1930s the contradictions of the administration's position were becoming increasingly clear. As missions entrenched their role in key public health sectors such as maternal and child health, the unwillingness of the colonial administration to pay for these services became ever more untenable.

Missionary maternal and child welfare services

At the same time that the colonial medical department was turning its attention to the poor state of maternal and child health across the Territory, missionary medical staff similarly sought to institutionalise and extend the services they offered towards expectant mothers and children. Maternal and child welfare had always been of concern to medical missionaries, although placed in the context of wider services and granted no special place – other than, perhaps, in the rhetoric and imagery of mission medical work espoused to promote its cause back in the Metropole. However, as international medical attention, and in particular as imperial public health concerns increasingly came to focus upon the potential benefits that could be offered by specialised services designed to target this particular group, missions were at the vanguard of attempts to create such services in Tanganyika.

The contribution of the missions to the particular health needs of women and children was not solely one of scale. The quality of the services created, and the model they provided for others, was also of great importance. The maternal and child welfare clinic of the Africa Inland Mission (AIM) was used as a model by the colonial state in its own designs for effective services in this field. The attempts by medical missionaries to educate traditional birth attendants in certain western principles of hygiene and cleanliness were later adopted by the state. As in the training of African medical staff generally, missions played a crucial role in the training of western-educated midwives. Missions, physically situated in the communities they served, were better placed to both understand and persuade local society of the benefits such services offered. By the 1930s, missions had firmly staked their claim to dominate the field of maternal and child welfare.

Perhaps the most significant of maternal and child welfare services in Tanganyika during the inter-war period were those established by the Africa Inland Mission in Tabora Province. The Mission was established in three sites in Shinyanga District: Kola Ndoto, Luhumbo, and Uduhe. Medical work was carried out on all three stations, but the main centre for medical services was Kola Ndoto, under the supervision of Dr Maynard, the wife of the resident priest. Dr Maynard had always undertaken maternity work as part of her medical service, but had attended women confined in their own homes rather than at an established and properly equipped centre. In 1926, a maternity home was built to provide adequate ante and post-natal care. The centre was built and paid for by the local native authority with Dr Maynard in charge. Thus although technically a Native Administration institution it was to all intents and purposes a mission facility, and was treated as such by both colonial and local administration.[25]

Table 8.2
Africa Inland Mission MCH work, Kola Ndoto, Shinyanga District

No. of	1926	1927	1928	1929	1930	1931	1932	1933
Births*	146	512	794	969	841	1,322	1,730	1,937

* These figures apply solely to the MCH centre at Kola Ndoto. Maternity work was also carried out at Luhumbo station under one of the mission nurses, but these figures were not recorded.

[Source: Shinyanga District Annual Report, 1931, 38, TNA 712; DMSS to Chief Secretary, 3 March 1934. The exact numbers between the Annual Reports and the DMSS vary slightly. For the period 1930-33, the difference is 7 births.]

Even before permanent buildings had been erected, Dr Maynard had supervised some 146 births and treated 3,000 infants and children – in addition to her general medical work which administered to over 26,000 outpatients (see Table 8.2).[26] The growth from this start was, given the size of the centre and in relation to other successful medical missions, exceptional.

Figures for the three Government clinics in Tanganyika are instructive: 1,287 confinements were attended to between 1930 and 1933. At the AIM clinic, Dr Maynard and her staff attended to 5,830 in the same period. A comparison with one of the most successful mission medical services in East Africa – those of the Church Missionary Society (CMS), in Uganda, under the capable leadership of Dr Albert Cook – similarly highlights the rapid success that Dr Maynard achieved. In 1928, nine years after the maternity and child health services had been initiated by the CMS, some 2,000 confinements were attended to in one central institution and twenty-four clinics. Dr Maynard attended nearly 800 after just three years of operation and in one clinic.

The Kola Ndoto Maternity Home became a model for maternal and child welfare facilities. Dr Maynard was consulted over the planning for a government clinic in Nzega in 1928. She advised on the building, the layout, the necessary equipment, and the potential costs of providing such a service. The Governor of Tanganyika declared that: 'the best possible little hospital should be built on the lines of that under Dr Maynard's charge in the Shinyanga District.'[27] Education, sanitary 'western' birth procedures, curative medicine for the sick, were all combined in the maternal and child welfare services, and the AIM Maternity Home at Kola Ndoto became the model for all the Territory.

Dr Maynard's clinic was pioneering not only in that it was one of the first such services to be established in Tanganyika, nor in its formal structural relationship with the local African community. It also undertook perhaps the first formal statistical survey of infant morbidity and mortality in Tanganyika. From 1 January 1927, the first thousand births were recorded, and monitored in the following years in order to establish some kind of benchmark for the success of the scheme. For the first three years of the survey, infant mortality was recorded to be a mere 10.5 per cent.[28]

Dr Maynard was also one of the first to train African midwives in order to extend services and make them more acceptable to the local community. In common with western perceptions of indigenous midwives in India, African birth attendants were widely felt to be a negative force for superstition and unhygienic practices, contributing to high mortality rates during birth. Training of Western-style midwives was regarded as an essential tool in the battle to promote maternal health. In 1927, five local Wasukuma women were being trained by Dr Maynard at the maternity home. The course lasted three years, and the first person to complete finished in 1929 – at which point eight African nurses were undergoing training. The uses to which such training was put were not limited to working under the direct supervision of Dr Maynard. Whereas some thirteen years later the British administration regarded unsupervised nurses and midwives with a great deal of suspicion, in 1930 three AIM-trained nurses had left the maternity home to get married. One nurse had already begun to undertake unsupervised maternity work in her chiefdom, and the other two were expected to follow suit. The local District Officer regarded these staff as the bedrock of district medical services in the future:

> Meantime Dr Maynard is taking in more girls for training. The trained nurse will form the nucleus of the District nursing staff in the future. The present Home cannot expand very much more and it will be necessary to find means of decentralising the work and this can be done through the medium of trained native nurses.[29]

The benefits of MCH services were thus spread out from the nucleus of Kola Ndoto from as early as 1930.

In 1927 the Church Missionary Society made an application to the colonial administration for financial support for six nurses. The Mission was to provide the cost of buildings, drugs and equipment, and requested £150 per year per nurse – half of the government salary of a health visitor. The nurses were to operate under the general supervision of the Director of Medical Services in the mission medical facilities and were recruited solely for the purpose of maternal and child welfare work.[30] By 1928, eight CMS

Table 8.3
Confinement figures at CMS Maternity Clinics, 1930-33

Name of Clinic	1930	1931	1932	1933	Total
Buigiri	**3**	**9**	**5**	**7**	**24**
Mvumi	**8**	**12**	**37**	**51**	**108**
Bukoba	**4**	**8**	**20**	**26**	**58**
Mpwapwa	**14**	**13**	**21**	**23**	**71**
Kilimatinde	**1**	**12**	**8**	**33**	**54**
Berega	**1**	**-**	**12**	**15**	**28**
Kongwa	**10**	**11**	**18**	**30**	**69**
Total Confinements	**41**	**65**	**121**	**185**	**412**

[Source: DMSS to ChfSec, 3 March 1934, TNA AN450 178/3.]

nurses were stationed throughout the diocese of Central Tanganyika. In comparison with the success of the AIM, the maternal and child welfare services created by the CMS seemed to have initially performed relatively poorly. Certainly the colonial administration regarded the CMS as representing a poor investment of state funds: over a four-year period government subsidies to CMS services amounted to £4,274. The AIM received only £800 in the same four-year period. Thus, a rough calculation of cost to government per birth was over £10 for the CMS, and a mere Sh.2 cents 74 for the AIM.[31] The Provincial Commissioner of Dodoma questioned the policy of providing state grants for failing clinics:

> ...it is evident that the cost per confinement is so prohibitive that the CMS must be told that the grants will have to be withdrawn in respect of all stations at which they cannot improve their figures.[32]

For the colonial administration, the key determinant of a successful service was 'value for money,' or in plainer terms, its cheapness.

By the mid-1930s, the tide seemed to have been turned. The cost-per-confinement for the CMS had almost halved by 1934 to £5/7/-;[33] and by 1938, some 2,085 confinements were attended to by CMS clinics (see Table 8.3).[34] As officials in the Medical Department noted: 'the popularising of a Maternity Clinic is notoriously uphill work,' and even Dr Maynard had struggled for years to get expectant mothers to enter the maternity clinic.[35] The Medical Department realised the difficulties in comparing mission maternal and child health services across the Territory: 'The outstanding success of Dr Maynard's activities is scarcely relevant, since there is no question of Dr Maynard being an alternative to the CMS.'[36]

The mission itself certainly regarded its maternal and child welfare services as something that would require time to become effective. Efforts to

Table 8.4
Confinements to Government and Assisted Clinics, 1938

Province	Clinic	Confinements	Total
Central Province (CMS)	**Berega**	**194**	
	Buigiri	**243**	
	Kilimatinde	**365**	
	Kongwa	**149**	
	Mpwapwa	**321**	
	Mvumi	**813**	**2,085**
Western Province (Govt)	**Kahama**	**437**	
	Nzega	**485**	**922**
Lake Province (AIM)	**Shinyanga**	**1,701**	**1,701**
Eastern Province (Govt)	**Dar es Salaam**	**103**	**103**
Tanga Province (Govt)	**Tanga**	**116**	**116**

[Source: Tanganyika *AMR* 1938, 34.]

establish clinics as thriving centres was 'a terribly up-hill task, on account of the crass ignorance' of traditional society.[37] The chief obstacle was, according to the Archdeacon, the influence of 'the old heathen midwives' who dominated the practice of giving birth.[38] The CMS nurses were still conducting the essential 'hard spade-work' in order to break down traditional notions and resistance to attending the mission clinics. The numbers attending the maternity clinics did not reflect, the Archdeacon claimed, the actual influence that the missionaries increasingly held. Increasing numbers of expectant mothers arrived at the CMS clinics during 1934, expressing a desire to be admitted for childbirth.[39] By the end of the 1930s, the CMS, alongside other mission clinics, was one of the main providers of maternal and child welfare in the Territory (see Table 8.4).

Maternity and child health services continued to evolve and expand throughout the Territory during the 1930s, although almost entirely under the sole province of the mission sector. The White Father's maintained clinics on Lake Tanganyika at Karema and at Kagondo; the Augustana Lutheran Mission established dedicated services in its hospitals at Ndolage and Singida; at Peramiho in southern Tanganyika the Benedictine sisters superintended confinements; the UMCA Hospital at Magila had a special branch for maternity work, supervised by the Sisters of the Sacred Passion; and the UMCA in Masasi District ran several maternity clinics, with a larger centre at Masasi Hospital.

Of course, mission maternal and child welfare services suffered from the same structural and personnel problems that affected all voluntary sector medical services. In 1939, confinement cases almost halved from the previous year in the Central Province when two CMS nursing sisters fell ill and were unable to work. The quality of medical staff also played a role in the effectiveness of the services. The CMS nurse in-charge at Rubungo, Bukoba, prior to 1933 was felt to be 'not altogether professionally competent', did not know the local language and was 'generally indolent'.[40] The arrival of a new nurse in 1933/4, Mrs Galbraith, seemed to restore momentum to maternal and child health, and a noticeable difference was seen within two months of her arrival. The success of Dr Maynard in all the medical facilities she built up was in large part the result of both her skill, and her popularity amongst the local community. In some cases mission clinics competed with others to minister to expectant mothers and children. The failure of the Rubungo clinic was ascribed to its close proximity to a Catholic clinic under the capable leadership of Dr Adams Clark, a gynaecologist, for example.

However, the key structural deficit that underlay the problems of the mission sector, and the factor that impeded better co-ordination and direction, was the failure of the state to adequately or systematically fund mission medical services in the pre-war period. The adoption of a grants-in-aid policy, and the post-war shift to greater integration of the various sectors of health care provision, was in some part a consequence of the key public health role the missions had played in maternal and child welfare.

Colonial funding of MCW services in the inter-war period

During the 1920s the colonial administration in Tanganyika was reluctant to set a precedent through the provision of funds for mission medical work of any kind. The Director of Medical Services outlined his fears in 1927:

> While I agree that every encouragement should be given by Government to Mission workers such as Mrs Maynard I think you will agree that very great care is necessary in creating precedents for granting financial assistance to Medical Missionary workers.[41]

The concern was that once government provided a grant to one mission, it would 'lead to similar demands from others'.[42] The administration was keen not to create 'a most embarrassing precedent'.[43] Grants were consequently made on an *ad hoc* and strictly non-recurrent basis. Applications for funds needed to be made each year, and prior grants were to be no guarantee of continued funding.

Although the administration was tremendously keen in its admiration of, and desire to support, the AIM facilities in Shinyanga, it was also eager to ensure that it did not set a precedent in funding its work. In 1927, the Acting DMS set out his unwillingness to be seen to support a mission hospital, whilst declaring his desire 'that Mrs Maynard's work should be assisted in every way.' He suggested that 'the Clinic should be fully equipped from the start and I suggest that the Government should consider the question of making a loan to the Native Authority.'[44] The work was, in effect, being subcontracted out by the Native Authority to a provider – in this instance the local mission. The state could argue, therefore, that it was supporting a service offered by part of the administration, not an external voluntary agency. It was a distinction that was little more than splitting hairs, and the colonial state was increasingly unable to maintain the fiction that it would not provide grants to missions for work it could not do itself. Significant resources were channelled into the Church Missionary Society maternal and child welfare services from the early-1930s, and sums of approximately £900–1,000 were made available annually for mission-run maternal and child welfare services in Tanganyika. By 1933, the Medical Department was ready to commit to regular grants for work of this kind:

> [T]his Department is prepared to consider sympathetically applications for assistance in special lines of work having a direct bearing on public health, such as maternity and child welfare, anti-venereal diseases, and yaws work, leprosy and hookworm and the like.[45]

Inevitably, the system of *ad hoc* grants became increasingly formalised over the course of the 1930s, and the administration came to realise that it could no longer rely on informal procedures.

The official policy of grants-in-aid from the post-war period was the result, in large part, of the work missions had undertaken in maternal and child welfare. Whilst the colonial administration could maintain the fiction to some extent that the 'curative' focus of medical missions and the use of medicine for evangelical purposes should exclude such services from official funding, the role of missions in public health campaigns and in the provision of services that the state realised fell under its own responsibility made the absence of official funding an increasing embarrassment. The emphasis from the mid- to late-1930s on social welfare in Africa, and in particular on health, contained in the Colonial Development Acts left the colonial state vulnerable to accusations of failing to do enough to fulfil its mandate of care. The work in maternal and child health showed the professionalism of medical missions; it revealed the contradictions in official colonial policy; and ultimately it led to a demand for greater integration of the Territory's medical services under a more unified direction through the use of grants-in-aid and increased state supervision over the use of those grants.

The sectoral advantage of the mission

Addressing the Imperial Congress in 1933, Dr Mary Blacklock acknowledged the important pioneering work done by missions in the field of maternal and child health services. However, she rejected the implication that the dominance of missions in this field reflected negatively upon the colonial states across the Empire:

> Now the fact that these services, particularly the welfare side, have so often been developed by voluntary workers, may be considered by some to reflect adversely on the vision and energy of the various Governments. We must remember, however, that the success of these services is very dependent upon the education of public opinion, and that Governments, unless supplied with a large 'propaganda staff', may find this task difficult.[46]

Missionaries, often regarded by colonial authorities as propagandists for European lifestyles – however much the missionaries themselves may have rejected that assessment – lived with the people they provided pastoral care for. They had a greater understanding of the social mores and values of their communities. The mission sector was ideal, in other words, for undertaking work of this kind: work that included a strong element of education and social reform of aspects of traditional life, as well as the medical side. The state was too far removed from this level of society, had too few personnel dedicated to this aspect of work, to effectively undertake the task of improving health services for mothers and children. The voluntary sector had an underlying sectoral advantage in its position, its structures, and its relationship to the community in which it was based.

The success of the AIM, in particular, lay in the close ties it held to the Native Administrations in Shinyanga, and respect accorded to it by the local population. The CMS was able to build up its own successes through slow and steady education and propaganda, through links established with local women, chiefs, and people of influence. The CMS Archdeacon in Central Tanganyika recognised the importance of building up confidence in the local community:

> The largest and most flourishing Maternity Centre at the present time in this Territory – where the number of confinements each year can be counted by the thousand [i.e. Kola Ndoto], had to work steadily and patiently for fifteen years before they could persuade a single woman to come into their hospital for confinement. I mention this as shewing [*sic*] that Maternity and Child Welfare work, though second to none in importance, is amongst the hardest which the Missionary Societies have attempted to accomplish.[47]

For the medical mission this issue of building up trust within a community over a long period of time was critical to the success or otherwise of that mission. The coercive powers available to the state were simply not available to the mission.

Whether the use of compulsion and a degree of force made the colonial state medical services any more effective, however, is doubtful. Attempts to promote the government maternal and child health clinic at Kahama in the late-1920s were significantly less sensitive than those in Shinyanga and Central Tanganyika Diocese. Few women had attended the clinic, and reports suggested that the sister-in-charge toured the local villages, ascertaining which women were pregnant and encouraging local chiefs to force women to attend the clinic for delivery. Even once at the clinic, women seemed reluctant to remain:

> I was told it was not uncommon for women to escape from the clinic even on their expected day of delivery, when they had made their way outside and gave birth in the bush.... I was told that women who had been delivered of one child in the clinic never presented themselves voluntarily for a second birth, but attended only after being sought out in the villages.[48]

In 1926 and 1927, 'considerable pressure was used', it was alleged, to the extent that 'husbands whose women refused to attend were beaten' on the order of the local chiefs.[49] In consequence, the clinic at Kahama suffered a poor reputation among the local community, and few attended from personal choice. The slow and steady model of mission services was not appropriate to the results-driven colonial administration, with its annual reports, targets, statistics and 'league table' approach to public health scheme evaluation. In contrast to the clinic at Kola Ndoto where 'everyone is a volunteer and women come from long distances,'[50] the government clinic had failed to build up a level of trust and acceptance within the community for its services. Such services were welcomed by the African communities in which they were situated, but only once they had become accepted as one of the options for health care amongst many. Where such services flourished, it was because the local missionaries had made efforts to make them acceptable, working within local customs and traditions to build that bridge of trust.

Living in the communities in which they served, missionaries were perhaps better placed to appreciate local obstacles to maternal and child welfare. In Ndanda, the Benedictine Sister Thecla sought to use traditional birth attendants as a way of importing western notions of hygiene and cleanliness without forcing women to attend the clinic. Sr Thecla realised that unmarried, and crucially childless, young women would not be acceptable to mothers giving birth, and thus concentrated on the older traditional attendants. The colonial state, when seeking to adapt this idea to increase the numbers of women attended to with western notions of childbirth and childcare, focused on the training of young, unmarried women – on the assumption that they were better educated, literate, and therefore more amenable to new ideas.[51] The resulting difficulties in getting them accepted were inevitable, and had been foreseen.

The assumption that the primary difference between missionary and colonial state medicine lay in the types of services it offered, ie. curative or preventive, has tended to hide more interesting differences between the two. The 'place' of each, its relationship to the African communities both claimed to serve, is perhaps one of the most important of these differences. Based within the communities, a permanent presence with an often longer history of work within a particular area, missions were in many instances better able to judge the more appropriate mechanisms for popularising the medical services they offered. Unlike western biomedical traditions in which decisions over treatment and care lay with the medical practitioner, in indigenous African healing traditions the initiative lies with the patient and the patient's family. The family of the sick or injured person would decide which form of treatment and practitioner amongst the plurality of systems available was most suitable. If a Tanganyikan chose to go to a mission clinic, it was a conscious choice that represented a perception that this healing system offered the best form of care for a particular condition.

Traditional birth attendants operated in the villages and settlements of Tanganyika before the arrival of the missionaries and colonial occupiers. Services offered by these representatives of 'western science' were therefore forced to compete not by replacing alternative forms of healing, but through building up levels of trust and acceptance in their comparative skill and success. In this, missionary medicine, particularly in the sphere of maternal and child health, held an advantage over colonial state medicine. It relied primarily upon education, and upon a holistic vision of health which encompassed both bodily and spiritual well-being, closer to traditional understandings of health and healing than the more overtly scientific paradigm under which the secular model operated. Far from shying away from offering a more preventive medical approach to the health problems of Tanganyika in the pre-war period, the missions incorporated such notions in their health, education, and even evangelistic work, and were arguably better placed and more successful in imparting western notions of preventive health than their secular counterparts. The sectoral advantage of the medical mission, most critically defined by the level at which it operated – as part of a community – is perhaps the sharpest difference between mission and colonial state models of western biomedical health care in this period.

Conclusion

In terms of overall numbers of African mothers attending the maternal and child health clinics in Tanganyika in this period, the numbers remain small. It is certainly the case that the successful clinics under the care of Dr Maynard and those of the CMS in Central Tanganyika Diocese succeeded in attracting expectant and new mothers. This acceptance, however, needs to be qualified. Many communities were left without immediate access, and even in areas where services were made available, their reach and overall use was certainly not exhaustive. The acceptance of a western biomedical advantage in this field was won slowly and partially. Reliance on indigenous traditions remained high, and missionary medicine – in all its forms and services offered – was never more than one option amongst many for the African population.

Nevertheless, given the short period in which maternal and child health evolved from early notions to effective services, and especially compared to the clinics offered by the colonial government, missions were relatively successful in this field. Moreover, the gradual rise of such services needs to be placed alongside the similarly slow evolution of such services in the United Kingdom, where they only began to make a serious impact from the mid- to late-1930s.

The dominance in maternal and child welfare services established by the missions did not result from a particular Christian regard for the place of the 'child' and 'mother', but because their position in local communities allowed the culturally intrusive public health message to be transmitted in a more sensitive and acceptable way. The esteem with which Dr Maynard was held, and the close relationship with the Native Authority, ensured a degree of local support that the colonial state would rarely be accorded. It was not simply a question of lack of commitment from the colonial state. The government clinics that did exist failed to perform anywhere near as adequately as those run by missions. As voluntary agencies without the extensive and often contradictory commitments of government responsibility, as long-term inhabitants in particular areas with very real commitments to raising living standards in those communities, the mission sector had an advantage over the colonial state that allowed it to undertake its public health duties more efficiently and successfully.

Medical missions were hamstrung in their effectiveness in many ways: through the underlying conflicting purposes to which this social mission was dedicated – healing of bodies or salvation of souls; by the poor funding mechanisms and consequent insecurity and instability that this conferred;

and through shortages of staff, medical equipment and drugs. As a sector, medical missions had little in the way of unified policy, and would compete with each other for the bodies and souls of the local communities. Yet, as with the voluntary sector now, missions were in many ways placed in a unique position in which to contribute to the health needs of rural African society. They provided a front-line service, perhaps not the most important of medical needs, but a vital one nevertheless. Their public health role, often undervalued or misrepresented, was of great significance in getting principles of western biomedicine accepted as a viable option in the African plural medical tradition. The arena of maternal and child welfare was one of many in which medical missions contributed, but it was an important one, and it positioned them as major players in the health services of Tanganyika, one that, post-1945, the colonial state could no longer ignore.

Notes

1. Quote from Secretariat Minutes (SecMins), Chief Secretary (Ch.Sec), 11 April 1929, Tanzania National Archive (TNA) 10721 Vol. I. Thanks are due to David Hardiman, Maureen Malowany, Shula Marks, and Debbie Gaitskill for comments on the original paper.
2. SecMins, 5 August 1937, TNA 450 692 Vol.1.
3. O. Akerele, I. Tabibzadeh and J. McGilvray, 'A New Role for Medical Missionaries in Africa', *WHO Chronicle*, 30 (1976), 175–80.
4. R.M. Titmuss, B. Abel-Smith and A.W. Williams, *The Health Services of Tanganyika: A Report to the Government* (London: Pitman Medical Publishing Co., 1964), 36–7.
5. I. Loudon, 'Childbirth', in I. Loudon (ed.), *Western Medicine: An Illustrated History* (Oxford: Oxford University Press, 1997), 209–16.
6. *Ibid.*, 213.
7. M. Balfour, R. Young & M. Scharlieb, *The Work of Medical Women in India* (London: Oxford University Press, 1929), 129–130.
8. J. Koponen, 'Population: a dependent variable', in G. Maddox, J. Giblin and I.S. Kimambo, *Custodians of the Land: Ecology and Culture in the History of Tanzania* (London: James Currey, 1996), 19–42.
9. Tanganyika *Annual Medical Report* (*AMR*) (1921), 83. Comparative child mortality figures for the UK at the time were approximately 25.1% mortality before the age of ten.
10. Tanganyika *AMR* (1922), 100.
11. *Ibid.*, 100; Tanganyika *AMR* (1924), 156.
12. Tanganyika *AMR* (1922), 100.
13. *Ibid.*, 100.
14. Tanganyika *AMR* (1924), 156.
15. Tanganyika *AMR*, (1925), 68.

16. *Ibid.*, 75.
17. *Ibid.*, 75.
18. *Ibid.*, 112.
19. *Ibid.*, 113. By the 1930s, individual shows were competing across the Empire for the Imperial Baby Week Challenge Shield. Ten certificates of merit were awarded throughout the Empire, and the Church Missionary Society clinic at Kongwa received one of these prized bits of paper in 1935.
20. It appears that by the late-1920s/early-1930s, the declining trend in population had been arrested, and population numbers had begun to rise again. Whether this was due to colonial maternal and child welfare services is debatable. The small reach of these services and limited impact in overall terms suggests that it was at best no more than a contributory factor. For an analysis of population trends and possible causes see: Koponen, *op. cit.* (note 8); G. Maddox, 'Environment & Population Growth in Ugogo Central Tanzania', in Maddox *et al.*, *op. cit.* (note 8), 43–65.
21. SecMins, ChfSec, 11 April 1929, TNA 10721 Vol.1.
22. SecMins, 30 March 1936, TNA 10834.
23. Director of Medical Services, *Post-War Development: Medical Department*, 8, TNA AN450 1179.
24. *Ibid.*
25. Colonial Tanganyika was, at this time – and in common with many parts of British Africa – administered through the system of Indirect Rule. Recognised 'tribes' were administered by legally constituted Native Authorities (NA) with responsibility for administration within the area of their jurisdiction. The NAs were expected to raise local taxes, keeping a proportion for the funding of essential services, including health.
26. Shinyaga District Annual Report, 1926, 30–2, TNA 712.
27. ChfSec to Provincial Commissioner (PC) Tabora, 5 October 1928, TNA 10834; PC Tabora to ChfSec, undated, TNA 10834; District Officer (DO) Nzega to PC Tabora, 11 October 1928, TNA 10834.
28. Shinyaga District Annual Report, 1930, 30, TNA 712. The main unit for measurement is generally the first five years of life, so the low figure of 10.5% would probably have risen. Nevertheless, it still represents a low infant mortality rate for the period.
29. Shinyanga District Annual Report, 1930, 30–1, TNA 712.
30. DMSS (Director of Medical and Sanitation Services) to ChfSec, 14 November 1927, TNA 10721 Vol.1; Bishop Chambers to DMSS, 14 November 1927, TNA 10721 Vol.1.
31. DMSS to ChfSec, 3 March 1934, TNA 10721 Vol.1.
32. PC Dodoma to ChfSec, 19 March 1934. TNA 10721 Vol.1.
33. SecMins, 7 March 1934, TNA 10721 Vol.1.
34. Tanganyika AMR 1938, 34.

35. PC Dodoma to ChfSec, 19 March 1934. TNA 10721 Vol.1.
36. SecMins, 7 March 1934, TNA 10721 Vol.1.
37. Archdeacon John Briggs, CMS, 20 July 1934, TNA AN450 178/3, 2.
38. *Ibid.*, 1.
39. *Ibid.*, 2.
40. Ag PC Lake Province to ChfSec, 14 April 1934.
41. DMSS to PC Tabora, 22 February 1927, TNA 10721 Vol.1.
42. SecMins, 27 June 1927, TNA 10721 Vol.1.
43. Ag DMSS to ChfSec, 7 September 1927, TNA 10721 Vol.1.
44. Ag DMSS to ChfSec, 7 September 1927, TNA 10721 Vol.1.
45. SecMins, DMSS, 4 December 1933, TNA AN450 178/3.
46. M. Blacklock, 'Health services for women and children', *Health and Empire*, 1 (1934), 31.
47. Archdeacon John Briggs, CMS, 20 July 1934, TNA AN450 178/3, 3.
48. SecMins, 30 March 1936, TNA 10834.
49. *Ibid.*
50. *Ibid.*
51. Interview with Dr Leader Stirling, Dar es Salaam, January 2000.

9

Curing Bodies to Rescue Souls: Health in Capuchin's Missionary Strategy in Eritrea, 1894–1935

Uoldelul Chelati Dirar

The chapter focuses on the role of health care in the missionary practice of Capuchins in Eritrea between 1894 and 1935. Their activity in this field is analysed with regard to its role in proselytising activities as well as in its interaction with local notions of health, disease and the body. On one side it is shown how, in conformity to a wider mission strategy, curing diseases was perceived as instrumental in acquiring new converts. On the other side it is discussed how little knowledge missionaries had of local medical traditions and how this knowledge was often flawed by stereotypes and prejudices.

Indigenous Christianity and missionaries

The region corresponding to the present state of Eritrea, the youngest African nation, has a very long history of missionary endeavours that goes back to the early contacts with Jesuits missionaries in the sixteenth century.[1] The continuity of this interest is also shown by a copious literature of travel[2] – sometimes of a highly imaginative nature[3] – that was kept alive also by an ancient tradition of pilgrimages of Orthodox monks to the main centres of Christianity.[4] Two main factors contributed to determine this strong missionary attraction to the region. On one side, the existence in the region, since the fourth century, of a lively autochthonous Christian tradition[5] and, on the other side, the strategic location of Eritrea and the Horn of Africa, which made it a potential gateway for further missionary penetration into Central Africa.[6] The ancient local Christian tradition was expected to provide a good platform for an easier evangelisation of Africa. In fact, missionaries believed that due to the common monotheist and biblical background, the followers of the Christian orthodox tradition could easily be converted either to Catholicism or to Protestantism. According to Catholic missionaries it was a matter of bringing back what they defined alternatively as heretics or lost brothers to the original pure *Ecclesia*.[7] On the

Protestant side the aim was to reform the Orthodox tradition, and this was expected to be achieved facilitating access to the Holy Testament by translating it into vernacular languages.[8] Both missionary groups perceived the conversion of Orthodoxes as a crucial step in the further spreading of Christianity in Africa. From this point of view the similarity of perceptions on both Catholic and Protestant side with regard to the missionary potential of the region is quite striking.[9] Both also perceived medicine as being of instrumental value in forging the first contact with the indigenous population and in obtaining their sympathetic reception.

At the same time, missionary activities in the region created a fascinating contradiction that does not appear to have much troubled either the missionaries in the field or their authorities in the metropolis, but which, to a certain extent, helps to make the Eritrean and Ethiopian cases peculiar in the history of Christian missionary endeavours in Africa. This was the anomaly of missionaries working among people whose conversion to Christianity dated back to the Apostolic period.[10] This contradiction left its mark on missionary activity in the region since early Jesuit endeavour in the sixteenth century and it helps to explain the relatively limited success of missionary penetration in the region.

This paper will focus on the role and use of health in the missionary practice of Capuchin fathers in Eritrea between 1894 and 1935. Priority has been given to Capuchin fathers because to extend it also to Protestant missionaries would have enlarged the analytical spectrum excessively and made the paper too general. The analysis of the activity of the Capuchins, who were Italian missionaries in an Italian colony, also provides an opportunity to analyse the interaction between colonial authorities and Christian missions in the domain of health. The rationale for choosing the period 1894–1935 as the chronological span of the present paper lies in the fact that, on one side, 1894 marked the arrival and official beginning of Capuchin activities in Eritrea, following the expulsion of the Lazarist fathers. This was an important development of missionaries activities in Eritrea as it meant the end of the presence of the French-based Congrégation de la Mission of St Vincent de Paul, better known as Lazarists, and the 'nationalisation' – in the sense of Italianisation – of Catholic missions in Eritrea.[11] On the other side the year 1935 is also a crucial date, as although it did not represent the end of Capuchins presence in Eritrea, it saw a radical change in Italian colonial policies that had a strong impact on health policy. The main factor in this was the fascist invasion of Ethiopia, which led to a substantial change in Italian colonial strategy in the region. This change can be noticed in the more active and organic involvement of the colonial state in all aspects of social policies, including in the health sector. After a brief summary of the main medical traditions and practices in pre-colonial society, the paper will deal with Capuchins' medical theories and practices in Eritrea and with their interaction with pre-existing local traditions.

Health, healing and medicine in pre-colonial society

There has been little historical research on nineteenth century's concepts of health and medicine in the region that corresponds to the present state of Eritrea. This is partially due to the fact that most of the relevant literature tended to focus on the Christian orthodox tradition of the Abyssinian highlands paying little attention to non-Christian areas. This is to a great extent the legacy of the general attitude of the so-called Ethiopicist scholarly tradition,[12] which tended to emphasise the written tradition of the region marginalising, at the same time, those cultures which were not inscribed into this tradition. It is, therefore, important to define pre-colonial medical knowledge and practice in Eritrea.

In the pre-colonial period it is possible to identify three main medical traditions which are: the Christian Orthodox, the Islamic, and a set of different traditions which I shall provisionally indicate as 'others'. It is, however, important to emphasise that this classification reflects more a need for clarity in the present study rather than a set of clear-cut distinctions that existed at that time. In people's daily lives the boundaries among those three traditions tended, and still tend, to be much more fluid and porous than such a classification would suggest. As discussed by many authors, popular choices in matters of therapies and therapists have a degree of creativity and flexibility that frequently transcend religious, ethnic or linguistic identities. Moreover, those choices have never been bounded by colonial administrative or cultural boundaries. In fact, as a rule, effectiveness and availability are the two main criteria that influence people's choice.[13] As a rule, effectiveness and availability are the two main criteria that influence choices.[14]

In this section there will be a broad description of indigenous concepts of health, healing, and therapy in the years immediately before the coming of missionaries to the region. Being mainly a broad sketch of pre-colonial local medical traditions, there will not be a discussion of complex issues such as changes in local therapeutic systems, nor transformations in local medical taxonomies, all of which would require a deeper diachronic perspective.[15]

The Christian tradition

With regard to the Christian tradition, Eritrea undoubtedly shares many aspects of the broader Abyssinian Christian tradition.[16] There was a commonality in religious and medical training, for although local churches and monasteries provided a basic education in literacy and a broad familiarity with religious literature, the only place where people could obtain a higher education was in Central Ethiopia. The town of Gondar was the main centre of Christian religious learning in the region where learned religious people as well as aspiring students used to gather.[17]

In the Christian society of the Abyssinian highlands the Church had a central role in defining and implementing social norms as well as in regulating the flow of daily life. Health and medicine belonged to this domain. Therefore, a preliminary step is the definition of health and medicine in this context, a definition that cannot be separated from environmental factors. In fact, in the climatically harsh and resource-poor environment of northeast Africa the Church played a crucial regulative role in determining working rhythms[18] and food-consumption, through the introduction of a strict religious calendar.[19] In this calendar a central religious as well as 'medical' practice was fasting, which could be considered as a local cultural marker reflecting the need to introduce some standard social behaviours in order to cope with extremely harsh environmental conditions.[20]

With regard to health and medicine the local Christian orthodox tradition had developed a very complex and sophisticated tradition in which the medical and religious dimensions were intertwined. In this context religion provided both the cultural framework for the definition of health and disease as well as the social actors in charge of curing and healing. This tradition developed a holistic approach based on the perception that health was embedded in a sound religious and social order and that disease was a perturbation of it. Moving from those assumptions it is possible to identify two levels in the local Christian medical tradition: aetiology and therapy. At an aetiological level disease is considered as an expression of disorder in the complex network of relations between individual and group, living and dead, human and divine which concurs with the definition of what we can tentatively and inadequately define as social order. Fetching from a wide and rich cultural tradition inclusive of Hellenistic, Judaic, and Arab contributions,[21] the definition of this order is based on the representation of a mythical past where, at the beginning, humans and spirits co-existed and interacted peacefully.[22] This idyllic order has been disrupted by human greed and lust. As a result, the original harmony has been substituted by hostility and anger and nowadays the only relation between the two is a negative one and sickness is the metaphoric as well as real locus of this encounter. Referring to Biblical passages,[23] the local Christian tradition identifies as a crucial factor for the development of this pattern of disorder the revelation of the art of writing to human beings by corrupted angels. Those former angels, now demons, used to strike in disguised form and the only protection against them is the use of talismans and prayers.[24]

Apart from very few diseases such as skin ailments and gonorrhoea which could be easily detected and cured at a purely pharmacological level,[25] the majority of illnesses were tackled by traditional aetiology at a dual level: the level of soul and the level of body. In this context, aetiology requires special expertise and a certain degree of specialisation. Having said that, therapy remains a social and collective exercise that involves the whole community to which the sick person belongs. In fact, if sickness is the locus of encounter between humans and demons or fallen angels, the triggering factor in attracting the demon's strike ultimately has to be found in the behaviour of the sick person within his community, which might have engendered irritation in some of its real or disguised members. Arguments in the market, rows about land, interrupting a spirit's siesta when fetching water, walking through the village in a provocative way, could all be causes for provoking a hidden demon. With the spectrum of diseases so ample and difficult to identify, specialisation was required and patients were recommended to make recourse to more than a 'practitioner.' However, in this holistic approach the quest for symptoms, though undertaken by the expert, involved the whole community that, along with observations, comments, and recollection of details of the social life of the victim, all contributed in the aetiologic enquiry.

When symptoms were identified the therapy began, involving a dual and parallel process aimed at healing the soul and curing the body. The therapeutic moment was probably the event that revealed the complexity of the cultural and social praxis underlying the concept of health, disease, and medicine in this tradition. Healing the souls was a spiritual process based on the use of images and words. Behind this practice there was the assumption that fallen angels, by revealing the art of writing to human beings, had caused the original rupture of harmony between human beings and spirits. The ultimate factor in creating disorder and re-establishing order has, therefore, to be found in the art of naming.

Names in fact, were considered to be an integral part of human beings and as such they could be the privileged target of negative forces through the evil eye (or *buda*), charming, or other devious practices.[26] For that reason when baptised, individuals were given two names, a public one and a secret one, which was only known to the closest members of the community.[27] Similarly, the agents of the invisible world were also believed to have their own secret names. By knowing this name, the evil that demons generate could be restrained. As a form of naming associated with writing, this special healing power was attributed to *däbtäras*, learned people trained in religious tradition but not fully fledged priests.[28]

Däbtäras, thanks to their mastery of writing and their religious education, were assumed to be able to see spirits and consequently have the power to move in that grey area created by the disruption of the original harmony between humans and spirits. *Däbtäras* acted as if inspired and assisted by God in their practice. This special protection enable them, to see spirits, identify them and neutralise their malign power by naming them. To this end they used to produce two kind of protective devices, namely books containing collections of protective prayers,[29] and a wide range of talismans and amulets. The first were produced for literate customers, while the second were for the majority of illiterate or semi-literate customers. Both books of protection and talismans were based on the principle that naming has a healing power. Through the listing and graphic representation of the names of God and of demons, *däbtäras* provided spiritual protection to the sick from the disruptive infiltration of demons.

Däbtäras were nevertheless often in an ambiguous position, as there was a fine and poorly defined line between ecclesiastical approval and condemnation. The Church acknowledged the therapeutic value of reading the Gospel and the *Psalms of David* when washing a sick person with holy water. It also tolerated reading about lives of saints or the *Homilies* of Michael. However, it disapproved of, though did not openly condemn, reciting the names of God for healing purposes and the resort to divinatory techniques.[30] Parallel and organic to the healing of souls was the cure of bodies. *Däbtäras* also had a rich and longstanding knowledge of herbalism, based in part on local experience and in part on medical treatises inspired by the Greek–Arab medical tradition – in particular the *Canon* of Avicenna, the *Thesaurus* of al-Khwarizmi, and the medical treaty of 'Ali ibn Rabbân.[31] This medical tradition, which had been codified in a written form since the fifteenth century, covered a wide spectrum of diseases ranging from migraine, cardiovascular, and respiratory problems to insomnia, amnesia, evil eye, anxiety, insanity, and spirit possession.

A crucial issue still not tackled by scholars dealing with the social history of the region is the level of social sharing of this complex, medical knowledge. In fact, as discussed by Helen Lambert with regard to Rajasthani popular therapeutics, there is a general tendency to assume that when there are complex and possibly written medical traditions, they are easily and uniformly available to the whole population.[32] However, in a context marked by a strong hegemony of orality over literacy, it remains to be assessed how much of this rich codified tradition was really accessible to the majority of the population and how much popular medicine relied rather on alternative and probably syncretistic practices.[33]

Cases of possession or problems related to mental diseases represent the best example of the complexity of the aetiological and therapeutic approach of popular medicine. In fact, the wide range of diseases that, for sake of brevity I will define as mental diseases, are normally tackled with a multifaceted approach based on the social identification of the source of unbalance. As mentioned earlier, this process involves not only patients but also their families and local communities at large. Once the problem has been identified, the therapeutic intervention depends on the complexity of the case.

The easiest cases are normally treated with a combination of pharmacological and thermal treatments. Many springs or thermal waters – known as *may chelot* – are believed to have therapeutic power. Normally, those springs are associated with the name of a famous local saint celebrated for his thaumaturgic powers. In Eritrea some fifty holy waters were in use till recent time and each of them was renowned for a specific therapeutic power.[34] What is worth mentioning is that the resort to these springs was not a prerogative of Christians alone; it was common to have Muslims enjoying their therapeutic benefits by simply renaming them in honour of a Muslim holy man.[35]

Another more complex aspect of healing, which to a certain extent includes many of the themes discussed up to now is associated with the tradition of *zar*, a tradition which is shared with different local variations through the whole of north-east Africa[36] and part of the Middle East.[37] *Zar*, which will not be discussed here in detail,[38] can be summarily described as a complex ritual of healing marked by possession often associated with phenomena of glossolalia, and based on a practice of ritual dances and singing. This ritual involves specialised healers, the sick person and its community, and imply also a codified set of actions, which has led scholars to talk in terms of a theatrical component.[39] Also, in the case of *zar* it has to be emphasised again, that this ritual can be defined as cross-religious as it involves both Christians and Muslims.

The Islamic tradition

Islam in Eritrea has a very long local presence that dates back to the early years of the Prophet Muhammad's preaching.[40] However, one of the strongest impulses to the Islamisation of Eritrea came much later during the nineteenth century, with the Egyptian penetration of the region and the spread of brotherhoods such as the Mirghaniyya and Qadiriyya from the Middle East.[41] The brotherhoods in particular encouraged the development of an esoteric form of religious practice – quite far from orthodox Islam – which affected also the approach to the issue of health and healing.[42] In fact, as mentioned earlier with regard to the Christian medical tradition, it is difficult to assess how much of the highly sophisticated Islamic medical tradition actually reached Islamic communities in the region. In Eritrea, similarly to the case of Hausaland discussed by Ismail H. Abdallah,[43] nineteenth century sources shows that little of that prestigious tradition became an actual part of a shared medical knowledge in the region. Islamic medical practices, rather than being based on the humoral tradition of the

Dar al-Islam, relied on the assumption that supernatural elements were to be considered the main actors both in diagnostic and healing process. Paradoxically it is possible to say that the main beneficiary of the 'official' Islamic medical tradition has been the Christian Orthodox society of the Abyssinian highlands, which, through translations from Arabic, incorporated it into its medical corpus.[44] With regard to the concept of health and the practice of medicine among Muslim communities, European sources of the nineteenth century report of a common use of amulets (*higiâb*) made with passages from the Holy Quran written on small pieces of parchment kept in leather boxes.[45] Those small amulets used to be worn on the arms or around the neck, never being removed. Again, this reveals a strong belief in the curative and protective power of words, being in this case sentences from the Holy Quran. In a society marked by the prevalence of orality, with a limited level of literacy, this practice is also evidence of a persistent perception of a 'magic' relation between writing and naming. Other common practices were divinatory rituals (*istikhâra*)[46] supported by an ancient local herbalist tradition, often shared with the Christian population.

Key personalities deputed to the application and transmission of this social knowledge for medical purpose were the *sheikh* (community or spiritual authority) or the *faqîh* (expert of Islamic jurisprudence or *fiq*). They were frequently revered particularly after their deaths, with their tombs becoming places of pilgrimage.[47] In fact, many of those *shekhs* were believed to have thaumaturgic powers due to their special holy spiritual status (*barâka*). However, what is striking in the literature of the nineteenth century is the fact that while such beliefs and practices were distant from or marginal to 'official' Islamic devotional practices, they tended to be shared by the population at large and had also many elements in common with Christian practices.[48]

Other medical systems

Certain communities, such as the Kunama and the Nara, were relatively peripheral to the main tradition of Abyssinian highlands. They lived in a different region, and they were outside the Semitic tradition linguistically and culturally. Both populations lacked a written tradition, and for this reason their religious beliefs and practices tended to be confined by the European regard to an area of autochthonous tradition that colonial and missionaries sources were inclined to classify generically and mistakenly as animist.[49] Nevertheless, both societies had and still have a highly developed herbalist tradition covering a wide range of illnesses. Unfortunately, we are limited in our discussion of those traditions by the fact that little ethnomedical investigation has been done so far in those societies, so that we still depend for our knowledge on the strongly biased colonial literature or on few, equally biased missionary sources.[50] It is nevertheless clear that these people had a fluid and pragmatic approach towards healing that allowed them to shift between different medical systems regardless of religious, regional, or economic identities.

Finally, when discussing issues of health and healing in the Horn of Africa in the nineteenth century, it is important to take into account the role played by political instability, warfare, and ecological imbalance in this region. A devastating sequence of conflicts, epidemics and famine ravaged the region through the second half of the century and into the early years of the twentieth century, leading to massive depopulation and to the dislocation of entire communities.[51] As will be discussed later, all those major troubles also had a direct impact on the very concept of health and healing, and affected missionary medical work in the region. In fact, often the main 'disease' was hunger and the main therapy or *materia medica* was food.

Missionary theory and praxis

It is in this complex and often hostile environment that both Catholics and Protestants competed fiercely and with different fortunes to establish missionary stations. Health issues played an important role in this competition, providing both an opportunity to offer free services to the neophytes as well as a powerful instrument of proselytism among the indigenous population. From this point of view the Eritrean experience falls into the paradigm developed by Megan Vaughan when she suggests that missionary doctors competed with local medicine in an effort to transform local societies, challenging them in one of their most vital aspects, the concept of body, health, and sin.[52] However, in the Eritrean case there is little evidence that this was done consciously and I would rather suggest that this relation might be defined in terms of an unconscious competition. In fact, as I will discuss in this section, on one side, health was considered as an area where missionaries could easily attract and contact local populations and from that point start their proselytising mission. On the other side, in spite of the admitted relevance of health and medicine as tools for proselytism, there is little evidence that missionaries made any real effort to understand the cultural complexity underlying local concepts of health, medicine and body.

Missionaries, both Protestant and Catholic, had engaged in healing from the inception of their activity in this region. The German Lutheran Peter Heiling, the first Protestant missionary to visit this region in the seventeenth century – is reported to have practised medicine at the royal court of Gondar,[53] and other missionaries such as Samuel Gobat and Johannes Ludwig Krapf of the Church Missionary Society obtained considerable success through their medical activity.[54] Similarly, the first Catholic missionary congregation active in the region in the nineteenth century – the Congrégation de la Mission or Lazarist Fathers – gave frequent medical assistance, and by the 1880s – through the services of nuns of the order of the Sisters of Charity – ran two dispensaries in the towns of Keren and Massawa.[55]

However, for the period covered by this paper the dominant missionary presence in Eritrea was that of Capuchin fathers. Their presence was strongly supported by the Italian government and by some representatives of the Italian Catholic intelligentsia, which was not at ease with the presence in the colony of missionaries of other nationalities as they were suspected of acting as agents of their respective governments.[56] For this reason, in 1894, the French Lazarists were expelled and the Protestant presence, which by this time had switched to the Swedish-based Evangeliska Fosterlands-Stifelsen – better known in Eritrea as the Swedish Evangelical Mission (SEM) – was increasingly marginalised. The latter were finally expelled in 1935.[57]

In discussing the medical work of the Capuchins it is crucial to identify the beneficiaries of their medical treatment as well as the approach they had to the organisation of health services. At the beginning of their presence in Eritrea there were three main beneficiaries: Italian settlers, Italian soldiers, and Eritrean communities. The initial Italian colonial plan to make of Eritrea a colony of settlers led to the establishment of a small community of Italian settlers scattered over the highlands. By this means, and through the use of large subsidies, the Italian state sought to divert the endemic flow of Italian immigrants traditionally attracted by the Americas or Australia to a territory under the political and economic control of the Italian state.[58] This plan did not enjoy the full support of important segments of the Italian entrepreneurial sector, which envisaged the development of a capitalist-oriented colonial agriculture.[59] In the end, the settlers, who were prevalently from the poorest rural areas of Italy, were sent to Eritrea without adequate planning and, moreover, with very few resources. The missionaries, in consequence, often beside their spiritual services also had to provide medical assistance to the settlers, at least in term of basic treatments.[60]

The army provided the other major Italian presence in Eritrea. Though Italian soldiers had their own medical facilities, the protracted and intense war between Italy and Ethiopia in the years 1894–7 saw a massive involvement of missionaries in spiritual and medical work amongst wounded Italian soldiers. This work reached its height with the Italian defeat at Adwa in March 1896, in which the Italian army was annihilated by the Ethiopian Army led by Emperor Menelik, with thousands of casualties on both sides.[61] In this context, the efforts of the missionaries were not motivated only by compassion or national solidarity, but were aimed also at using medicine as an opportunity to contact and possibly redeem a segment of the Italian population that was traditionally pervaded by anticlerical and even atheistic feelings.[62] Through the dispensation – often surreptitiously administered – of the extreme unction to the moribunds or through the patient and careful assistance to the wounded, Capuchin missionaries tried systematically to re-claim lost Italian souls to their flock.[63]

The last and, for the sake of this presentation, more important section of the population that was the object of missionary medical attention were the Eritreans themselves. In the period from 1894 to the close of the first decade of the twentieth century, there were many obstacles to such work and Capuchins were faced with a situation of great political and social instability. There were repeated droughts, protracted warfare, and internal anti-colonial rebellions, all of which made of Eritrea an unsafe territory for missionaries, so that their work was discontinuous and precarious.[64] There were also material and human constraints on their activity. Because of this, their medical work was extemporary and lacking any organic link with their global missionary strategy. There were no clear instructions to missionaries to undergo medical training or to carry medicines with them, and such work appears to have relied on the initiative of individual missionaries. Moreover, the absence of reliable statistical data makes it hard to assess its impact on the region. Lastly but not least, it has also to be stressed that in those years personal health was in itself a 'mysterious intangible enemy'[65] for the missionaries, as malaria, sunstroke, and other maladies claimed the life of many of them and forced many others into premature retirement. In particular a heavy toll in missionary lives had to be paid to keep operational their stations of Assab on the Red Sea, and Barentu in the western lowlands, which were notorious for their insalubrious climate. All of this prevented any substantial gains for the Capuchins in the early years of their presence in Eritrea.[66]

A substantial change can be noticed starting from 1912 when Monsignor Carrara took over the leadership of the Capuchin mission in Eritrea. He organised the mission in a more structured way and launched a more aggressive proselytising campaign. This included a more systematic approach towards medical work.[67] Beside a renewed and more intense missionary effort among the Orthodox and Islamic communities, a particular attention was now given to populations such as Kunama, Blin, and Mensa', which were relatively more peripheral with regard to both traditional highlands and colonial centres of power. I have already discussed the religious and social status of the Kunama in the nineteenth century. The case of Blin and Mensa' is much more obscure and complex. Originally Christian, they had been alienated by the political instability and warfare of the nineteenth century, and as a result they had either converted to Islam or maintained a vague and superficial Christian practice, in the process losing much of their original Christian identity.[68]

The main missionary efforts of the early twentieth century focused on those populations, which is also a sign of the fact that the consolidation of colonial rule and the 'normalisation' of the territory were reducing missionaries' chances to gain a hold among the Christian Orthodox and the Islamic segment of the population.[69] Moreover, the missionary literature of those years shows clearly that those populations, and particularly the Kunama, as will be discussed later, were perceived as the embodiment of the perfect stereotype of missionary expectation. However, in a broader perspective, this impressive Catholic missionary revival cannot be understood properly without connecting it to the papacy of Pope Pius XI (1922–39),[70] who had ignited a season of missionary zeal in which, for the first time in the Catholic tradition, the issue of medical missions was discussed as a structural component of missionary endeavours. In his famous encyclical *Rerum ecclesiae*, published on 28 February 1926, the Pope sanctioned the moral duty of healing as a key component of missionary evangelical efforts. A direct result of this new attitude toward missions – and medical missions in particular – can be seen in the fact that in those years, for the first time, medical manuals specifically designed for missionaries were published,[71] medical courses tailored for missionaries were opened,[72] and also detailed statistical studies on the impact of diseases and morbidity on missionary activities were carried out.[73] These new efforts to revivify Christianity through missions and medicine were publicised through media events, such as the impressive Missionary Vatican Exhibition that was held in Rome in 1925 to celebrate the Jubilee, in which a whole section was dedicated to medical issues, with the declared aim of arising missionary enthusiasm among visitors either in terms of recruitment or financial support.[74]

A very interesting source that sheds light on the unfolding of those events in the Eritrean context is the by-weekly missionary magazine *Annali Francescani*, published in Italy and widely distributed in parishes and other Franciscan networks with the aim of disseminating information about Franciscan missionary endeavours and, ultimately, to raise financial support from its readers.[75] Through this magazine it is possible to follow the main lines of missionaries activities in Eritrea and also to reconstruct missionaries' perception of their fieldwork. It is significant that one of the main subjects of reports coming from Eritrea in those years was the Kunama population. In missionaries' perception the Kunamas seemed to fit into the stereotypes of the backward, hopeless, and eternally childish African tribe waiting for missionary enlightenment.[76] To win the Kunama to the Catholic flock, missionaries adopted a strategy of itinerant proselytism by touring from their stations, from village to village. In this effort, medical assistance was clearly defined as the key instrument in contacting those populations and winning their hearts. To this end, instructions were given to missionaries to always carry with them basic medicines for the most common diseases such as malaria, eyes diseases, and skin infections.[77] In fact, these illnesses were relatively easy to cure both in terms of medical skills and pharmacological and medical equipment and such treatments were expected to have a strong impact on the Eritrean population.

Contemporary sources reveal a fierce struggle unfolding among Capuchins, Protestants and Muslims to win the allegiance of the few remaining potential proselytes, with health becoming one of the main areas of this competition. Capuchin missionary sources of those years clearly state the urgency of providing more qualified medical assistance in order to contain the advance of rival groups. The Swedish missions in particular were accused by the Capuchins of taking unfair advantage of their stronger network of financial and logistic support from the motherland.[78] The competition with the Protestants was described in terms of rivalry between cultural systems similar in their common Christian foundation, but divided by different confessions. Ironically enough, Protestants were often vehemently accused of making an instrumental and not genuinely Christian use of their medical services.

The other main rival to Capuchin missionary endeavours in those years appears to have been Islam. Contemporary missionary sources frequently describe Islam in terms of a corrupted and barbarian religion, and accuse it of winning the hearts of the local population resorting to superstitious practices. As an example of this practice missionary often mention the use of amulets and talisman containing short passages from the Holy Qur'an.[79] In the competition with Islam differences were much more marked and no room appears to have been left for any possible conciliation. For complex historical reasons Christian orthodoxes appear to have been marginal in this competition and were not the main target of missionary medical zealotry. This can be partially explained by the fact that in Eritrea, as in the rest of Africa, Christian missionaries considered Islam their fiercest and most dangerous rival.

Missionaries and colonial health

A final point which deserves attention in the discussion of missionary theory and practice of medicine, is their interaction with colonial authorities. Relations between Catholic missionaries and the Italian colonial administration were never straightforward, due to the projection in the colony of the traditional rivalry between State and Church in the Italian liberal state.[80] Many colonial civil servants had strong liberal and secular convictions,[81] which in some cases could give room to openly anticlerical attitudes. This generated a pattern of uneasy relations marked by repeated attempts, on the missionary side, to establish a more organic and structural relation with the colonial administration and an ambiguous series of responses by the administration.[82] This pattern can be detected also in the field of medicine. In fact, according to the Royal Decree of 30 December 1909, note 845,[83] nobody was allowed to practice medicine in the colony if not provided with a formal medical training, which had to be certified officially. This provision applied to areas in which medical facilities provided by the colonial medical service were available, which meant all main urban centres and many villages. However, the text was ambiguous and appeared to have been devised mainly to protect the medical rights of European patients living in the colony rather than of the entire population. A further element of ambiguity was introduced by article 391 of the same law, which called for some degree of respect for indigenous medical traditions, so far as they were not patently detrimental to the maintenance of health and hygiene, and with the assumption that such remedies were availed of only by indigenous patients. At the same time, colonial legislation – at least in its formal expression – appeared to be conscious of the complexity of medical systems present in the colony and it was also quite careful in delineating clear boundaries for areas of medical intervention along racial or, more subtly, 'cultural' divides. In this respect, missionary medical services were sanctioned primarily as a frontier activity in peripheral areas where the colonial administration had not established its own hospitals or clinics. Otherwise, due also to the lack of a consolidated tradition of Catholic medical missions in the colony, missionaries were allowed to operate in colonial medical institutions only as nurses – an area of work associated in particular with Catholic nuns, as was common in Italy at that time.

The predominance of the colonial state over Catholic missionaries in the health sector is revealed also by the amount of medical literature produced by the two institutions in the field of tropical medicine. On the missionary side only two significant publications can be noticed. The first one is a short manual of medicine and surgery for use by missionaries and rural parishes, published in 1924.[84] The second is a more ambitious treaty of tropical medicine for missionaries which, however, was published only in the post-colonial period, in 1957.[85] On the other side, the massive involvement of the colonial state in the health sector is paralleled by an impressive scientific production, which is attested by the publication of ten different journals and bulletins and 197 articles and monographs dealing with tropical medicine.[86] Two aspects deserve particular attention in those publications. The first is the fact that it is possible to notice a direct correlation between the increase in the Italian population in the colony and the growth of interest in medical issue. Evidence of this is the fact that 135 of the above-mentioned 197 scientific contributions were published between 1930 and 1938 when there was renewed fascist interest in colonial expansion, due to the military preparation for the impending fascist invasion of Ethiopia in 1935, and the subsequent massive effort for the occupation and colonisation of the territory. This all led to an impressive increment of the presence of Italians in the region. Secondly, in the colonial medical literature we can detect an attempt to co-opt the local population in the colonial medical discourse. This is reflected also in the publication of bilingual manuals aimed at the technical and 'ideological' training of Eritreans in the health sector, though always in a subordinate position, in observance to the principles of racial prestige.[87]

Apart from addressing medical issues according to European aetiological perspectives, these manuals also pursued two other important goals. First, they attempted to develop through a translation in Tigrinya – one of the most widely spoken Eritrean languages – an indigenous medical vocabulary reflecting European concepts of body and health. In this, they sought to redefine indigenous perceptions and representations semiologically and, therefore, structurally. This literature included also a short but ideologically dense introductory section, which openly called for the abandonment of local medical practices and which urged Eritrean nursing personnel to act as propagators of civilisation and progress among their fellow compatriots.[88] This call for a medical crusade was made even more explicit in the manuals compiled for Eritrean midwives in which special emphasis was placed on the 'privileged' role that women were expected to play in society by procreating and raising children.[89] Colonial medical literature is openly nurtured by a strong feeling of superiority and by a clear perception of medicine not only as a branch of sciences but also as a cultural force through which to assert European superiority over colonised populations.[90] However, what is less evident but rather expressed in form of nuance is the fact that this dismissive feeling of superiority seems to refer also to missionary medical practices which both legal regulations and sundry contemporary sources tend to define as amateur medicine.

Missionary education and health

The predominant role of the colonial state in the health sector was partially balanced by the fact that missionaries were allowed, and to certain extent invited, to play a major role in the education of Eritreans. In fact, until the coming of Fascism, budgetary constraints, together with a deliberated refusal to allow the formation of an educated local élite, had led to a neglect in substantial investments in this sphere by the Italian colonial state. This area was left as a prerogative of Catholic missionaries who designed the curricula, provided the teaching staff, and also drafted the teaching material.[91] Therefore, it is in the domain of education that it is possible to detect another significant dimension of missionary interaction with the colonial state in the field of health. In fact, all the teaching material drafted by the Capuchin missionaries, between 1912 and 1939 included a section on hygiene and basic health notions, and one on superstitions. Drafted both in Italian and in Tigrinya, these materials deserve particular attention not only from an educational perspective, but also as part of the campaign launched by Capuchins to win souls by curing bodies. In them, we find clearly expressed, a structured missionary challenge to local belief systems and therapeutic practices.

Firstly, the section of these manuals dealing with hygiene and health classified diseases according to the aseptic medical concepts of the Western tradition. Banal diseases like cough or flu were deliberately listed together with other more complex, and in the local perception, more frightening and culturally connotated maladies such as epilepsy, fainting, or convulsions. A neutral scientific description, together with basic remedies, was provided for each of these diseases. Secondly, the textbooks sought to substitute local concepts and praxis of health and medicine with European ones. This attitude was most evident in the section on hygiene, which was generally marked by a strong eugenic discourse, where hygiene was described as:

> [T]he science which teaches us how to keep ourselves healthy. Health is a treasure, but to maintain it we have to fight against filth. Filth is the source not only of physical diseases but also of moral diseases; it is clear evidence of rudeness and incivility. The civilisation of peoples is rooted in cleanliness. Therefore children must learn to love cleanliness.[92]

However, in suggesting behavioural models those manuals were also generating unsolvable contradictions. In fact, the main emphasis in the definition of hygiene was on the centrality of healthy living spaces, more precisely of houses defined along parameters and standards unlikely to be met by the majority of the Eritrean population, which was mainly destitute and either living in rural areas or squeezed into segregated urban spaces.[93] To this regard, there seems to be some similarities between the eugenic concept of urban space theorised and partially implemented by Italian colonial authorities in urban areas and the representation of healthy spaces in mission textbooks. In fact, colonial administrators also tended to represent Eritrean indigenous districts as places that: 'for congenital dirtiness and lack of any sense of hygiene [are] frequently a repository of viral and infectious diseases.'[94]

Some of those themes were already anticipated and embedded in missionary teaching materials by 1916. However, there is an important area where the eugenic discourse developed by the Italian colonial administration in the late 1930s clashed with missionary strategies. In fact, there was tension over the racial regulations that were experimented in the colony from 1936, and introduced as the Racial Laws in 1938, as these discriminated against the offspring of mixed couples – *meticci* in the Italian literature[95] – who represented a privileged field of social and religious intervention for Catholic missionaries, particularly in urban areas.[96]

A second important section of these textbooks – under the heading of 'Errors and Prejudices' – deals with beliefs about the evil eye, charms, and the protective and therapeutic value of amulets. Interesting enough, the main targets of this mission literature were practices attributed primarily to Muslims. One of the textbooks states:

> Amulets, from the Arabic *hamlet* (pendant), are all sorts of objects kept around the neck or on the body that are believed to provide protection against witchcraft, spells and other evils. Those hamlets are particularly common among Mohammedans and they are in the form of stones, rings, pieces of paper and other objects all bearing sentences from the Quran or magic formulas. It is not even worth demonstrating that these things are the result of human credulity and superstition.[97]

It is notable that Orthodox Christians are omitted from such statements, even though they shared similar views and practices. It is also notable that the missionaries presented as examples of superstition notions the alleged bad luck brought by breaking mirrors or scattering salt,[98] popular believes common in Italy but not in Eritrea. In this respect the Capuchin missionaries appear to have been carrying over to their civilising and medical crusades in Eritrea conceptual models and strategies rooted in their experience of struggle against 'paganising' popular culture in their motherland.

The interaction with local cultures

Up to now, the main focus of the discussion has been on indigenous and missionary concepts and practices of medicine as separate phenomena. However, it is important to analyse patterns of creative interaction between the two. This may help us towards a better understanding of crucial issues such as the interpretation and retention by local populations not only of concepts related to health, but also, in a broader perspective, of important Christian dogmas like the resurrection of soul and the definition of sanctity.

On the missionary side, there was a failure to comprehend the complexity of local concepts of health and medicine and a tendency to dismiss them in terms of primitive beliefs and superstition. A sort of cultural blindness prevented any grasp of the dense network of symbolic values that underlay local medical practices. In the case of the Orthodox tradition, there was a shared culture rooted in the Judaic–Christian tradition, with many practices that were echoed in 'unofficial' practices in the Italian countryside. Despite this, the missionary literature seemed largely unconcerned with Orthodox medical practices. The main reason for this attitude lies in the fact that the Orthodox Church was at this time on the defensive, and therefore not seen as a major competitor. Mission propaganda was directed primarily at forces that were seen to constitute the greatest obstacle to the expansion of Catholicism, namely Islam and the so-called 'primitive' religious cultures. Islam was subjected to a particularly violent critique, with its medical practices being stigmatised as backward and also as a source of moral and spiritual corruption. Others were depicted as stereotypical African 'savages'.[99] The Kunama people who, from 1914 onwards, were the object of intense Catholic missionary efforts, were described as 'our poor savages' or generically 'our poor Kunamas'.[100] Missionary activities among them were defined in terms of the:

> [W]ork of redemption from errors and superstitions and an uplift to the first stages of Christian civilisation and also a work of conquest as, otherwise, those poor savage would be continuously lured by Protestants who want to make them sons of Luther and by Muslims who would be happy to make them followers of Muhammad.[101]

The missionaries ridiculed rituals involving possession and trance as cheap stratagems staged by shrewd individuals to get free food from the community and avoid their community work and daily routine.[102] The overall Kunama perception of health and medicine was dismissed in patronising terms as a congeries of childish superstitions.[103]

The Capuchins also misjudged the set of reasons behind popular use of the medical facilities they provided. Their literature is full of triumphant reports of frequent and numerous visits by local people to missionary stations and the enthusiastic gatherings around missionaries during their visits to remote villages. Sick people are reported to have come to them begging for medical treatment, which missionary sources interpreted as evidence of the success of their strategy.[104] However, when these reports are examined carefully, it is evident that the kind of treatments requested and administered were limited predominantly to the treatment of skin infections, extraction of spines, and administration of tablets against malaria or other forms of fever. It appears that in Eritrea, as in other parts of Africa – as is clear from various other studies – mission medicine was preferred to local therapy in a pragmatic and selective way, based on principles of effectiveness, cheapness and a relatively easier availability of missionary medical treatments.[105]

This pragmatism can explain the striking absence of Capuchins' healing intervention from the sphere of mental diseases as well as from the wide range of illnesses that were considered related to a more complex level of intervention, and that normally required the involvement of *däbtäras* or other similar experts. It is apparent that in the more complex and socially connoted aspects of health, Eritreans still resorted to their traditional therapies. Often, the missionaries achieved their greatest success in medical work at times of particular social or economic crises, when the failure or collapse of local mechanisms of crisis-management gave them a comparative advantage. This was true in the case of the famines, droughts, and epidemics that repeatedly ravaged the social landscape of Eritrea in this period. A case in point is the devastation experienced in the years 1918–21 as a result of the combined effect of drought and the long term consequences of the Spanish Influenza which ravaged great a part of the world. Missionary sources reveal clearly that, in that tormented time of devastation and destitution, the very meaning of health and medicine had changed radically. Reports such as those of *Annali francescani* drew an appalling picture of Eritrea, with thousands of starving people in the countryside wandering in search of food, trying to move to urban areas and often collapsing on their way. In this context it appears evident that health was equivalent of nourishment and, consequently 'medical' intervention consisted mainly of providing food to starving people.[106]

On the whole, the missionaries failed to change patterns of belief and gain converts on a large scale through their medical work. On the other side, local communities exploited, quite cleverly, the chances presented by the increased offer of medical services brought by the arrival of missionaries, limiting their level of interaction prevalently to the technical dimension and generally rejecting the religious and proselytising aspect associated with it. From this point of view, again, Eritrea shows a behavioural pattern that confirms Ranger and Arnold's analysis of colonial and missionary medicine in colonial Africa.[107] Evidence of this attitude can be found in many missionary sources. For instance, there are complaints from missionaries stationed in Assab about Afar people who used to send their children to the missionary station to get food or medical treatments and then withdrew them without allowing them to stay in the mission and attend its school. Similarly, a missionary stationed among the Kunama population, reported of his proselytising efforts:

> [T]hey listen to you carefully and they appear doubtful when we say that God does not make rain, provide wheat, or send locusts, but they burst out with laughter when we describe them Hell, which corresponds to saying 'Poor Father, he wants us to have only one woman, wants to prohibit us to go with other [women]'.[108]

Medical man or holy man? The case of Angelico da None

As a conclusion of this discussion on Capuchin missionaries' medical endeavours in Eritrea, I would like to focus on the activity of the Capuchin missionary, Father Angelico da None, which could be considered paradigmatic of the many contradictions described in previous pages. The relevance of this missionary is due to the fact that he was one of the first Capuchin fathers to develop medical work as a central component of his missionary activities. To a certain extent Father Angelico da None embodied and also anticipated the new consciousness of the Catholic church about the relevance of medical missions in missionary strategy, which has been discussed in previous pages.

Born on 6 May 1875 in the village of None (province of Turin) Father Angelico after receiving his religious training, opted for missionary activity and was sent to Eritrea in March 1914. From the very beginning, he insisted on the necessity of providing basic medical training to all missionaries. He himself had some broad knowledge of hygiene, first aid, and pharmacology, due to the fact that his brother owned a pharmacy in the village of None.[109]

In his writings Father Angelico made clear that the theology of *curate infirmos*, which was later elaborated in an organic way by Pope Pius XI, had to be one of the main pillars of missionary proselytising strategies.[110] Medical intervention was described as a privileged ground from which to mount a challenge to both local beliefs and Islam.[111] According to contemporary sources and also his biographers, the success of Father Angelico's missionary strategy in Eritrea – particularly in the area of Keren, where he was based for a long time – was impressive and was openly acknowledged by Catholic authorities and held up to be an example of successful missionary work.[112]

As pointed out with a certain amount of pragmatic cynicism by Father Angelico da None himself, an important element in his success in proselytising was the ravaged situation of Eritrea at that time. Indeed, the crisis of 1918–21 was particularly severe in the area of Keren,[113] where he worked. In a report under the explicit title *Non tutti Mali Vengono per Nuocere* (Not all Evils Come to Harm) Father Angelico openly stated that:

> [T]he famine which has tried our people so hard may, to a certain extent, be defined as a flagellation by God, but at the same time it can be described as

an expression of his mercy, through which he has attracted to himself many souls.[114]

However, the same missionary sources disclose a more complex reality and a wider range of reasons for the success of Father Angelico's missionary exploits. In fact, it appears that more than the display of Western medicine and the provision of food, what really earned the Capuchin father the respect of the Eritrean population was the spread of a belief in the thaumaturgic power of his hands. It seems in certain respects that in the perception of his patients Father Angelico had been incorporated into the model of the holy man of both the Christian and Muslim traditions. This came about as a result of his tireless efforts to help sick and disadvantaged people, and in particular because he was in the habit of placing his hands over the people he was curing.[115] Therefore, his acceptance and success among local communities was due not so much to his status as a Catholic Capuchin missionary but rather to his assimilation into a local therapeutic model. This is confirmed by the way the local chief of the village of Mahelab, *käntiba*[116] Mohamed Bula introduced him to his fellow villagers:

> 'People of Mensa': the Catholic *sheikh* who will cure the plagues and diseases of whoever would like to take advantage of his expertise has arrived from Keren. He will do this for no charge. With my permission he will come here to the village of Mehelab once a month and will stay here for a few hours. He has to be respected as a benefactor of our tribe. This is what we *Kantiba* Mohamed Bula order to you.[117]

In his prominent essay 'The Work of Art in the Age of Mechanical Reproduction', Walter Benjamin, discussing the mutated rules regulating the accessibility to Art in the industrial society through the introduction of serial reproduction, used the metaphor of modern medicine. According to Benjamin, modern medicine, by breaking the aura which surrounded magicians and traditional doctors with an appearance of closeness, has somehow increased the distance between patient and doctor.[118] The case of Father Angelico, I would say, shows an opposite development in which the aura has been re-established through a creative redefinition of Western therapeutic procedures and their reception through their adaptation into a local framework of medical practices. This can be considered as a metaphor of the complex relationship between medical missionary intervention and indigenous medical knowledge.

Notes

1. A recent extremely detailed study on those relations in H. Pennec, *Des Jésuites au Royaume du Prêtre Jean* (Paris: Centre Culturel Calouste Gulbenkian, 2003).
2. C.O. Crawford (ed.), *Ethiopian Itineraries, circa 1400–1524* (Cambridge: Cambridge University Press, 1958); C. Conti Rossini, 'Geografica I. L'Africa orientale in carte arabe dei secoli XII e XII. II Carte Abissine. III Gli itinerari di Alessandro Zorzi', *Rassegna di Studi Etiopici*, iii (1943), 167–99; B. Hirsh, 'Cartographie et Itineraires: Figures Occidentales du Nord de l'Ethiopie aux XV° et XVI° Siecles', Paper presented at the 9th International Conference of Ethiopian Studies, Moscow, August 26–9, 1986
3. An example of this is the myth of the so-called 'Prester John', a Christian king who was allegedly living surrounded by pagans somewhere in Abyssinia. This myth polarised the imaginative attention of generations of European Christians and played a crucial role in arousing missionary interest over the region. On this and similar themes: F. Alvarez (edited by C.F. Beckingham and G.W.B. Huntingford), *The Priester John of the Indies* (Cambridge: Cambridge University Press, 1961); C. Conti Rossini, 'Leggende geografiche Giudaiche del IX Secolo (Il Sefer Eldad)', *Bollettino della Reale Società Geografica Italiana*, ii (1925), 160–90; C.E. Nowell, 'The Historical Prester John', *Speculum*, xxviii, 3 (1953), 1–11; G. Melville, 'Le Prêtre Jean Figure Immaginaire du Roi Sacré', in A. Boureau and C.S. Ingerflom (eds), *La Royauté Sacrée dans le Monde Chrétien, Colloque de Rayaumont, Mars 1989* (Paris: 6, École des Hautes Études en Sciences Sociales, 1992), 81–90.
4. E. Cerulli, *Etiopi in Palestina*, 2 vols (Roma: Libreria dello Stato, 1943–7); R. Lefevre, 'Roma e la Comunità Etiopica di Cipro nei Secoli XV e XVI', *Rassegna di Studi Etiopici*, i (1941), 71–86; R. Lefevre, 'Note su Alcuni Pellegrini Etiopi in Roma al Tempo di Leone X', *Rassegna di Studi Etiopici*, xxi (1964), 16–26; R. Lefevre, 'Presenze Etiopi in Italia prima del Concilio di Firenze del 1439', *Rassegna di Studi Etiopici*, xxiii (1967–8), 5–26; G.S. Khoury, *The History of the Ethiopian Community in the Holy Land from the Time of Emperor Tewodros II till 1974* (Jerusalem: The Ecumenical Institute for Theological Research Tantum, 1983).
5. Sergew Hable Sellase, *Ancient and Medieval Ethiopian History to 1270* (Addis Ababa: Addis Ababa University Press, 1972), 97–105. Please note that for Ethiopian and Eritrean names there is no notion of surname; full names are therefore listed where appropriate.
6. D. Comboni, *Piano per la Rigenerazione dell'Africa proposto da D. Daniele Comboni, Missionario Apostolico dell'Africa Centrale* (Torino: Falletti, 1864); J.L. Krapf, *Travels, Researches, and Missionary Labours, during an Eighteen Years Residence in Eastern Africa* (London: Trübner, 1860), 24.

7. G. Sapeto, *Viaggio e Missione Cattolica fra i Mensâ i Bogos e gli Habab con un Cenno Biografico e Storico dell'Abissinia* (Roma: Sacra Congregatione Propaganda Fide, 1857), 260
8. G. Aren, *Evangelical Pioneers in Ethiopia* (Stockholm: EFS, 1978), 42–4.
9. Uoldelul Chelati Dirar, 'The Nile as a Gateway for Missionary Activity in Abyssinia', in H. Erlich and I. Gershoni (eds), *The Nile: Histories, Cultures, Myths* (Boulder: Lynne Rienner, 1999), 139–49.
10. In fact, the earliest spread of Christianity in the region is dated back to the beginning of the fourth century; see Sellase, *op. cit.* (note 5), 24.
11. Lazarist fathers were expelled under allegation of fomenting anti-colonial feelings among the local population. On this episode see: C. Marongiu Buonaiuti, *Politica e Religioni nel Colonialismo Italiano (1882–1941)* (Milano: Giuffrè, 1982), 50–2; C. Betti, 'Missionari Cattolici Francesi e Autorità Italiane in Eritrea negli Anni 1885–1894', *Storia Contemporanea*, v–vi (1985), 905–30; C. Betti, *Missioni e Colonie in Africa Orientale* (Roma: Studium, 2000).
12. According to different scholarly traditions the terms 'Ethiopisants', 'Ethiopicist' and 'Ethiopianists' have been used with more or less interchangeable meaning. On this issue see: B. Tafla, 'Interdependence through Independence: The Challenges of Eritrean Historiography', in H.G. Marcus (ed.), *New Trends in Ethiopian Studies, Papers of the 12th International Conference of Ethiopian Studies, Michigan State University 5–10 September, 1994* (Lawrenceville: Red Sea Press, 1994), 497–514.
13. T.O. Ranger, 'Godly Medicine: The Ambiguities of Medical Mission in Southeast Tanzania, 1900–1945', *Social Science and Medicine*, xvB (1981), 261–78; G. Prins, 'But What was the Disease? The Present State of Health and Healing in African Studies', *Past and Present*, 124 (1989), 159–79; D. Arnold, *Colonizing the Body: State Medicine and Epidemic Disease in Nineteenth-Century India* (Berkeley: University of California Press, 1993), 2–44; M. Vaughan, 'Healing and Curing: Issues in the Social History and Anthropology of Medicine in Africa', *Social History of Medicine*, vii (1994), 283–95.
14. J. Orley, 'Indigenous Concepts of Disease and their Interaction with Scientific Medicine', in E.E. Sabben-Clare, D.J. Bradley, and K. Kirkwood (eds), *Health in Tropical Africa During the Colonial Period: Based on the Proceedings of a Symposium held at New College, Oxford 21–23 March, 1977* (Oxford: Clarendon Press, 1980), 127–34.
15. Key references to this issues remain S. Feierman, 'Change in African Therapeutic Systems', *Social Science and Medicine*, xiiiB (1979), 277–85; and J. Janzen, 'Ideologies and institutions in the precolonial history of Equatorial African therapeutic systems', *Social Science and Medicine*, xiiiB (1979), 317–26.

16. With Abyssinian Christian tradition I am referring here to the broad cultural and religious tradition shared among the prevalently Semitic-speaking Christian populations of the highlands of the present states of Eritrea and Ethiopia.
17. Teshome Wagaw, *Education in Ethiopia* (Ann Arbor: University of Michigan Press, 1979), 11.
18. A. Pollera, *Lo Stato Etiopico e la Sua Chiesa* (Roma: SEAI, 1926), 295–9.
19. Dejene Aredo, 'How Holy are Holidays in Rural Ethiopia? An Enquiry into the Extent to which Saints Days are Observed among Followers of the Orthodox Christian Church', in R. Pankhurst, A. Zekaria and T. Beyene (eds), *Proceedings of the First National Conference of Ethiopian Studies* (Addis Ababa: Institute of Ethiopian Studies, 1990), 165–76.
20. I. Taddia, *L'Eritrea colonia* (Milano: Franco Angeli, 1986), 153; J. McCann, 'History, Drought and Reproduction: Dynamics of Society and Ecology in Northeast Ethiopia', in D.H. Johnson and D.M. Anderson (eds), *The Ecology of Survival: Case Studies from Northeast African History* (London: Lester Crook Academic Publishing, 1988), 283–303.
21. On those influences a key reference remains the work of Claude Sumner: C. Sumner, *Ethiopian Philosophy*, 5 vols (Addis Ababa: Addis Ababa Central Printing Press, 1974–86). On this issue in relation to healing see also J. Mercier, *Ethiopian Magic Scrolls* (New York: George Brazille, 1979), 8–10; R. Cacciapuoti, 'Medicina e Farmacologia Indigena in Etiopia', *Rassegna di Studi Etiopici* i, 3 (1941), 323–29.
22. For this section I draw heavily on the fascinating work of Jacques Mercier, see particularly J. Mercier, *Le Roi Salomon et les Maitres du Regard: Art et Médecine en Ethiopie* (Paris: Editions de la Réunion, 1992); J. Mercier, *Arts that Heals: The Image as Medicine in Ethiopia* (New York: Prestel, 1997).
23. For instance Enoch 15:8; Jubilees 10: 8–9.
24. Mercier, *Arts that Heals, op. cit.* (note 22), 46.
25. Cacciapuoti, *op. cit.* (note 21), 323–29.
26. *Ibid.*
27. Pollera, *op. cit.* (note 18), 315.
28. Ayele Tekle-Haymanot, 'Le Antiche Gerarchie dell'Impero Etiopico', *Sestante*, ii, 1 (1965), 61–7; B. Tafla, 'Titles, Ranks and Offices of the Ethiopian Orthodox Tawahdo Church: A Preliminary Survey', *Internationale Kirchliche Zeitschrift*, lxxvi, 4 (1986), 293–306.
29. S. Strelcyn, *Prieres Magiques Éthiopiennes pour Délier les Charmes* (Warszawa: Panstwowe wydwnictwo naukowe, [Rocznik Orientalistyczny, T. XVIII], 1955).
30. Mercier, *op. cit.* (note 21), 12–13.
31. S. Strelcyn, *Médecine et Plantes d'Ethiopie: Les Traités Médicaux Ethiopiens* (Warszawa: Panstwowe wydawnictwo naukowe, 1968), 22.

32. H. Lambert, 'The Cultural Logic of Indian Medicine: Prognosis and Etiology in Rajasthani Popular Therapeutics', *Social Science and Medicine*, xxxiv, 10 (1992), 1069–76. I am particularly grateful to David Hardiman for bringing to my attention this extremely interesting article.
33. A stimulating discussion of the relationship between the written and oral tradition in the Abyssinian region in D. Crummey, S. Sishagne, and D. Ayana, 'Oral Tradition in a Literate Culture: The Case of Christian Ethiopia', Paper presented to the International Symposium on *Unwritten Testimonies of the African Past*, University of Warsaw, 7–8 November 1989; and J. McCann, 'Literacy, Orality, and Property: Church Documents in Ethiopia', *Journal of Interdisciplinary History*, xxxii, 1 (2001), 81–8.
34. G. Tresca and S. Fameli, 'Appunti di Etnomedicina Eritrea', *Annali di Medicina Navale*, serie I, xxi (1965), 1–40.
35. *Ibid.*
36. I.M. Lewis, *Ecstatic Religion* (Baltimore: Penguin Books, 1971); R.J. Natvig, 'Liminal Rites and Female Symbolism: The Egyptian *Zar* Possession Cult', *Numen*, xxxv (1988), 57–68; J. Boddy, *Wombs and Alien Spirits: Women and the Zar Cult in Northern Sudan* (Madison: The University of Wisconsin Press, 1989); I. Lewis, A. Al-Safi and S. Hurreiz (eds), *Women's Medicine: The Zar-Bori Cult in Africa and Beyond* (Edinburgh: Edinburgh University Press, 1991); S. Kenyon, 'Possession and Change in Eastern Africa', *Anthropological Quarterly*, special edition (spring 1995); G.P. Makris, *Changing Masters: Spirit Possession and Identity Construction among Slave Descendants and Other Subordinates in the Sudan* (Evanston: North Western University Press, 2000).
37. L. Kapteijins and J. Spaulding, 'Women of the *Zâr* and Middle-Class Sensibilities in Colonial Aden', *Sudanic Africa*, v (1994), 7–38; T. Battain, 'Osservazioni sul Rito *Zâr* di Possessione degli Spiriti in Yemen', *Quaderni di Studi Arabi*, xiii (1995), 117–30. For a detailed and updated bibliography of Arabic texts dealing with *zar*, see R.J. Natvig, 'Arabic Writings on *Zâr*', *Sudanic Africa*, ix (1998), 163–78.
38. There is quite a rich literature on the phenomenon of *zar* in Eritrea and Ethiopia. To mention just some of them: M. Griaule, 'Mythes, Croyances, et Coutumes du Bégamder (Abyssinie)', *Journal Asiatique*, ccxii, 1 (1928), 95–6; M. Griaule, *Le Livre de Recettes d'un Dabtara Abyssin* (Paris: Institut d'Ethnologie, 1930); M. Leiris, 'Le Culte des Zars à Gondar (Ethiopie Septentrionale)', *Aethiopica*, ii, 3–4 (1934), 96–103, 125–36; M. Leiris, 'La Croyance au Génies "Zâr" en Ethiopie du Nord', *Journal de Psychologie Normale et Pathologique*, xxxv, 1–2 (1938), 108–25, these articles and others are now collected in M. Leiris, *La Possession et ses Aspects Théâtraux chez les Ethiopiens de Gondar* (Paris: La Sycomore, 1980); C. Conti Rossini, 'I Camminatori sul Fuoco in Etiopia', *Rassegna di Studi Etiopici*, iii, 1 (1943), 94–110; W. Leslau, *Documents Tigrigna (Ethiopien septentrional): Grammaire*

et Textes (Paris: C. Klincksieck, 1941); W. Leslau, 'An Ethiopian Argot of People possessed by a Spirit', *Africa*, iii, 19 (1949), 204–12; A. Young, 'Why Amhara get Kureyna? Sickness and Possession in an Ethiopian *Zar* Cult', *American Ethnologist*, ii (1978), 567–84; H.S. Lewis, 'Spirit Possession in Ethiopia: An Essay in Interpretation', *Proceedings of the Seventh International Conference on Ethiopian Studies, April 1982 Addis Ababa* (Addis Ababa: Institute of Ethiopian Studies, 1984), 419–27; M. Lawson, *Unambiguous Communication: The Pragmatic Function of Zar Possession among the Amhara of Ethiopia* (Chicago: The University of Chicago Press, 1987); E. Pellizzari, *Possession et Thérapie dans la Corne de l'Afrique* (Paris: l'Harmattan, 1997); A. Palmisano, 'Etiopia: Suono e Parola Divina nei Culti *Zar*', *Africa* (Rome), lvii,1 (2002), 471–501.

39. Leiris, *La Possession et ses Aspects*, *ibid.*, 55.
40. J.S. Trimingham, *Islam in Ethiopia* (London: Frank Cass, 1952), 44.
41. E. Cerulli, 'Sull'Islam in Eritrea', *Oriente Moderno*, xxx (1950), 208–15; F. Constantin, *Les Voies de l'Islam en Afrique Orientale* (Paris : Karthala, 1987).
42. Trimingham, *op. cit.* (note 40), 224.
43. I.H. Abdallah, 'Diffusion of Islamic Medicine in Hausaland', in S. Feierman and J.M. Jahnzen (eds), *The Social Basis of Health and Healing in Africa* (Berkeley: Los Angeles University Press, 1992), 177–94; by the same author, a more detailed discussion of this theme in *Islam, Medicine, and Practitioners in Northern Nigeria* (Lewiston: Mellen, 1997).
44. M. Rodinson, *Magie, Medicine et Possession à Gondar* (Paris: Mouton, 1967), 54.
45. W. Munzinger, *Studi sull'Africa Orientale* (Roma: Ministero Affari Esteri, 1890), 94–6, 114–27, 140–2.
46. A. Pollera, *Le Popolazioni Indigene dell'Eritrea* (Bologna: Cappelli, 1927), 256–9.
47. Trimingham, *op. cit.* (note 40), 152–59, 242–7.
48. Munzinger, *op. cit.* (note 45), 250–1.
49. Trimingham, *op.cit.* (note 40), 218.
50. To now, one of the main authority on this subject remains the outdated A. Pollera, *I Baria e i Cunama* (Roma: Reale Società Geografica, 1913), which is often flawed by imprecision, misunderstandings, as well as bias. A poignant discussion of Pollera's ethnographic work can be found in B. Sorgoni, *Etnografia e Colonialismo* (Torino: Bollati Boringhieri, 2001), 54–67. For more updated research on Kunama society during Italian colonialism, see G. Dore, 'Prassi Coloniale e Africanistica: L'Organizzazione Sociale dei Cunama della Colonia Eritrea', Seminario di Etnologia, Materiali di Didattica e di Ricerca, Cà Foscari, Venezia, 1994–5.
51. R. Pankhurst, *The History of Famine and Epidemics in Ethiopia, Prior to the*

Twentieth Century (Addis Ababa: RRC, 1985), 67–9; J. McCann, *People of the Plow* (Madison: University of Wisconsin Press, 1995), 90–3.

52. M. Vaughan, 'Healing and Curing: Issues in the Social History and Anthropology of Medicine in Africa', *Social History of Medicine*, vii (1994), 283–95: 295
53. R. Pankhurst, 'The Beginnings of Modern Medicine in Ethiopia', *Ethiopia Observer*, ix (1965), 114–69.
54. *Ibid.*
55. Ample reports of this activity in the monthly bulletin *Annales de la Congrégation de la Mission* published in Paris by the *Congrégation de la Mission* better known as Lazarist.
56. The very coming of Capuchin fathers in the colony was the result of a long negotiation between the Vatican and the Italian state, which culminated with the expulsion of Lazarist French missionaries in 1895. A detailed reconstruction of this episode in Buonaiuti, *op. cit.*(note 10), 63–6; C. Betti, 'Missionari Cattolici Francesi e Autorità Italiane in Eritrea Negli Anni, 1885–1894', *Storia Contemporanea*, v-vi (1985), 905–30; C. Betti, *Missioni e colonie in Africa Orientale* (Roma: Edizioni Studium, 1999).
57. Buonaiuti, *op. cit.* (note 11), 207–13
58. Yemane Mesghenna, *Italian Colonialism a Case Study of Eritrea (1869–1934)* (Lund: Lund University, 1988), 101–5.
59. O. Confessore, 'La "Rassegna Nazionale" e la Politica Coloniale Crispina (1893–1896)', *Rassegna Storica del Risorgimento*, x (1967), 3–36.
60. R. Rainero, *I Primi Tentativi di Colonizzazione Agricola e di Popolamento dell'Eritrea (1890–1895)* (Milano: Marzorati, 1960), 114.
61. F. da Offeio, *I Cappuccini nella Colonia Eritrea* (Roma: Ss Concezione, 1910), 70–85.
62. On anticlerical feelings among Italian soldiers, see particularly R. Morozzo Della Rocca, *La Fede e la Guerra, Cappellani Militari e Preti Soldati, 1915–1919* (Roma: Studium, 1980).
63. da Offeio, *op. cit.* (note 61), 92.
64. Particularly on anti-colonial resistance see T. Negash, *No Medicine for the Bite of a White Snake: Notes on Nationalism and Resistance in Eritrea 1890–1940* (Uppsala: University of Uppsala, 1986).
65. M. Jennings, 'The Mysterious Intangible Enemy', *Social History of Medicine*, xv, 1 (2002), 65–87.
66. da Offeio, *op. cit.* (note 61), 49.
67. M. da Nembro, *La Missione dei Minori Cappuccini in Eritrea, 1894–1952* (Roma: Istituto Storico Cappuccino, 1953), 284.
68. Pollera, *op. cit.* (note 46), 153–77; K.G. Roden, *Le Tribù dei Mensa: Storia Legge e Costumi* (Stockholm: Evangeliska Fosterlands-Stiftelsens Förlags, 1913); Trimingham, *op. cit.* (note 40), 242.

69. A. da Bergamo, 'Nuove speranze', *Annali Francescani*, lx, 12 (1929), 381–2.
70. U. Bertini, *Pio XI e la Medicina per le Missioni* (Roma: Unione Missionaria del Clero in Italia, 1930), 46.
71. B. Nicola, *Piccolo Manuale di Medicina e Chirurgia Teorico–Pratica: Ad uso dei Missionari – Curati Rurali – Infermieri* (Torino: Marietti, 1924).
72. Bertini, *op. cit.* (note 70), 81–4.
73. M. Boldrini and A. Uggè, *La Mortalità dei Missionari* (Milano: Vita e Pensiero, 1926).
74. Bertini, *op. cit.* (note 70), 48.
75. In the earlier period the bulletin *Annales de la Congrégation de la Mission,* published in Paris by the Lazarist fathers, had a similar purpose.
76. Ezechia da Iseo, 'I selvaggi del Gash-Setit', *Annali Francescani*, lii, 5 (1921), 135–7.
77. da Nembro, *op. cit.* (note 67), 284.
78. Mauro da Leonessa, 'Verità dolorosa', *Annali Francescani*, li, 10 (1920), 233–4.
79. A. da None, 'La Nuova Stazione di Halhal', *Annali Francescani*, lii, 31(1922), 441–3.
80. A very detailed discussion of this issue in Marongiu Buonaiuti, *op. cit.* (note 11), 45–8.
81. A broad discussion of Italian colonial administrators' backgrounds can be found in G. Dore, 'Giovanni Ellero: Un Funzionario nell'Impero d'A.O.I. Amministrare e Conoscere nell'Eritrea e nell'Etiopia d'Età Coloniale', in G. Dore and Uoldelul Chelati Dirar (eds), *Carte Coloniali: I Documenti Italiani del Fondo Ellero* (Torino: Harmattan Italia, 2000), 3–25.
82. Uoldelul Chelati Dirar, 'Church and State Relations in Eritrea: Missionaries and the Development of Colonial Strategies, 1869–1941', *Journal of Modern Italian Studies*, viii, 3 (2003), 401–20
83. *Bullettino Ufficiale della Colonia Eritrea*, 2 (13 January 1910).
84. Nicola, *op. cit.*, (note 71).
85. F. Canova, *Manuale di medicina missionaria* (Torino: SEI, 1957).
86. Detailed bibliographic references to this literature in M. Girolami and G. Scotti, *Contributo dell'Italia alla Conoscenza della Nosografia dell'Africa* (Roma: Istituto poligrafico dello Stato, 1963), 9–20.
87. Examples of this effort are A. Ciotola, *Nozioni di Medicina Pratica ad Uso degli Indigeni (Me'enti deqi Hager nay Zekhone ftun afawes felTet)* (Asmara: Tip. Fioretti, 1932); A. Ciotola, *Nozioni di Ostetricia, Ginecologia e Pediatria, per le Assistenti Levatrici Indigene* (Asmara: Tip. Fioretti, 1934) A similar text had been published in Tigrina in 1928 by the Swedish Mission and it was a translation of a famous Swedish medical text: C.M. Groth (translated into Tigrinya by T. De Pertis), *Manuale di Ostetricia (*Asmara: Missione Evangelica, 1928*).*

88. Ciotola, *Nozioni di Medicina Pratica, op. cit.* (note 87), I–II.
89. Ciotola, *Nozioni di Ostetricia, Ginecologia e Pediatria, op. cit.* (note 87), III.
90. A detailed critical discussion of this theme in Roy MacLeod's introduction to R. MacLeod and M. Lewis (eds), *Disease, Medicine and Empire* (London: Routledge, 1988), 1–18.
91. Tekeste Negash, *Italian Colonialism in Eritrea (1882–1941)* (Uppsala: University of Uppsala, 1987), 80–6.
92. Missione Cattolica (ed.), *Manuale di Letture Scelte Italiane–Tigray ad Uso delle Scuole Indigene* (Asmara: Tipografia Francescana, 1916), 296. Author's translation.
93. U.C. Dirar, 'From Warriors to Urban Dwellers: Ascari and the Military Factor in the Urban Development of Colonial Eritrea', *Cahiers d'Etudes Africaines*, xliv (3), 175 (2004), 533–74.
94. A. Cimmino, 'Igiene Coloniale', in AA.VV., *Corso di Ingegneria Coloniale* (Napoli: Pironti, 1938), 38. Author's translation.
95. G. Campassi 'Il Madamato in Africa Orientale: Relazioni tra Italiani e Indigene come Forma di Aggressione Coloniale', *Miscellanea di Soria delle Esplorazioni*, (1987), 219–60; L. Goglia, 'Sul Razzismo Coloniale Italiano', *Materiali di Lavoro*, ii–iii (1991), i (1992), 97–115; G. Barrera, *Dangerous Liaisons: Colonial Concubinage in Eritrea, 1890–1941* (Evanston: Northwestern University, 1996) (PAS Working Paper, 1); B. Sorgoni, *Parole e Corpi* (Napoli: Liguori, 1998); N. Labanca, 'Il Razzismo Coloniale Italiano', in A. Burgio (ed.), *Nel Nome della Razza: Il Razzismo nella Storia d'Italia, 1870–1945* (Bologna: Il Mulino, 1999), 145–64; R. Iyob, 'Madamismo and Beyond: The Construction of Eritrean Women', *Nineteenth-Century Contexts*, xxii, 2 (2001), 217–38.
96. P. Giandomenico, 'Salviamo il Meticcio', *Annali Francescani*, lx, 11 (1929), 347–8; M. da Leonessa, 'La Spinosa Questione degli Italo-eritrei', *L'Antischiavismo*, xl (1927), 192–6.
97. M. Cattolica (ed), *Manuale di Istruzione ad Uso degli Indigeni* (Asmara: Tipografia francescana, 1912), 125.
98. A.M. di Nola, *Lo Specchio e l'Olio* (Bari: Laterza, 2000), 99.
99. A. da Bergamo, 'Nuove Speranze', *Annali Francescani*, lx, 12 (1929), 381–2.
100. da Nembro, *op. cit.* (note 67), 222.
101. E. da Iseo, 'I Selvaggi del Gash-Setit', *Annali Francescani*, lii, 5 (1921), 135–7.
102. Missione Cunama, 'Tra i Cunama: Ossessione o Trucco?', *Annali Francescani*, lii, 4 (1921), 110–2
103. Missione Cunama, 'Tra i Cunama: Alcune Superstizioni del Popolo Cunama', *Annali Francescani*, lii, 1 (1921), 24–6; P. da Bergamo, 'Tra I Cunama: Usinè (streghe)', *Annali Francescani*, lii, 8–9, 30 (1921), 236–38.
104. da Nembro, *op. cit.* (note 67), 284.

105. Orley, *op. cit.* (note 14), 127–34.
106. C. Carrara, 'Dolori e Lutti nella Missione dell'Eritrea', *Annali Francescani*, li, 13 (1920), 306–7.
107. Ranger, *op. cit.* (note 13), 261–78; D. Arnold, *Imperial Medicine and Indigenous Societies* (Manchester: Manchester University Press, 1988), 17.
108. P. Pio da Bergamo, 'Tra i Cunama: Difficoltà e Speranze', *Annali Francescani*, lii, 8–9, 30 (1921), 236–8.
109. A. Rossi, *Servo di Dio P. Angelico da None (Pittavino Matteo) Cappuccino Servo di Tutti* (Bra: Vice-Postulazione, 1983), 47.
110. da Nembro, *op. cit.* (note 67), 284.
111. A. da None, 'La Nuova Stazione di Halhal', *Annali Francescani*, liii, 15 (1922), 441–3.
112. da Nembro, *op. cit.* (note 67), 263; Rossi, *op. cit.* (note 109), 45.
113. A. da None, 'Un Pò di Restituzione', *Annali Francescani*, li, 7 (1920), 161–3.
114. P. Angelico da None, 'Non Ogni Male Viene per Nuocere', *Annali Francescani*, lii, 23–4 (1921), 679–80.
115. C. da Chaux de Fonds, *Padre Angelico da None* (Torino: Vice-Postulazione, 1970), 64. More biographic details in C. da Chaux de Fonds, *Abba 'Ngelico* (Torino: Tip. Scaravaglio, 1962).
116. The title *käntiba*, originally designated the chief of districts and later was used to indicate the major of a town. In Eritrea *käntiba* became common also as purely honorific title except than among the Habab and Mensa people where it was used to indicate the chief of a village or community: A. Tekle-Haymanot, *op. cit.* (note 28), 61–7; C. Conti Rossini, *L'Abissinia* (Roma: Cremonese, 1929), 165.
117. da Chaux de Fonds, *Padre Angelico da None*, *op. cit.* (note 115), 85. Author's translation. It is interesting and also revealing the fact that the Capuchin father is basically represented as a 'Catholic' *sheikh*.
118. W. Benjamin, 'The Work of Art in the Age of Mechanical Reproduction', in W. Benjamin (edited by H. Arendt), *Illuminations* (New York: Harcourt: Brace and World, 1968), 211–44.

10

The Social Dimensions of Christian Leprosy Work among Muslims: American Missionaries and Young Patients in Colonial Northern Nigeria, 1920–40

Shobana Shankar

Here the role of mission medicine in the British campaign to control leprosy is considered. The case of the emirates of colonial Northern Nigeria draws attention to the social relations of medical work, not only between European and African, Christian and Muslim, but also within colonial circles and indigenous communities. The campaign exposed the different interests of administrators and missionaries, who were North American and somewhat removed from colonial government. For their part, patients were largely migratory young men. This chapter argues that although local social dynamics were often misread in mission sources, they influenced the direction that medical care took in this region of Africa.

Introduction

Leprosy stands alone in the history of medical missions for several reasons. Given the importance of the disease in the Bible, it is little wonder that Christian missionaries saw work among leprosy sufferers as a special calling. By the twentieth century, Christian organisations led the worldwide leprosy relief campaign, bringing together missions, the medical community, voluntary societies, colonial government, and local authorities in Africa and Asia. This collaboration brought attention to sufferers among colonised peoples and made leprosy no longer solely a Christian concern but a critical matter of colonial-era public health.[1] As Megan Vaughan rightly notes, 'No other disease called forth the resources required for institutionalization on a large scale.'[2]

Though scholars have explored the significance of leprosy missions in blurring lines between medical and religious healing and between imperial mandate and Christian evangelism, research on the cultural and social dynamics of the campaign is just beginning. The perspectives of sufferers themselves, collected in oral interviews, have provided some information about the perceptions and impact of medical efforts in practice.[3] Yet even in patient-centred studies such as Eric Silla's *People Are Not the Same* about leprosy sufferers in Mali, missionary attitudes towards leprosy sufferers and efforts to convert them receive more consideration than the perspectives of the largely Muslim populace on Christian medicine.[4] This tendency, in part a reflection of mission sources, creates the impression of a stark dichotomy between Christian missionary power on one side and Muslim patients' subjecthood on the other.

This essay focuses on the mission leprosy campaign in another region of Muslim Africa – the emirates of British Northern Nigeria – to suggest that Muslim–Christian relations in the medical sphere were complicated and changing. These interactions occurred in the context of missions' intensification of medical work as a way of breaking down restrictions on Christian evangelism to Muslims, imposed by British colonial authorities until the early-1930s.[5] By the middle of that decade, Christian societies worked with Muslim Native Administrations (NAs) to operate facilities for the segregation of leprosy sufferers, thus planting the beginnings of centralised government healthcare in the region.[6] Finding similar medical situations and openness to Christian medical missions among Muslim rulers in Northern Nigeria and Sudan in this period, one historian mentions that Muslim authorities in Omdurman gave financial support to keep open a Church Missionary Society (CMS) hospital.[7]

Neither missions nor political authorities – British colonial and NA – exercised complete control over the leprosy campaign. Local actors, including sufferers, their families and communities, had some degree of power to either relocate to mission institutions or to remain there and recommend or discredit Christian medicine to their neighbours and friends. This discussion therefore considers the many interests that shaped the leprosy campaign in Muslim Nigeria in the 1930s, with a focus on the British Empire Leprosy Relief Association (BELRA), the most important Christian society in Northern Nigeria, the North American Sudan Interior Mission (SIM), and sufferers themselves. The goal here is to re-examine the extent to which colonial power and western medicine determined the leprosy campaign as a voluntary and hopeful one for Africans who entered segregation facilities, as Vaughan and others have discussed with different emphases.[8] As this essay seeks to illustrate, social relations, not only between Europeans and Africans but also within African societies and European circles, influenced the direction of medical work in colonial Northern Nigeria.

'Empire suffering': leprosy control in British Africa and the case for medical missionaries to Muslims

Struck by the calculation that 'there are more lepers under the British flag than there are under any other political grouping,'[9] government and medical authorities aggressively promoted leprosy relief throughout the Empire in the 1920s. An important first step was the establishment of the British Empire Leprosy Relief Association (BELRA) in 1923. According to the Association, treating the health of the peoples within British domains represented a matter of good government. In this, leprosy control took priority, despite the disease's limited contagiousness, for 'the humanitarian, the patriotic and the Christian aspects of the task.'[10]

This campaign came after decades of disagreement and debate over the formation of an official policy on leprosy. As Sanjiv Kakar has discussed, the causes and modes of leprosy transmission continued to provoke debate in the late-nineteenth and early-twentieth centuries. Although Armauer Hansen isolated the bacillus, *mycobacterium leprae*, in 1873/4 and rejected heredity as the cause of leprosy, questions remained about how it spread and, consequently, the efficacy of confinement of sufferers. The growing popularity of the germ theory strengthened the arguments of those in favour of isolation, despite the prevailing belief in heredity among some. In the midst of ongoing disagreements, pro-segregation elements among British officials and local elites worked together to establish asylums in India. Christian workers indirectly helped their cause, for they had their own interest in leprosy sufferers; the Mission to Lepers, founded in 1874, led the effort in establishing several colonies.[11] With little government support forthcoming, these institutions, mainly mission-run, which segregated sufferers, became standard in India, from whence leprosy research and measures were exported to other colonies.

The Calcutta School for Tropical Medicine and Hygiene stood at the centre of this Empire-wide leprosy campaign. Its head, Sir Leonard Rogers, developed an injection of chaulmoogra oil in 1915, and Dr Ernest Muir, his colleague and successor at the School, held the job of visiting leprosy asylums in India to promote the use of the new medicine.[12] Chaulmoogra proved to be somewhat difficult to obtain, and a few years later, Rogers experimented with combining it with hydnocarpus oil in the form of sodium salts. This new combination therapy, under the trade name of Alepol, was considered an advance because of the convenience of its powdered form and it was subsequently promoted for use throughout the colonies.[13] By the time Muir toured leprosy institutions in Nigeria and other African colonies to publicise the improved medicines and leprosaria model in the 1930s, he had determined that the oils were often ineffective and, in some cases, actually harmful. Nonetheless, medical practitioners continued to administer the oils, the more effective use of sulphone being still some ten years away. While drug research continued, segregation of leprosy sufferers remained the prescribed biomedical practice well into the 1960s.

The introduction of the new leprosy measures in Nigeria and many of the other African colonies occurred as a centrally managed affair. Before the 1920s, British officials in Nigeria had tended to work on a provincial basis with the support of NAs, though colony-wide legislation may have existed.[14] These efforts largely depended on the willingness of local officials to provide funds to establish segregation facilities outside of towns. In the Southern Provinces of Nigeria and non-Muslim areas of the North, missionaries regularly worked with British Residents to house and care for leprosy sufferers. In the Muslim areas of Northern Nigeria, where missionaries were barred, lazarets were established and essentially served as rural locations for the distribution of alms to perhaps 100 or so leprosy sufferers. Government segregation was hardly systematic or widespread.

After the establishment of BELRA, the situation began to change. Medical research within African colonies was prioritised, perhaps to parallel the kind in India. In 1926, an anonymous beneficiary bequeathed a sum of £5,000 through the Medical Research Council, affiliated with BELRA, for the establishment of a 'Tropical Medical Research Fund' stipulated for use in Kenya or Nigeria. The Colonial Office and the respective administrations were expected in return to establish a hospital-based medical post in pathology and clinical investigation and encourage local government eventually to take on the work itself.[15] The Council recommended that:

> [C]utaneous ulcers, their classification, aetiology, prophylaxis and treatment, should be chosen as the subject of investigation. They [the advisory committee] believe that this is a question of high importance, and one urgently requiring thorough investigation such as should be possible with the special opportunities provided by this scheme.[16]

Though the level of research undertaken in Africa never approached that in India, BELRA maintained its interest in the identification, classification and treatment of ulcers, divided into two kinds: leprotic and trophic. The Association advised that the second type, occurring most commonly in leprosy sufferers who had become non-infectious or 'burnt-out', should be cared for in asylums for infectious cases until humane conditions for the disabled were available.[17]

BELRA also emerged as the chief organiser of medical missionary efforts to combat leprosy in Nigeria. The same year that the Association proposed the establishment of research work, it negotiated an agreement between the

Figure 10.1
An old leprosarium church at Yadakunya, Nigeria, now a TB ward.

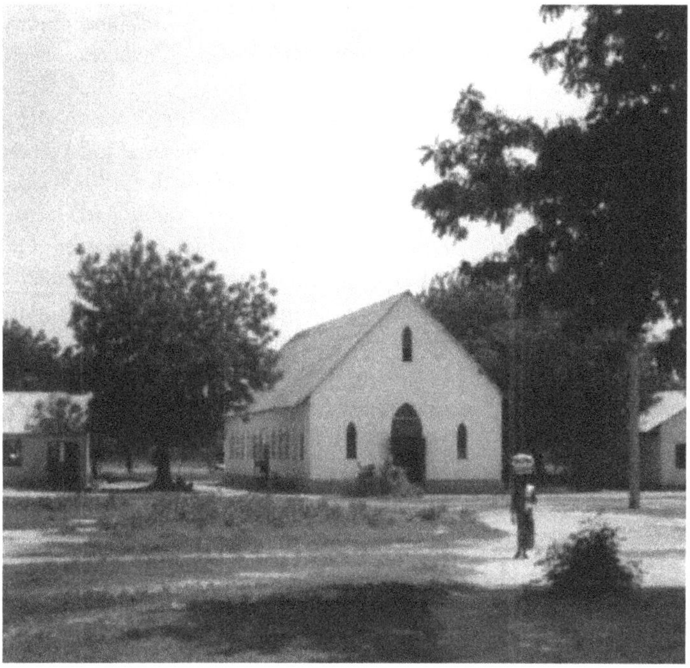

United Missionary Society and authorities in south-eastern Nigeria for the opening of a leprosarium at Itu, where the number of residents reportedly increased by a hundred-fold in one year.[18] This co-operation no doubt facilitated the 1928 negotiation of a jointly managed leprosarium between the Church of Brethren Mission, a North American Mennonite society, and the Muslim NA at Garkida, a religiously mixed area in the northern province of Adamawa.[19] In 1934, BELRA worked with the NA to open the leprosy settlement at Sumaila in the predominantly Muslim province of Kano. Sumaila's European staff included missionaries who were the first to work officially in Kano after the British occupation of Northern Nigeria.[20]

In 1929–30, T.F.G. Mayer conducted an intensive study of leprosy in Nigeria. Some of his findings about the leprosy campaign were reported in BELRA's *Leprosy Notes* in 1929, and the Government of Nigeria issued an extensive report on the distribution of the disease in Nigeria, with detailed maps, the following year. Mayer assessed the situation in the colony rather positively, praising the NAs for their active participation in leprosy relief. Commenting on the local bottling of hydnocarpus oil shipped from India and the land made available for patients who chose to relocate to segregation facilities, he found a spirit of self-help alive and well in Nigeria.

Yet Mayer bemoaned the shortage of medical personnel and referred to the Muslim provinces in stating that 'certain highly infected areas are closed to missionary effort.'[21]

It is true that in provinces like Kano, medical infrastructure and staff were sorely needed. In 1928, for example, the only hospital for Africans in Kano city had just one 'first tour Medical Officer, with no knowledge of Hausa or experience of handling African Staff and Native patients, and a second tour Nurse.' His touring had stopped entirely because the Officer had to be on site, and the NA hospital had not yet been completed.[22]

Kano's problem seemed to be common throughout the African territories. Sir Leonard Rogers voiced a concern similar to Mayer's: 'the paucity of indigenous medical training in tropical Africa is a handicap as compared with India.'[23] In a separate statement, he suggested that the way to advance leprosy work in Africa, where finances were limited, was through grants to missionary and other doctors who promoted voluntary segregation and sufferers' self-support on special leprosaria land, which Africa was seen to possess aplenty.[24]

BELRA advocated a clearly pro-missionary position and saw the ban on Christian medical workers in territories such as Muslim Northern Nigeria as a detriment to the establishment of medical facilities. Mayer went even further to associate Islam with the spread of leprosy in his lengthier report, entitled *Distribution of Leprosy in Nigeria with Special Reference to the Aetiological Factors on which it depends.* He postulated several modes by which leprosy contagion entered into Nigeria, highlighting ancient migrations and especially the negative influences of the trans-Saharan trade in which Muslims in Northern Nigeria were particularly active. Further, he commented on the 'indifference' in the North, perhaps 'due in part to Mohammedan "fatalism"', illustrated by the practice 'from Kano eastwards' of giving 'two or three cowries as alms to lepers in the hope that the donors might be fated to escape the disease'.[25] Mayer mentioned several other key points: the relative absence of leprosy among 'pagans' who isolated themselves from the predations of Muslim slave-raiders; the annual month-long fast during Ramadan as a factor contributing to decreased immunity; and the high prevalence of syphilis – evidence of sexual promiscuity 'well-recognised as favouring the spread of leprosy' – among Muslim Hausa as compared to its absence in the Southern Provinces.[26]

Missionary involvement in leprosy relief came to be seen not only as an economic necessity but also a moral one. Yet the medical mission agenda in the Northern Provinces of Nigeria differed slightly from the efforts in other colonised areas where Christian missionaries had already had a presence but were encouraged to increase their medical work. Christian missionaries had to make their reputation in Muslim Northern Nigeria as medics associated first and foremost with leprosy. Moreover, while missionaries in the emirates would resemble others in approaching leprosy as partly a curse of moral laxity, secular and Christian observers aimed to use medical missions to combat an Islamic worldview that they perceived as despotic and backward – a cause of poor health and hindrance to reform. Medicine became the answer for such practices as the giving of alms that prevented sufferers from seeking to change their physical health and social status. A critical component of the leprosy campaign in Muslim Nigeria therefore would be missions' efforts to rehabilitate sufferers and foster their independence.

New institutions in the fight against leprosy: American missions and provincial leprosaria in Northern Nigeria

In 1936, the Nigerian government published yet another report on leprosy relief in Nigeria, this time geared towards maximising limited medical resources and carefully defining a target patient population. Dr Muir, acting as the Medical Secretary of BELRA, wrote the report after touring leprosy facilities and attempting to assess the state of general public health work throughout the colony. He felt that leprosy should be considered a key disease to be combated with a long-range policy of voluntary segregation and centralised leprosaria.[27] In addition to a blueprint for co-operation between missions, colonial government, and NAs, Muir laid out new guidelines for the careful selection, classification, and arrangement of patients.

Muir identified the presence of a majority of 'ex-leprosy' patients as the chief problem in Nigeria's institutions – these he defined as disabled persons who were no longer infectious. In certain facilities, like the government's settlement in Maiduguri, a predominantly Muslim city near Lake Chad in the extreme northeast of the Northern Provinces, the doctor found that the overwhelming presence of sufferers described as 'dole receivers who are content to receive shelter and provision and have no desire to recover' had suffused the entire character of the place.[28] Several of the sites he visited in the Muslim emirates of Northern Provinces, including those at Azare and Katsina, were deemed to be hopeless because of the infirmity of the majority of their populations. Kano's new BELRA-assisted Sumaila settlement was, however, a favourable exception in the North.

The report proposed that central provincial settlements should be formed under the daily management of missionary staff who had thus far run institutions such as Itu economically and efficiently. The medical personnel, to include a lay worker in the absence of nursing sisters, would screen patients who were treatable and whose recovery might attract others. Muir advised:

> [T]here should especially at first be predominantly hopeful cases who come voluntarily with the object of recovery. If the majority of patients are of the disfigured and disabled type, who have no hope of or interest in recovery, then the morale of the settlement will be rendered hopeless and development on the right lines be found utterly impossible.

The most welcome leprosy sufferers would have the highly infectious type of the disease but still be 'capable of being rendered physically strong and healthy… to undertake a fair amount of work.' Of special interest were expectant mothers in this latter category, whose newborns could be isolated from the infectious patients at the camps. As an extra measure:

> [A] certain number of intelligent young patients in the milder stages of leprosy should be admitted not only with the object of treatment, but also that they may undergo special training in the recognition, treatment and prevention of leprosy.[29]

Muir's logic reflected the then current thought, based on improved microscopic technology, that leprosy sufferers in the earlier phases of the illness carried more bacilli and were more infectious than those who had had the disease for longer.[30] A young, productive, and reproductive population in isolation meant more chance of success with oil injections, greater self-sufficiency and lessening numbers of new infections. Muir made a special point of mentioning young children in his report, describing leprosy almost as a kind of childhood illness. 'Those infected in early childhood,' he wrote, '…are chiefly responsible for spreading the disease to the next generation.'[31]

In his conclusions about the prospects for improving leprosy relief, the doctor sounded optimistic about collaborative work and the social and cultural climate on the ground. He even aimed to counter the negative impressions about Muslim attitudes towards leprosy, such as Mayer's:

> I have heard it said that the people in the Northern Provinces of Nigeria are callous regarding leprosy, suggesting that this is a characteristic of the people as a whole. I disagree with this opinion; the Somaila [sic] Settlement disproves it. The reason for the apparent callousness is that such camps as those at Katsina and Maiduguri have been begun on the wrong lines.[32]

Muir did not see a problem of Muslim attitude, rather one of Muslim practice. He wanted to replace lazarets, and with them, the practices of begging and alms-giving, with self-contained residential settings that minimised costs and interrupted intercourse between leprous communities and wider society. Thus, the medical ideology of segregation translated into the socio–economic logic of self-sufficiency and hopefulness.

Muir's report provided the opportunity for Christian societies' official takeover of leprosy institutions. In the Northern Provinces, four missionary bodies negotiated contracts with Muslim NAs, with the former typically responsible for daily management and medical staffing and the latter agreeing to provide land, accommodations, and regular allowances to patients.[33] Of the four, the first in leprosy work, the American Brethren continued at Garkida colony. SIM, headquartered in Toronto and later in the United States, took responsibility for Provincial Leprosaria in Kano, Katsina, and Sokoto in 1937 and later in Bauchi, Niger, and Ilorin-Kabba (Egbe). Sudan United Mission (SUM), also an interdenominational society, worked in Maiduguri and Mkar. The CMS already had a presence in Zaria and extended its work to the leprosy settlement established earlier by the government.

This opportunity came somewhat unexpectedly to Christian missions in Northern Nigeria. Missionaries had, of course, known the importance of medical work and had provided treatment since the early 1900s, but medical work was, by and large, undertaken locally as need and individual interest arose. SIM, for one, had conducted dispensary work at its stations in non-Muslim parts of the Northern Provinces, mostly in treating 'ulcers, guinea worms, rheumatism, venerial [sic] diseases, itch, and septic wounds,' and 'the accommodation of those without lodgings and who, on account of the loathsome nature of their diseases would not be welcomed nor allowed elsewhere.' In certain locations, SIM missionaries assisted British Residents with the isolation of leprosy sufferers.[34] For its part, the CMS conducted medical work as well and opened the first Christian hospital in a Muslim area when the Mission moved from Zaria to Wusasa in 1929.[35] Yet only in 1927 did colonial authorities begin to consider how to incorporate medical missions uniformly into official health work, a co-operation that was to begin with government inspection of mission sites and support for centres where trained medical staff worked.[36]

If Muir and BELRA gave a great boost to medical missions in Nigeria and in the Northern Provinces especially, the explosive growth of the leprosy work of the North American Christian societies would not have been possible without the sponsorship of American Mission to Lepers (AMTL). Later known as American Leprosy Missions, this organisation was based in New York City and grew out of its early roots in Presbyterian missions and as the US Committee of the British Mission to Lepers, the primary Christian society working in India. AMTL became an interdenominational and independent organisation in 1917, though it continued to work closely with the Mission to Lepers in India.[37] The American society's focus grew quickly beyond India, however; in 1930, when it extended its 'Invitation to Affiliate with the Mission to Lepers', it supported leprosy stations in China, Japan, Korea, Palestine, Persia, Siam, Sumatra, the United States, Northern Rhodesia, and South Africa.[38]

It was at a meeting of AMTL in New York in November 1930 that the connection between SIM and leprosy missions seems to have been made. Dr Albert Helser, working for the Brethren at the Garkida leprosy settlement, and Dr Thomas Lambie, SIM missionary in Ethiopia, were both present. After some time in Southern Sudan with the United Presbyterian Board of Foreign Missions, Dr Lambie established the Abyssinian Frontiers Mission that he joined with SIM around 1927. Mission work, including leprosy relief, was begun in Ethiopia in 1927, with Lambie establishing a close friendship with Ras Tafari (Haile Selassie), when he was still Regent. Dr Lambie later became an advisor to Emperor Selassie and gave up his American citizenship for Ethiopian in 1934.[39]

AMTL, like BELRA, promoted a nationalistic spirit in its worldwide campaign against leprosy. As AMTL President William Jay Schieffelin put it at the November 1930 meeting:

> [T]he United States is no longer the small isolated country that it was one hundred fifty years ago. It is a world power, with vast foreign interests and dependencies, to which our men and women go, not only as travellers, but as business and church representatives, as officials and government workers.... Owing to improved means of transportation, the whole world today has the wanderlust, particularly Americans.[40]

Unlike the British organisation, the American one had no relationship to government; its emphasis lay in linking American and Christian purpose. A representative of the Presbyterian Board of Foreign Missions spoke at the meeting about the uniqueness of AMTL in reminding the audience that leprosy 'must be treated by an agency that can cut across all geographical and denominational lines and deal with one common problem around the world.' He noted that 'religious boards would not do that'. Yet leprosy work represented the ultimate expression of Christian mission for, as Dr Lambie said of his Ethiopian experience, 'the leper can do nothing in return.'[41]

The influence of Dr Lambie and the growth of AMTL no doubt had a significant impact on the leprosy work of Dr Helser in Northern Nigeria. Helser left the Brethren to join SIM in 1936,[42] and Lambie visited the region around this time. Perhaps borrowing from the strategy used in Ethiopia, SIM at this time began cultivating close friendships with emirs and other Muslim rulers in Northern Nigeria.[43] However, the American missionaries tended to operate independently of the British colonial government, which was in fact a source of frustration for the authorities.[44] A vast majority of SIM missionaries came from rural areas of the Midwestern states of the USA. Given the differences in educational and class background, British officials found little in common with SIM missionaries and concluded that they were extremely religious and narrowly focused on their evangelical pursuits. Nonetheless, the government was dependent on the Mission's personnel and financial resources and could not too closely control SIM attempts to impart its brand of Christian culture to the leprosaria residents.

Social dynamics of the leprosaria: young, male and mobile

Though the leprosy settlement was the site of constructing or 'engineering' a social microcosm, medical missionaries and government authorities could not entirely control this process. As mobile people who may have begged for a living or moved to NA lazarets when they were opened, sufferers' willingness and ability to relocate, avoid relations with non-leprous people, and submit themselves to new authorities in fact played a significant part in the shaping the character and success of the leprosaria in becoming self-sufficient isolation centres.

Not long after SIM's takeover of the leprosaria in 1937, the population of the provincial leprosaria became overwhelmingly male, preventing the settlements from ever really becoming microcosms of mainstream Hausa society. In June 1939, just six months after the Kano leprosarium was moved from Sumaila to Ya da Kunya, a village closer to the city of Kano, nearly sixty-five per cent of all inmates were male, a proportion that remained fairly consistent through the 1940s. Intriguingly, the statistics of the period before June 1939 suggest that females were at first willing to move to the Leprosarium but quickly found it unsuitable. In December 1938, 105 females accounted for nearly half of the total 225 patients; within six months, the male population swelled from 120 to 209 and became more than two-thirds of the total. The population of females, meanwhile, had increased by only twenty or so persons. The patients were also young, 20-year-olds representing the overwhelming majority among males and females. By 1940, this age group made up forty-three per cent of the whole settlement at Ya da Kunya, with one in four inmates being a man in his twenties.[45]

While the youthfulness of the leprosaria population conformed to Muir's recommendation, several factors may have had a greater impact than the authorities' designs alone. Elderly, and severely disabled leprosy sufferers were less able to move easily. Indeed, the elderly, once at the camp, often deserted. One man who had come to Katsina Leprosarium after his disease had advanced to the point where treatment was impossible fell by the road in an attempt to leave the mission to return home to die. A missionary remarked, 'This was not unusual for it seems that many wish to go home to die, some even die on the road home.' The man was brought back to the camp, where a young Nigerian Christian stayed with him until he died.[46] Officials also actively worked to remove 'old cases' cluttering up the leprosaria, relocating them if possible still on the grounds but away from the busiest areas of the centres.[47]

Women faced unique hardships in that medical officials and missionaries sought to isolate children – both infected and healthy – from parents who had the disease.[48] Although mothers allowed their babies to be weighed and examined, they resisted being separated from them.[49] To remedy this situation, European and American nursing sisters occupied themselves with developing closer relations with women and young children. Their duties specified visitations with women, attendance at deliveries, and playing with children.[50]

SIM missionary Martha Wall, a registered nurse, wrote that without this time together, 'we might lose women patients as well as the hope of saving babies.'[51] Wall recounted a feast for the opening of the crèche she had planned with the help of Husaina, a Hausa woman helper. The missionary became despondent when she saw that Husaina, who prepared the food, remained unresponsive and cold to her; moreover, mothers and their children stayed away until they eventually arrived nearly two hours after the scheduled time of the party. 'Word had gotten around the camp that the white doctor was planning to take their babies away by force.'[52] This kind of sentiment proved strong, and women frequently left the settlements rather than face the continuing pressure to give up infants. Even before they arrived at the leprosaria, mothers who suffered from leprosy frequently faced the prospect of losing their children to relatives who took advantage of their powerlessness. One woman's struggle with leaving behind several children with her husband, after the death of two others in infancy, suggests that many female leprosy sufferers may have come to mission institutions hoping to flee family mistreatment, only to find the same lack of sympathy from the whites.[53]

The suggestion here is not that young men always stayed at the camp and did not run away, but that even if they did leave, others like them arrived in their place to keep the sex ratio firmly in favour of males. Some studies have suggested that the disease may be more prevalent in males. Others have found that more men tend to present themselves for treatment.[54] Further research on gender and leprosy is required, but the data available here suggest that socio–cultural factors, conscious efforts on the part of missionaries and officials and perhaps the course of the disease itself may have simultaneously worked to bring more young men than others to the leprosaria.

For their part, SIM did not explicitly identify the male orientation of the institutions in their descriptions of the leprosaria community; nor did the Mission portray life at the colonies as typical of a Hausa village. Rather, as befitting the young population that tended to come to them, SIM missionaries emphasised the new life offered at the leprosaria. They were places where leprosy sufferer could find that 'somebody cares for him, and will do everything possible to give him a fresh start and a new lease of life,' wrote Albert Helser.[55] 'Teach him from the Bible,' Helser advised, 'that no disease is beyond God's power to cure.'

The leprosaria were therefore first and foremost productive, highly systematised and efficient medical–residential communities that signified them as 'western medical institutions', as distinct from sanctuaries or almshouses. Kakar identifies a similar shift in India somewhat earlier, in the late-1880s. Above all, this institutional transformation conveyed to residents and visitors that leprosy sufferers, with merely a small degree of investment and assistance from local rulers, could be self-reliant and satisfied.

To maintain themselves, residents of the camps were expected to work diligently, another possible reason for the absence of older people. Gangs of male patients built the residences, latrines, bathing places, and incinerators needed for the new communities. After these were built, inmates did repairs and maintenance. In each camp, specialised craftwork began, with patients working as blacksmiths, weavers, and carpenter to make tools, bandages, and furniture on site. Women and older girls spun thread on distaffs for the bandages. Children performed odd jobs in cleaning and hauling.[56] Patients worked as launderers, police, animal keepers, schoolteachers, and watchmen at the camp's market.

Medical procedures created still more jobs, albeit ones that were considered more desirable than those mentioned above. 'Cleansed' people administered injections, dressings, and other treatment. Assistants helped doctors in amputations and other leprosy-related surgeries as well as unrelated procedures, including circumcisions, and deliveries. They also attempted to treat and record a range of other conditions, including bone decay, eye troubles, and 'diseases of interest to public health' such as bilharzia, chicken pox, gonorrhoea, malaria, syphilis, and sleeping sickness. Some residents prepared smears for blood, stool, gland puncture, urethral, and vaginal tests, and others maintained medical records. [57] Laboratory workers, typically longer-term residents who tended to be Christians, received training from missionary medical staff.

The regimen of injections itself reinforced the principles of self-sufficiency and the patient hierarchy of the leprosarium. At 8am, at least two days weekly, patient–nurses supervised the formation of an assembly line at the dispensary where sterilised instruments lay on a table. Each person receiving medication moved from the missionary doctor or nursing sisters, who took temperatures and wrote patients' numbers and dosage on a piece of paper, to the injection patient-nurses who administered the oil into any of twelve different places on the body from the chest to the knees.[58] Missionary staff avoided – as far as possible – physical contact with leprosy patients, and, in some cases, did not even open doors.[59] One nurse inserted two needles into the bodily area selected for that day's treatment, another injected the hydnocarpus oil, another massaged the area, another applied ointment to the surface of the skin, and the chaulmoogra oil was administered by a final nurse.

This routine, though represented in mission propaganda as a formal and impersonal drill, cultivated familiarities, between missionaries and certain patients and between patients themselves. Patients in positions of authority over other residents gained greater visibility with the missionaries and colonial officials who visited the leprosaria; these special individuals included nurses and policemen who represented the rest of the community during special occasions.[60] During regular medical inspections, especially the treatment of ulcers, patients had to submit themselves to the scrutiny of native dressers and missionary medical staff, 'with their dressings off, exposing what the other day had been hidden under bandages,' wrote Martha Wall.[61] In a confessional mode, patients who lived at the leprosaria were expected to reveal themselves without modesty or shame. This emotion, known as *kunya* in Hausa, is significant not simply between sexes but also for social inferiors, youngsters and between certain family members – such as first-born children and their parents. The medical encounter therefore forced new kinds of relationships between strangers, and interactions amongst Africans were just as, if not more, notable than the relations between foreign missionaries and Northern Nigerians.

In these social dynamics, though hierarchies existed, SIM workers claimed that all patients were treated equally and need only avail themselves of the opportunities for self-betterment. The medical superintendent at Kano, Dr Edwin Harris, could have been back in the United States and was probably writing for an audience there, when he described the community at Ya da Kunya in the vein of the American dream: 'Any one is free to advance to a better position by improving the quality of his work especially by learning to read and write. The latter accomplishment insures a man or woman a good job.'[62] Self-sufficiency had intertwined with competition and opportunities for western education and employment.

Alongside initiative and industry, fairness was another dimension evoked in mission sources. A 'democratic' system operated at the leprosaria, according to SIM reports that spoke of residents choosing a head of each quarter, like a *mai unguwa* in Hausa wards or neighbourhoods, from amongst themselves. Another individual apparently served as chief representing all the leprosy sufferers in dealings with the missionaries. This leader and a council composed of Muslims and Christians together dealt with 'any trouble that [arose] in camp'.[63]

Missionaries stressed that religion especially was a matter of personal choice for all and was not a bar to presenting a Christian witness successfully through medicine. Indeed, Helser remarked that 'Mohammedans and pagans alike rejoice to see the power of God manifested through science and beyond science in the cleansing of the lepers.'[64] Conversion resulted from personal choice, and no coercion was brought to bear, either on Christians who held open-air services 'on their own initiative' or on Muslims. Dr Harris admitted that the missionaries had conformed their expectations somewhat to the setting: 'In accepting the restricted work phase of testimony as found in a Moslem leper colony, we have learned to be satisfied with quality of growth of the individual Christian.'[65]

The individual who came under the missionaries' scrutiny in the leprosaria and succeeded in the new regime was, more often than not, a young man. Men in their late-teens and early-twenties apparently had fewer attachments and were therefore able to take advantage of a 'new life' that included work for white missionaries and education in their system of learning. Yet they also had to be willing to break with social customs and formalities that were rewritten in the context of the leprosaria, codes that younger men may have wanted to escape. Yet how voluntary involvement in this new system actually was can only be better understood through an examination of the narratives and experiences of patients themselves.

The experience of the leprosaria: coming of age or cleansing?

From what kinds of backgrounds did leprosaria patients come? What changes did they experience in coming to the mission institutions and after they left? The lives of leprosy sufferers, explored through oral sources and read alongside missionaries' testimonies, help illustrate the contradictions in the stated aims and actual functioning of the settlements. The leprosarium was not intended to be a place of permanent relocation, only a treatment and rehabilitation centre. The long duration of treatment by injections and the work that one had to undertake to live at the leprosaria, however, militated against an easy relocation upon discharge. Although the settlement appeared to mirror 'real life', with its work, schooling and community life, it was not, in fact, a way of life that patients would have experienced before coming, nor likely to experience after leaving.

As with many young Hausa men, a good number of those who became leprosaria residents were attending Qur'anic school when the disease began to show itself. Many of them hailed from rural backgrounds and were involved in *almajiranci,* itineration in search of or with a teacher. Students and often teachers too live on alms, though pupils may pay their way by supporting their teacher through earnings and farming. Rural youth may find themselves working closer to or in bigger cities through this system, returning home to help their families during the year with planting or harvesting.

Those who contracted leprosy did not necessarily experience immediate changes in their lives. Sale Tomas, from a village in Dambatta north of Kano city, was diagnosed with this disease at the age of six while studying at a Qur'anic school in his home village and remained there until the age of thirteen, when he travelled to his grandfather's village for treatment and to teach. The disease did not cause any deformity until his late teens. 'That's why I was sent to hospital,' he remembered. 'Before that time, nobody would guess.' The increasing disability impaired his ability to farm and perform other heavy manual work, but he may have had students who provided help on the farm.

The impairment to one's ability to work prompted sufferers to leave off educational pursuits and undergo more intensive treatment, but mission medicine appears not to have been the first choice for sufferers and in many cases only a last option. Sale's experience of waiting until his body had deteriorated is not uncommon, and even after the introduction of western drugs, leprosy sufferers tried herbal remedies after the appearance of skin lesions and other telltale signs.[66] The remedies that were mentioned included an unpleasant-tasting infusion of the bark of a particular tree. Indeed, most former patients recollected the herbal remedies with distaste and preferred the injections.

Failing these remedies, the decision to send a child or admit oneself to the mission leprosaria was made, usually after families and communities had learned something of the Christians' reputation for healing. The missionaries made trips specifically to find sufferers but these did not always attract sufferers to return to the leprosaria on the spot. Rather, people made decisions after hearing about the news of successful healing. The father of Hamza Zubairu, a patient at the Katsina leprosarium, took his young son for leprosy treatment after a woman in their village in Katsina described the missionaries' treatment of her daughter's burns.[67]

Another former patient reported a similar experience that brought him to the Kano Leprosarium, where he received injections for five years. As a young man, he had taken an injured girl who had fallen from a height to an itinerant Christian missionary at his village of Tasa, south of Kano City.[68] He was diagnosed with leprosy when the American saw his hand. Missionaries had held religious classes at Tasa as early as 1936 and thus built a reputation there gradually. Moreover, the Emir of Kano formally approved the instruction and sent the District Head to explain the meetings to the Tasa chief;[69] within two years, medical and preaching visits from Tasa to nearby villages began regularly.[70] The support of emirs generally helped convince people of the acceptability of trying the mission medicine, and they made regular visits to the leprosaria to meet with residents and installed representatives to live at the mission sites. It is also the case that many former leprosy patients emphasise communal or authorities' sanction, suggesting that they themselves were not solely responsible for or acting improperly by relocating to the mission leprosaria. Indeed, the involvement of fathers as escorts to the mission institutions suggests the sense of compulsion and the idea that resistance would have signalled disobedience.

Though former patients implied that the leprosaria represented a last resort, they did not perceive the institutions as places of exile. Parents had tried every other remedy available, and leprosy was clearly a serious enough condition that warranted extraordinary measures. The difficulty came after youths had spent many of their formative years at leprosaria away from home. Physical disability was not solely the cause of scorn or shame, for sufferers had remained within communities taking indigenous therapies. Rather, leprosaria residents had missed the Islamic educational experiences with their peers and working alongside their male family members on the farm. Families expected no contribution from their leprous kin. The separation that leprosy segregation efforts had imposed created a cultural and social distance that became insurmountable.

Many former patients returned home after treatment but later went back to the mission. At Ya da Kunya, those cured of leprosy built homes in a special section of the facility reserved for cured workers. Others, like Malam Sale, became educators and undertook outreach efforts to draw more patients to the leprosaria. Still others entered government service. Cured sufferers tended to live a migratory existence, particularly those who converted to Christianity, attended Bible school and became itinerant evangelists. Strikingly, amongst Christian Northern Nigerians, few of these former leprosy sufferers were identified to an outside researcher as such. Leprosy in family histories rarely enters discussions as a topic of casual conversation or as part of the 'received' history of the Christian community. Rather, information about sufferers' conversion is discussed rather cautiously and as a matter of speculation rather than certainty.

What is not emphasised in leprosy sufferers' recollections is leprosy as a medical condition and the process of treatment at the mission institutions. In contrast, disease and 'cleansing' predominate in mission depictions of patients' experiences. 'Cleansing' did not only mean arrested leprosy; missionaries often actually wrote about worsening cases and relapses. Rather, their notion of treatment encompassed changing attitudes towards the illness and especially the ability of people to surmount it through modern medicine. Missionaries also wrote of the growing sympathy and action on behalf of leprosy sufferers among Muslims as a result of their interaction with Christians as a facet of this 'cleansing'. As illustration, Helser offered a story about the arrival of a severely deformed leprosy sufferer in Kano. A Muslim worker fetched her water and 'patiently helped what he could and then and went and bathed and washed his clothes.' The missionary noted that 'many who saw this true Christ-like spirit marvelled at the change in this Mohammedan helper.'[71]

The transformation described in missionary accounts differs from that experienced and observed by Northern Nigerians. Europeans and Americans stressed the volition and actions of the individual – diseased, healthy, converted, or unconverted – who came to see leprosy as controllable and not as a cause for judgment. This was not simply a Christian view but one characteristic of the medical missionary who combined faith in God and faith in science and believed that Muslims and 'pagans' too could understand the distinction.

Northern Nigerians also made a connection between leprosy and western culture, though they recognised the leprosaria as having deeper implications beyond the religious and scientific. They perceived relations in the leprosaria experience within the social relations and avenues of mobility in colonial Northern Nigeria. Whether Christian or Muslim, former leprosy sufferers became associated with Europeans in the popular imagination. Having lived among missionaries, leprosaria patients had shared a degree of intimacy with westerners that was unknown to most Northern Nigerians. The ability to read Roman script singled out those residents who had spent a relatively lengthy time in the mission institutions. Leprosy sufferers, regardless of their religious affiliation, held the reputation as workers or clients of Europeans and as Christians, a designation they often could only shed gradually after moving back into their communities.

Missionaries understood that literacy and work were the greatest attractions, after medicine itself, that they could offer Northern Nigerians, but they did not seem to grasp the effect of literacy on a person's social status. Helser related the following anecdote about how 'Mohammedans find Christ':

> After spending an hour reading selected passages [from the Bible] and exchanging comments, the Mohammedan cried out, 'I believe!' and fell down on his face before his Lord and Savior. After both [missionary and convert] offered prayers of thanksgiving that another name had been written in the Lamb's Book of Life, the new convert looked up and said, 'Have you got anything for me to do?' The face of the missionary fell. Is it possible this

man is a 'rice Christian?' The new convert saw his expression and said, 'Man of God, you do not understand. I do not want work about your place here, nor do I want you to give me any money for work I might do anywhere, but as a Christian, there must be something for me to do.' This was one of the times when a missionary's heart overflowed with joy. Then the new convert was told that he could take some Bibles along with him, back to his district, and start to teach the Mohammedan teachers in his area.[72]

Missionaries identified such individuals as 'scribes' who filled the special all-male reading classes held regularly at leprosaria. The westerners saw these men as well-to-do Muslims who read and wrote Arabic and were religious scholars.[73] In their writings, especially those for wide circulation at home, mission sources prioritised these men's experience of education, clearly highlighting the immersion of those they saw as the more influential Muslims among the leprosaria population. Yet they did not see that a good many of these men were Qur'anic students who had become disabled in the course of their education, aimed to continue in the new system under the Europeans and were able to better their positions in some measure through western education.

Scholars' relying on missionary sources alone would not see many the social complexities of the mission leprosaria experience, because of Christian writers' tendency to emphasise the religious dimensions and interiority of sufferers' experiences. Medical missionaries rarely had the chance to see patients outside the sphere of the leprosarium, clinic or hospital; they identified their social standing within this medical and mission milieu and not within 'indigenous society'. It is therefore only the medical missionaries' perspective to see the leprosaria as recreations of villages and 'traditional' communities. Rather, former patients' perspectives suggest that the leprosaria were seen as camps for migrants, in the physical and social sense.

It would be inaccurate to characterise the movement to the leprosaria as wholly voluntary, as medical and missionary authorities did. While these Northern Nigerians certainly had more volition than sufferers forced into segregation in other parts of Africa, they describe a complex lifelong process in which economic survival, family relationships, and social status were critical factors. Living at the leprosaria was just one episode in dealing with the disease, but oftentimes it altered the course of a person's life thereafter. More than 'learning to be lepers,' residents of the leprosaria developed social networks connecting them to the colonial economy. In that regard, they shared similar experiences with others whose experience of western culture was not strictly medical: clerks employed in government service and 'houseboys' of Europeans. The identities of leprosy sufferers did not always continue to be defined in terms of their illness for educational background and economic means outweighed other factors as young men came of age and ceased to be patients of the leprosaria.

Conclusion

Around 1939, the situation of young people in the leprosaria led to complications in the working relationship of the NAs and the SIM. When the news of the removal of children or attempts to do so by missionaries reached the Emirs of Kano and Katsina, they objected and expressed worries about the vulnerability of leprosy sufferers and their children. Muslim leaders feared that missionaries were using medicine as a means of converting Muslims to Christianity. The government wanted to insert the following clause into the certificates of occupancy for all mission sites:

> No Mohammedan children shall be taught religion by the Mission, whether with or without the consent of the parents. Second, Adults may be taught religion by the Mission if they come asking for it without persuasion.[74]

SIM objected vehemently, to the extent that leading missionaries threatened to pull the society out of the leprosaria.[75] In the end, stipulations on children's education only applied to the leprosaria, but the tensions between the emirs and SIM persisted for several decades.

By the late-1940s, the sulphone drug Dapsone began to replace the oil injections, and, around the same time, the NA and the missions attempted to decentrised the leprosy work by establishing Leprosy Segregation Villages (LSVs), run by African dispensers. The leprosaria continued to offer inpatient treatment while LSVs presented an alternative. While injections required many years of treatment, as many as ten or more, even sulphone oral therapy lasted one or two years. Thus, patients in the LSVs had experiences similar to leprosaria residents in that they remained at the villages to work and to farm.

Though the leprosarium way of life gradually disappeared, the SIM institutions had lasting effects on medical experience in the Muslim areas in Northern Nigeria. Rarely did the efficacy of therapies or the power of the government decide a person's course of medical treatment. Familial and community commitments and pressures factor heavily in such circumstances. Benefits must outweigh the costs, and those in need of medical attention still do see hospital medicine as a last resort, especially since the subsidised care of the leprosaria became steadily less common and payment is usually required upfront. Perhaps most importantly, the medical sphere continued to be the site of Muslim–Christian interaction, though Muslims gradually entered medical fields. Nonetheless, Nigerian Christians replaced missionaries in many of their health programmes, giving continued truth to the idea that western medicine is a Christian occupation.

Notes

1. M. Worboys, 'The Colonial World as Mission and Mandate: Leprosy and Empire, 1900–1940', in R. MacLeod (ed.), *Nature and Empire: Science and the Colonial Enterprise, Osiris*, 15 (2000), 207–18.
2. M. Vaughan, *Curing Their Ills: Colonial Power and African Illness* (Stanford: Stanford University Press, 1991), 95.
3. S. Kakar, 'Leprosy in India: The Intervention of Oral History', *Oral History* (Spring 1995), 37–5.
4. E. Silla, *People Are Not the Same: Leprosy and Identity in Mali* (Oxford: James Currey, 1998).
5. C.N. Ubah, 'Christian Missionary Penetration of the Nigerian Emirates, with Special Reference to the Medical Missions Approach', *The Muslim World*, 77 (1987), 16–27.
6. S. Shankar, 'Medical Missionaries and Modernizing Emirs in Colonial Hausaland: Leprosy Control and Native Authority in the 1930s', *Journal of African History*, forthcoming (2007).
7. R. Schram, *A History of the Nigerian Health Services* (Ibadan: Ibadan University Press, 1971), 235–6.
8. Vaughan, *op. cit.* (note 2), 78; J. Iliffe, *The African Poor* (New York: Cambridge, 1987), 214–29.
9. F.H Brown, '"Some Questions of Empire Suffering": A Year of Progress', *Leprosy Notes*, 5 (April 1929), 1–3: 2.
10. *Ibid.*
11. S. Kakar, 'Leprosy in British India, 1860–1940: Colonial Politics and Missionary Medicine', *Medical History*, 40 (1996), 215–30.
12. *Ibid.*, 226–7.
13. R.G. Cochrane, 'The Use of Alepol in the Treatment of Leprosy', *Leprosy Notes*, 5 (April 1929), 15–16.
14. For a full review of leprosy measures in colonial Northern Nigeria before the 1920s, see Shankar, *op. cit.* (note 6).
15. Benefaction for Research in Tropical Diseases, 1 March 1926, Public Records Office (hereafter PRO), CO 583/146/4.
16. W. Fletcher of Medical Research Council to Officer Acting for the Governor, 11 April 1927, PRO, CO 583/146/4. For details of the position's salary, see, in the same file, Chief Secretary to L. Rogers of the Medical Research Council, 3 December 1926.
17. R.G. Cochrane, 'Treatment in Leprosy: Complications and Sequelae', *Leprosy Notes*, 1 (Jan. 1929), 5–9.
18. G. Thomson to Secretary, 30 December 1927, 1–4, PRO, CO 583/156/2; Secretary to Thomson, 30 April 1928, PRO, CO 583/156/2.
19. Thomson to Secretary, 16 September 1929, PRO, CO 583/167/3; Secretary

to Thomson, 30 April 1928.

20. W.A. Lambert, My Life with the Lepers, manuscript of book, n.d., 11, University of Birmingham Library Special Collections (hereafter Birm Spec Coll), ACC 118 F1.
21. T.F.G. Mayer, 'The Anti-Leprosy Campaign in Nigeria', *Leprosy Notes*, 6 (July 1929), 30–4: 32.
22. Extracts of Medical and Sanitary Report, Kano Province Annual Report 1928, n.81-4, Kano History and Culture Bureau (hereafter KHCB), SNP/9043/1928/Vol.II/82.
23. L. Rogers, 'Training Leprosy Workers', *Leprosy Notes*, 5 (April 1929), 21–2: 22.
24. L. Rogers, 'Voluntary Leper Colonies and Clinics,' *Leprosy Notes*, 4 (January 1929), 10–12: 11.
25. T.F.G. Mayer, *Distribution of Leprosy in Nigeria with Special Reference to Aetiological Factors on Which it Depends* (Lagos: Government Printer, 1930), 3–4.
26. *Ibid.*, 4–5, 7.
27. Leprosy in Nigeria: A Report on Anti-Leprosy work in Nigeria with suggestions for its development by Dr E. Muir, Medical Secretary, BELRA (Lagos: Government Printer, 1936), Arewa House Archives (hereafter AHA), POR/A17.
28. *Ibid.*, 3.
29. *Ibid.*, 6–7.
30. Kakar, 'Leprosy in British India', *op. cit.* (note 11), 226.
31. Muir, 'Leprosy in Nigeria', *op. cit.* (note 27), 10. Oral evidence that people in Hausaland shared this view of children's vulnerability to the disease. Indeed, skin problems among children, related and unrelated to leprosy, appear to have been a chief reason for Muslims' visits to mission dispensaries.
32. *Ibid.*, 19.
33. See, for example, SIM's contract with the Kano NA. Notes on Leper Settlement Agreement, Kano Lep Misc 1936–1945, SIM Archives (hereafter SIMA).
34. Annual Report for Nigeria and French West Africa 1911, 3, SIMA, Annual Reports: Nigeria and French West Africa 1911–1945, EM-1.
35. A. Baikie (ed.), *Wusasa: Souvenir Pictorial Presentation with a Brief Historical Introduction* (Zaria: Falcon-Jones, n.d.), 7.
36. D. Alexander to Secretary, 11 October 1927, 3, PRO, CO 583/156/2.
37. 'World Map of a Compassionate Christian Service,' American Leprosy Missions, Inc., *c.*1954?, Union Theological Seminary Special Collections (hereafter UTS), Pamphlets 1348.
38. 'An Invitation to Affiliate with the Mission to Lepers', c. 1930, UTS, Pamphlets 1348.

39. T.A. Lambie, *A Doctor Without a Country* (New York: Fleming H. Revell Co., 1939); *A Doctor Carries On* (New York: Fleming H. Revell Co., 1942).
40. *Leper News*, 26 (November 1930), UTS, Pamphlets Lepers, A-Bo, 5.
41. *Ibid.*, 1, 3.
42. R. Hickey, *Christianity in Borno State and Northern Gongola* (Nigeria, 1984), ch. 3.
43. Though his stay in the region was brief, Dr Lambie accompanied his SIM colleagues on visits to Muslim District Heads. See 'Peaceful Invasion of the Northern Emirates of Nigeria', *The Sudan Witness*, 14 (January–February 1938).
44. 'Religious Tolerance', précis of replies from Residents to Secretary's Confidential Memorandum No. 1.5533/188, 15 September 1930, AHA, no. 5333.
45. These statistical data are found in reports in the following files located at SIMA: Kano Leprosarium Miscellaneous Reports and Info (hereafter Lep. Misc.) 1937–1945, SR-19/A, Kano Lep. Misc. Reports and Info 1946–1951, SR-19/A, and Katsina Lep. Reports 1938-1945, SR-21/A. It is important to note that the proportion of males reported at the Katsina settlement in the 1940s was lower than at Kano, generally about fifty-five percent. The total Katsina population hovered near 320 while Kano statistics fluctuated from the high three hundreds to the five hundreds. While only further research, including comparative data from Sokoto, can provide more insight about age and gender in the camps, the size of Ya da Kunya can provisionally be attributed to the importance of Kano city as a populous center of regional trade, religious learning, and administration. Perhaps further research will reveal how seasonal migration, employment opportunities, and surveillance measures factored into the leprosaria demographics.
46. Katsina Lep. Half-Yearly 1940 Report, 1–2, Katsina Lep. Resumes, 1938–1945, SR-20A. Interviews with Sale Tomas, 16 June 2001, 12 August 2001, Kano, Nigeria.
47. Katsina Provincial Leprosy Board, Half Yearly Meeting, 2–3, SIMA, Katsina, Lep. Misc. 1946–1947, SR-20.
48. Extracts from Dr Entner's letter, 9 September 2002, 2.
49. Report for Resident Kano, 1937, SIMA, Kano Lep. Misc. Reports and Info 1937–1945, SR-19/A, 5.
50. Typescript entitled 'Nursing Duties at Kano Leprosy Settlement,' n.d., SIMA, Kano Lep. 1936–1945, SR-18/A.
51. M. Wall, *Splinters from an African Log* (Chicago: Moody Press, 1960), 99.
52. *Ibid.*, 99, 102.
53. Interviews with Dije Yahaya, 22 April, 2001, 29 April 2001, Kagadama, Nigeria.

54. See, for example, E.S. Peters and A.L. Eshiet, 'Male–Female (Sex) Differences in Leprosy Patients in South Eastern Nigeria: Females Present Late for Diagnosis and Treatment and Have Higher Rates of Deformity,' *Leprosy Review*, 73 (2002), 262–67.
55. A.D. Helser, 'God Has Heard the Leper's Cry', *The Sudan Witness*, xv, no. 2 (March–April 1939), 7.
56. This material is drawn from leprosaria reports for the first ten years of the work, 1937–47, in the relevant station files of the SIMA.
57. Kano Lep. Half-Yearly Report 1940, 3.
58. Kano Lep. 1st Quarter Report to AMTL, 2.
59. Interview with Anna Beveridge, 24 June 2002, Sebring, FL, US. Ms Beveridge, a nurse, stated that this policy changed later although she does not mention a specific point in time. Marge Cummins, whose husband was a doctor, was at the Niger Leprosarium in the 1950s and 1960s, and commented negatively on government doctors who would not touch the patients. By that time, the availability of effective treatment and further research had presumably reduced fear of contagion on the part of those who knew about current thinking on the topic. Interview with Marge Cummins, 25 June 2002, Sebring, FL.
60. Excerpts from Dr Entner's letter, 9 September 1938, SIMA, Katsina Lep. Settlement Misc. 1937–42, SR/20.
61. M. Wall to friends, August 1939, 2, Katsina Lep. Settlement Misc. 1937–42, SR-20.
62. Typescript entitled Kano Leper Settlement, SIMA, Kano Lep. Misc. 1936–1945, SR-18/A.
63. Katsina Lep. 1st Quarter Resume 1941, 1–2, SIMA, Katsina Lep. Resumes 1938–1945, SR-20A; Kano Lep. 1st Quarter Report 1941 to AMTL, 2, SIMA, Kano Lep. Resumes 1937–1945 SR-19/A.
64. Helser, *op. cit.* (note 55), 9.
65. Kano Lep. Settlement, 2nd Quarterly Report, 30 June 1938, SIMA, Kano Lep Resumes 1937–45, SR-19/A, 2.
66. Interview with Hamza Zubairu, 22 April 2001, Roni, Nigeria, 22; Sale Audu Tomas interviews, *op. cit.* (note 46).
67. *Ibid.*; interview with Usman Karkarna, 6 June 2001, 12 June 2001, Kano, Nigeria.
68. Interview with Idi Ahmadu, 6 June 2001, Kano, Nigeria.
69. D. Talbot to C.G. Beacham, 18 July 1936, SIMA, Correspondence, Dr A. Helser 1936–56, CH-2, CH-3/A.
70. See 'Touring Notes from 1938 and 1939', SIMA, Kano Reports 1933–45, SR-18/A; Kano Lep. 3rd Quarter Resume 1947, SIMA, Kano Resumes 1946–66 SR-18.
71. A.D. Helser, *The Glory of the Impossible* (New York: Evangelical Publishers,

1940), 44–5.

72. *Ibid.*, 88.
73. See, for instance, 2nd Quarterly Report, Kano Lep Settlement.
74. Notes on the Kano Leprosy Board Meeting, 19 July 1939, SIMA , Kano Leprosarium 1936–1945, SR-18/A, 2.
75. G. Playfair to A. Helser, 3 September 1939, SIMA, Helser, A.D. 1939 (July–December) CH-2A.

11

Administering Leprosy Control in Ogoja Province, Nigeria, 1945–67: A Case Study in Government–Mission Relations

John Manton

Interactions between a Roman Catholic Mission and colonial and international bodies concerned with leprosy control in Nigeria between 1945 and 1967 are traced in this chapter. It identifies an increasing bureaucratic complexity in missionary medical work, seen in the development of a sophisticated epidemiological apparatus to serve information and planning needs of international public health organisations, in contracts to run medical enterprises on behalf of the state, and in the accountability of missionary enterprises to local communities. Finally, it outlines how the Roman Catholic Church maintained control of institutional investments when much of the colonial engagement with Africa was in retreat.

On 21 February 1956, a new general hospital was opened at Ikom in eastern Nigeria. Although it had been financed by the state, it was to be managed by Roman Catholic missionaries. The venture represented a new type of relationship between voluntary agencies and the state in the implementation of development and welfare work in Nigeria, replacing the system of largely informal negotiations and tendering for service provision that had existed hitherto. The occasion provided an opportunity for those present to reflect on the direction and progress of Nigeria at a time when a new constitutional and political accommodation was being reached between Nigerian nationalists and the British colonial regime.

The opening address was given by Dr Michael Okpara, Minister of Health for the Eastern Region of Nigeria.[1] Okpara made the significance of this new form of institutional relationship clear from the outset in his speech.[2] The central role of Government, which provided £25,000 of the £30,000 needed to construct the hospital, was emphasised, while the role of the Church was described variously and somewhat inconsistently as 'providing the houses for the principal staff' and '[having] supervised the construction and undertaken to run the hospital'. The contractual nature of the relationship was stressed, and it was insisted that '[to] ensure efficient maintenance the running of the hospital has for the present been handed to the Catholic Mission', who would be expected to be dutiful and faithful stewards 'so long as they are required to do so'.

From Okpara's viewpoint, the hospital formed part-and-parcel of an expanded rural health service, integrated with Government-led policies on preventive medicine. The priority for preventive medicine in the Ikom area was seen to be in leprosy control, which for much of Ogoja Province had before that time been entrusted to the Roman Catholic Mission, staffed by lay doctors from Ireland, Britain, and Italy, and by doctors, nurses, and administrators from an Irish missionary order, the Medical Missionaries of Mary. The influence of the Catholic Church in Ogoja Province had been on the increase since the appointment of Mgr Thomas McGettrick, an Irish St Patrick's Missionary priest, as Prefect Apostolic of Ogoja in 1940. The level of this increase can be gauged from the elevation of the Prefecture to full diocesan status and the consequent consecration of McGettrick as Bishop of Ogoja in 1955.

In the same issue of *Catholic Life*[3] which reported Okpara's visit to Ikom, letters were published from patients in Ogoja and Obudu Leper Settlements congratulating McGettrick on his newly elevated position. From Ogoja, where the leprosy settlement had been in operation since 1945, Adariku, representative of the outpatients, wrote: 'had it not been for your mercy to lepers, we would not have dreamed of the treatment; we get free today... without you most of us would be rotten ever since in the graves',[4] while Benedict, representing the patients at Obudu, noted that:

> [Since] your absent [*sic*] of nearly a year ago there were crying from many patients who thought that they could not see you again. They were only cooled down when they heard you were not leaving them but was going home for your Consecration... the pride we felt for your Consecration exceeded expressing. The good work and your skilful responsibilities were noticeable in Ireland and that is why your Consecration was possible.[5]

Benedict's letter finished 'Viva la Eire', offering a 'small lamb for your entertainment'. A similar offering was made by leprosy patients in Ogoja, while the people of the parish of Kakwagom, which also housed a Roman Catholic Mission leprosy clinic, gave £5.

These divergent indications of the level of trust vested in the Roman Catholic Mission, by nationalist politicians and by rank-and-file Catholics, and the differing degree to which the mission could be said to have earned the support of various groups in Nigerian society are symptomatic of social and political transformations taking place throughout Africa in the late-1950s and early-1960s. On this unpredictable terrain, the northern Ogoja Leprosy Control Scheme was an active participant in the shaping of the new accommodation between Nigerians and expatriates taking place at local, regional, and national level across the country. This leprosy scheme was administered for the Nigerian and Eastern Region Government and the people of Ogoja Province by the mainly Irish Roman Catholic Mission (RCM), in a blurring of the categories of administrator, missionary, and development expert typical of the late-colonial period.

In this paper I will describe the interaction between government and mission in the provision of a particular welfare service ostensibly under the auspices of the post second world war programmes for colonial welfare and development. My scrutiny will focus on the technical aspects involved in framing and implementing leprosy control policy, in the crucial years of constitutional change, Africanisation, and decolonisation just before and after Nigerian independence in October 1960. However, any consideration of the problems faced and the strategies employed by mission churches and missionary welfare provision in the period of decolonisation must proceed from an awareness of the evolution of missionary services and institutions. More specifically, we must pay attention in the first place to the nature of the service being provided, and the character of the providers of this service.

Leprosy stands in a unique relationship to the history of the western biomedical encounter with European imperialism. Irene Brightmer suggests that the profile of the European response to the prevalence of leprosy in a variety of colonial settings led to situations in which leprosy was constructed as 'different'[6] in character to other diseases. Any consideration of colonial and post-colonial approaches to leprosy must therefore be prefaced by an understanding of the circumstances in which leprosy came to be thought of as 'different', and of the impact this construction had on interactions between Europeans and colonial populations.

Furthermore, the hierarchical clerical forms of Catholic mission, as distinct from the various Protestant missions more broadly prevalent in British colonies, had a decisive impact on the development of leprosy control in Ogoja. More specifically, this development is predicated on the intricacies of the relationship between Catholic canon law[7] and the practice of medicine, and on the position of religious women in Catholic mission. These must be explicated in order to grasp some of the crucial issues in the chronology of Catholic missionary healthcare.

With this in mind, I shall attempt to outline the profile of and approach to leprosy in Ogoja before 1945, and the development of Catholic thought on medicine and the role of religious sisters and nuns in the broader Irish missionary enterprise, before continuing with a comparison between early patterns of expansion in the RCM Ogoja Leprosy Scheme in the 1940s and the growth and consolidation experienced in the late-1950s and early-1960s.

For the later period, I will examine the impact on the RCM Ogoja Leprosy Control Scheme of changing case-finding and treatment regimes, developed with the input of international organisations such as the British Empire Leprosy Relief Association (BELRA), United Nations International Children's Emergency Fund (UNICEF) and the World Health Organisation (WHO). Political and constitutional changes in Nigeria also had a crucial impact on the strategies available to and employed by Catholic missionaries in their attempts to maintain institutional continuity and stability. Transformations in the nature of the effective contract between mission and government, as hinted in Okpara's speech, altered the context in which Catholic missionary welfare services were provided, and in the case of leprosy control, interacted with fundamental technological and capacity changes to create a complex and, at times, fraught medical politics needing careful negotiation from all parties. Examined from the viewpoint of missionaries, this process sheds light on an important and largely neglected facet of the processes of decolonisation and the politics of independence in Nigeria.

The historic entity referred to here as Ogoja Province comprised the part of Cross River State north of the Cross River, the area around Afikpo in Abia State, and most of what is now Ebonyi State. It lies in the north-east of the former Eastern Region of Nigeria. The area contained within the current boundaries of Cross River State, centred on Ogoja town, exhibits an extraordinary linguistic diversity, the result of a complex settlement pattern and a high degree of mutual local isolation.[8] The extension of British colonial control in this area dated from about 1910, and infrastructural development lagged behind much of the rest of the Eastern Region. By 1940, when Monsignor McGettrick first came to Ogoja, there was still only one road. As he writes:

> In the old days Ogoja was called The Lost Province'. It was really a traceless praierie [*sic*]... There were cycle tracks to Obudu and Ikom.... Your best friend was a good walking stick; even a push cycle was not much use as the paths to the towns were worn deep by the feet of the thousands that tramped them.[9]

As late as 1958, the Willink Commission, convened to enquire into and allay the fears of minorities in the run-up to independence, writes in its introduction to the Eastern Region that 'little more need be said of Ogoja than that it is remote, poorly served by communications and, except for the two western Divisions, Abakaliki and Afikpo, divided into many small tribes.'[10] Sklar, presenting a portrait of the party political scene in Nigeria around 1960, writes of Ogoja that it 'presents a linguistic medley which is yet undocumented in its entirety'.[11]

More recent work has cast some doubt on the previously accepted judgement that the separate and dispersed groups inhabiting the eastern Divisions of Ogoja, Obudu, and Ikom 'recognised no inter-group association whatsoever'.[12] Though it is often the case that the languages of neighbouring groups are mutually unintelligible – a fact which does not preclude communication or trade.[13] Sandy Onor has traced common memories of eighteenth-century resource-motivated migrations among different groups in the north and the south of the region. At the same time, the independence of villages and groups within the area necessitated a protracted campaign of village-by-village military conquest, lasting from 1891 to 1909.[14]

Thus, it comes as no surprise that for colonial administrators and missionaries alike, the people of Ogoja Province resisted easy categorisation. The variation in local approaches to leprosy remained equally opaque to early observers. An intriguing document from 1895 reports the remark of an Ikom chief, referring to European visitors as 'those leprosy infested people who are addicted to speak [*sic*] through their nostrils'.[15] However, the construction of stigma with regard to leprosy is often taken to be a function of the impact of the same Christian missions which were eventually charged with alleviating the plight of leprosy sufferers in Nigeria. To see why this might be so, we must examine the way in which the bind between mission and leprosy came to be articulated in colonial contexts.

Remarking on the Ghanaian case, K. David Patterson notes that '[leprosy], because of the fear and revulsion it evoked in Europeans, attracted much more attention than its public health importance or the possibilities for successful therapy could justify.'[16] The interest of Governor Hugh Clifford[17] in leprosy in Ghana, leading to attempts to assess its prevalence in 1913, was mirrored in Eastern Nigeria. In Ogoja, the earliest mention of leprosy dates from 1910 and 1911, when successive medical officers reported inconclusively and in contradictory fashion on the local incidence of the disease, in response to a proposal from Calabar that 'leper establishments' be set up in administrative districts. W. Stewart Snell, reporting in 1910, comments that 'there is a good deal of leprosy in this district… the native knows the disease.'[18] The following year, his replacement, A.W.H. Grant, reported that the disease was rare and that consequently a leprosy centre would not be needed.[19]

This portrait of the contradictions in the approach of early colonial administrators to leprosy tallies well with Brightmer's outline of how the structure of nineteenth-century interactions between Europeans and Africans, largely urban and trade-based, limited European contact with

African leprosy sufferers. This fact, combined with leprosy's low mortality rate in comparison with cholera, plague, smallpox, typhus, and yellow fever, led to a situation in which 'secular medicine and research showed little interest in the disease and effectively left it to the missions'.[20] This 'accidentally'[21] transformed leprosy into a disease with a different, religious character, as is borne out by the history of leprosy control in Ogoja.

Before the institution of formal leprosy control services for northern Ogoja Province in 1945, leprosy patients from Ogoja banded together in small camps or travelled out of the Province to seek treatment in one of the established centres such as Itu and Mkar. By the late-1920s Dr Harry Hastings, of the Church of Scotland Mission, began leprosy work in connection with his hospital at Uburu, in the Afikpo Division in the south-west of Ogoja Province.[22] In 1933, Hastings expanded the scope of his work, attending outpatient clinics at Osu Edda, where a number of clan-based leprosy villages had assembled, seemingly under the sponsorship of a local leader.[23] This development was favourably commented upon by Ernest Muir in his report on anti-leprosy work in Nigeria in 1936,[24] and seems to have provided the template for clan-based settlements later adopted at Oji River (Onitsha Province) and Uzuakoli (Owerri Province).[25]

The attractiveness of new treatment opportunities is demonstrated by an early account of the impact of leprosy control schemes and the scale of the local leprosy problem in Ogoja, given in a 1934 official letter discussing a leprosy camp at Abakaliki. It is stated that a count in Ogoja and Ikom Divisions returned an incidence of leprosy of 7.4 per thousand, which could be generalised as a seven per thousand incidence province-wide, or upwards of 5,000 leprosy sufferers among a population of 725,000. Of this number, 529 are noted as having joined settlements, of which 66 were at Uburu (among a total population of 233), 46 at Abakaliki (among 62), 150 at the Dutch Reformed Church settlement at Mkar, Benue Province (where treatment was also available under the supervision of a medical doctor), and 267 at Itu.[26] The fact that patients from these divisions were seeking to address their problems in this way attests to a degree of local recognition of the significance of leprosy, and a consciousness of what means were available for altering the condition of the leprosy sufferer, though attempts to establish the pattern and distribution of such consciousness remain speculative.

Indeed, it remains difficult to discern the motivations behind the apparently spontaneous leprosy settlements, such as that at Abakaliki and those discovered by Hastings at Osu Edda, from official correspondence. The complexity of patterns of incidence of leprosy, degree of stigma suffered, and levels of access to local resources by groups of sufferers is readily acknowledged by Muir.[27] While it is clear that the existence of effective treatment motivated many sufferers to travel to newly-organised settlements under the care of European medical personnel, it is less clear whether locally organised leprosy settlements represented a response to expulsion of leprosy sufferers from their communities or an agreed procedure guaranteeing sufferers access to land and resources.

The original plans for the RCM Ogoja Leprosy Scheme were developed in the 1940s, in response to a growing recognition of the need for organised and cost-effective means of dealing with Ogoja's leprosy sufferers. There was still little sense of the prevalence of leprosy, estimates varying between five per thousand throughout Nigeria[28] or the figure of 7.4 per thousand quoted previously, and about five per cent in Ogoja Province, or 37,500 among a population of three quarters of a million.[29] As the Roman Catholic Mission had more personnel in northern Ogoja than any other missionary group, and only one doctor served the Province at this time,[30] McGettrick was invited to provide leprosy services. He asked Dr Joe Barnes, an Irish Catholic doctor who had previously worked in another Catholic hospital in Nigeria, to take charge of the work. Barnes arrived in 1944, followed by three nuns from the Medical Missionaries of Mary in 1945.

The particularities of Catholic health services in the Nigerian context owes much to a combination of their Irish vintage and the hierarchical organisation of Catholic missionary enterprise in general. The evolution of the RCM Ogoja Leprosy Scheme demonstrates this clearly. An understanding of the roots of this scheme in what has been characterised as a 'missionary movement'[31] in Ireland in the early years of the twentieth century will serve to illuminate our appreciation of the missionary character of what increasingly became a government welfare service. Furthermore, the developing role of women religious[32] in Irish Catholicism through the nineteenth and early twentieth centuries is of crucial importance in understanding the part the Medical Missionaries of Mary played in the RCM Ogoja Leprosy Scheme.

The involvement of women Catholic religious in institutional healthcare in Ireland had evolved hand-in-hand with the growing 'devotional revolution'[33] during the nineteenth century. The foundation of St. Vincent's Hospital in Dublin in 1834 by the Sisters of Charity, complemented five previously extant Protestant voluntary hospitals in the city[34] and betokened a new relationship between Catholic religious and the Irish public. Contributing to and building on a new religious sensibility in Ireland in the second half of the nineteenth century, when Catholic religious enjoyed a much greater degree of visibility, and a more institutionalised and ritualised expression of Catholicism replaced a locally-focused peasant religiosity,[35] institutional innovations by women religious did much to bring the Catholic Church in line with nationalist politics and aspirations in pre-Independence Ireland. By 1900:

> [T]he result was, first of all, an outwardly more devout population that [practised] its religion in impressive new churches and educated its children in an entrenched Catholic school system and, second, the proliferation of a network of Catholic social welfare institutions such as hospitals, orphanages, refuges, and reformatories.[36]

With regard to the role of women religious in the practice of medicine, the early-twentieth century presented a variety of contradictory trends in Canon law. A prohibition on religious providing assistance in childbirth and attending women in maternity homes, dating from 1901, was augmented in 1917 by the publication of the *Code of Canon Law*, forbidding the practice of medicine and surgery by religious.[37] While nursing sisters were encouraged by papal declaration to take state examinations after 1911,[38] the lifting of the prohibition on religious sisters practising as maternity nurses and midwives did not come about until 1936, an event which also signified the liberalising of dispensations for medical and surgical practice.[39]

At the same time as these prohibitions were creating difficulties for the nascent movement towards missionary Catholicism building steam in Ireland, a number of women were developing strategies to combine religious commitment with a medical vocation. Acting as a bridge between the institutional innovations of the nineteenth century, and the internationalist aspirations fostered by the Irish missionary movement which was reaping the benefits of British colonial expansion by superseding French Catholic missionary presence in British East and West Africa, women such as Mother Kevin in Uganda, Agnes McLaren and Margaret Lamont, Scottish converts to Catholicism who trained as doctors and harboured missionary aspirations, and Mary Martin, a wartime Voluntary Aid Detachment (VAD) nurse and 1920s missionary worker in Nigeria, all attempted to secure opportunities to blend medical missionary aspirations with a vocation to religious life.

From the Nigerian point of view, the success of Mary Martin and her supporters in founding the Medical Missionaries of Mary (MMM) in Port Harcourt, Nigeria in 1937, and attracting strong episcopal support in Africa and in Ireland, set the scene for the involvement of women religious in the administration of the RCM Ogoja Leprosy Scheme. Close in age and social background to many of the priests of the St Patrick's Missionary Society (Kiltegan),[40] the MMM worked in close association with Kiltegan priests both in Nigeria and in Ireland.[41] The support and involvement of the MMM was vital to the early success and continued development of the Ogoja Leprosy Scheme, decisively influencing the character of the scheme so carefully elaborated by Dr Joe Barnes.

In its early years, the RCM Ogoja Leprosy Scheme relied on the principle of segregation, with Barnes' claim that 'the control of leprosy depends on the isolation of all infectious cases'.[42] His proposals envisaged the scheme as an adaptation of the Nigerian Government proposals, and resisted the notion of home segregation of patients, insisting that leprosy control must be universal for the area of coverage. Building on this principle, the design of the scheme purported to completeness and effectiveness through the offices of a variety of institutions, staff and infrastructural supports, and propaganda. From the point of view of isolation, the scheme was divided into leper hospital, leper village, leper asylum, and the home. Each would have its own function in the project of leprosy control.

Barnes envisaged a medical staff of two, complemented by a nursing staff of two, a laboratory technician, and clerks.[43] The medical officers would see to the patients in the hospital and the 'model village', trying out the best treatment available and reporting to the Senior Leprosy Officer, Lagos, as well as examining new cases in the isolation villages. The nurses would be responsible for training African staff for the maintenance of isolation villages and for hygiene in the villages, but would reside apart from the village itself in order to underpin the isolation rule of the scheme as a whole. Barnes also envisaged a large African staff as the 'privates' of the leprosy control 'army', responsible for injections, record-keeping, and reporting.[44]

Propaganda was to blend medically inflected exhortation, examples of cure, and religious and pastoral intervention. The principles taught at HQ were to be disseminated among the general populace of Ogoja, and the gratitude of the cured leper was seen as one of the most powerful weapons in the propaganda armoury. The District Officer was seen as the second rank in the enforcement of local co-operation once this was secured in theory by the principal medical officer. The Sisters, through the mechanism of education and women's meetings, would see to it that the importance of adopting and caring for the children of lepers was appreciated at a local level, while the priest would counter local religious beliefs, whether Christian or traditional, regarding the stigma associated with leprosy. It was envisaged that these campaigns would be ongoing and repeated.[45]

The role of the MMM at the heart of the pastoral life of leprosy segregation villages was clear from the outset. An horarium provided as part of the regulation of convent life in Ogoja in 1945 demonstrates the judicious infusion of the secular with the spiritual which the MMM strove for, blending prayer with medical and house duties, setting time for walks and social work. Their activity in the work of the Legion of Mary, a Dublin-based world-wide Catholic lay organisation under the spiritual direction of professed religious, was envisaged as an integral part of the ideal segregation village, as depicted in the 1947 film, *Visitation: The Film Story of the Medical Missionaries of Mary*.[46] Among Europeans present in Ogoja, the MMM maintained the most intimate relations with the leprosy settlements and villages. However, the division of labour in Catholic evangelism often precluded them from taking a more active evangelical role. As Joseph McGlade notes:

> The story of the work of Irish sisters on the missions is always the same, and yet almost always without limit in its variety. In brief, the sisters do nearly everything which does not require the power of orders.[47]

It is perhaps unsurprising then that the medical establishment seemed less a site for evangelism than a locus of new technologies and interventions in the social order, and that the focus of missionary staff often seemed to be on perfectibility of medicine as charity as well as on the personal spiritual journey. In this respect, it could be said that the MMM were engaged in self-consciously transforming medicine as well as mission – as the MMM silver jubilee publication states:

> [I]t is no use having a hospital, clinic or dispensary without at the same time looking into the real needs of the neighbourhood, because medical care that does not integrate this battle against ignorance would be unrealistic and too academic.[48]

Elizabeth Barnes, who went to Ogoja as a doctor to join her husband Joe between 1948 and 1951, recalls that 'the administration of... the villages was very good... it worked very well, considering the whole thing was done on a shoestring'.[49] The medical scale and reach of the project continued to increase throughout the period from 1945 to 1960. McGettrick notes a threefold increase in the number of resident leprosy patients cared for in the period 1949 to 1954, from 2,336 to 8,100, while there was a similar degree of increase in the number of leprosy consultations, to 32,000.[50] At the same time, the level of co-ordination between leprosy services across the Eastern Region in Nigeria remained very much *ad hoc*. Zachary Gussow describes a general process by which:

> [A] loose arrangement existed between governments, international scientific associations, leprosy conferences, a few private foundations, and a vast network of voluntary agencies, all of which conferred occasionally to discuss policies. Within this informal structure, there was a less than satisfactory agreement about leprosy and little coordinated effort among leprologists and health planners.[51]

A description eminently applicable to Nigeria.

This loose arrangement began to tighten through the 1950s, and the first meeting of the Central Leprosy Board, held in July 1950 in Lagos, represented the culmination of six years of effort to set up an expert advisory body on leprosy control to assist Government in the framing of leprosy control policy. It was hoped in this way to consolidate the hitherto haphazard and scattered insights and developments in leprosy control technologies and procedures. The effects of having such a central forum were immediately apparent in the discussions minuted from the meeting. There was much discussion of the meaning of the concept of 'leprosy control', the degree to which missionary bodies should be funded in their efforts from Government coffers, and the appropriateness of segregation. The notion that there were still a number of competing models of segregation, as proposed by Dr MacDonald of the Itu Leprosy Settlement, was rejected, and it was pointed out that Itu was an exceptional case, owing its success as much to 'the personality and initiative of Dr MacDonald' as to its efficacy as a system in itself. It was agreed for the most part that sulphones were the most appropriate treatment for leprosy in Nigeria, and specifically diamino diphenyl sulphone (DADPS). While the issues debated were of a wide-ranging and often peculiarly local nature, we see already the emergence of various principles regarding leprosy control projects.

The principle of constituting leprosy services on a provincial basis was effectively ratified by this meeting and by the subsequent inaugural meeting of the Eastern Region Leprosy Advisory Board in May 1951. It was also agreed at an early stage that funding for provincial leprosy settlements would be provided by central and regional government, while local government, in whatever form it might take, would undertake to run local and rural leprosy control services.[52] It was decided that colonial welfare and development funds would be allocated according to the incidence of leprosy in a province, the degree of co-operation of local authorities and communities – with the proviso that funding might be available to encourage this co-operation in the first place – and the qualifications and efficiency of the staff to be engaged in provincial leprosy control.

In the Eastern Region as a whole, leprosy was thought to be on the decline in the 1950s, and retrospective statements by historians such as Ralph Schram and leprologists such as Stanley Browne underline this perception. Schram's intimation that the institutional care of leprosy was on the decline through the 1950s[53] tallies with the tendency towards outpatient treatment of leprosy, which accompanied new theories in disease eradication sponsored throughout the developing world by WHO. Browne claimed in 1970 that leprosy had been in decline in Eastern Nigeria since before the advent of mass sulphone treatment in the late-1940s.[54] Both claims are borne out more by the experience of the areas under Government programmes than under voluntary agency programmes, but the perceived success of the former gave a fillip to those who maintained the case for increased funding and resources for the mission-run areas.

By mid-1952, it was clear that the highest incidence of leprosy was in Ogoja Province,[55] and at the encouragement of Dr Freeman, the representative of the Catholic Mission and of the RCM's Leprosy Control Scheme in Ogoja, a resolution was passed to call on Government to increase contributions to voluntary agencies involved in leprosy control. By 1953, the possibility that UNICEF would provide specific leprosy drugs was seen as freeing up potential funds for the expansion of voluntary agency leprosy control, and as this possibility came to fruition in the next few years,[56] government aid to voluntary agencies increased substantially. The commitment of government to this form of funding was underlined by its inclusion in proposals for 1956–60 development proposals.[57] Support from local government was noted to be on the increase, and the efficacy of the various advisory bodies in securing advantageous trading and warehousing conditions for leprosy-related projects helped streamline the ongoing development and expansion of leprosy control.

The impracticality of conducting a full population survey as an adjunct to leprosy control had been acknowledged by Barnes in 1945. Issues of cost and consent were cited, and in the circumstances of the time, it had been decided to grow the work from seed, gradually establishing complete coverage. An important boost in the effort to extend this coverage was received in the shape of the UNICEF-funded yaws treatment surveys undertaken in Eastern Nigeria from 1954. The procedure for yaws surveys entailed an initial treatment survey (ITS) followed by more complete resurveys and penicillin treatment, ensuring a house-to-house coverage.[58] On the basis that surveys attempted to identify skin lesions this was integrated with case discovery for leprosy, and cases of leprosy discovered in this way were referred to leprosy settlements across Eastern Nigeria throughout the late-1950s and early-1960s.

The effect of the increase in funding and resources can be seen in startling fashion from figures presented to the Eastern Region Leprosy Advisory Board meeting in 1959. The report on Ogoja Province shows that in the Abakaliki Division alone, eight new treatment centres had been opened, bringing the total number to twenty and reaching the greatest number of patients of any divisional service in the Eastern Region. In Ogoja Division, a new segregation village was opened alongside ten new treatment centres, bringing a further 1,000 patients under treatment, while Ikom saw the opening of seven new treatment centres visited weekly by a Nursing Sister, as a result of a new road facilitating access to the north of the Division. The utility of the UNICEF yaws survey in case discovery was acknowledged, and great things were hoped for when the mobile field unit attached to this survey visited Ikom during 1959.[59]

By 1961, independence had seen a re-organisation of the provinces in the Eastern Region. Ogoja Province had been divided in two, with the old Divisions of Ogoja, Obudu, and Ikom in the new Ogoja Province, while the Divisions of Abakaliki, Obubra and Afikpo were in the new Abakaliki Province. The three Divisions of Ogoja Province, and the Abakaliki Division of Abakaliki Province were under the RCM Leprosy Control Scheme, and this area was re-designated the North-Eastern Control Zone. A report on leprosy control for 1960, published in 1961, shows that of 32,303 patients under treatment for leprosy in the six zones of the Eastern Region, 17,807, or fifty-five per cent were in the relatively under-populated North-Eastern Region.[60] The growing preponderance of this region in the figures was accounted for by case-discovery by the initial and re-survey teams employed in the Yaws Eradication Scheme piloted by UNICEF since 1954.

While mission statistics had been collated from the outset, to serve the information demands and requirements of the Church at the level of individual orders and dioceses as well as the Vatican, the need to formally compile statistical returns for UNICEF and for the Government leprosy service prompted a rethink in how mission medical services were organised and imagined. These effects are most clearly appreciated by comparing patterns in the development of the northern (ie. RCM) Ogoja Leprosy Scheme from its earlier years with patterns from the period 1956–63.

The accounts in particular demonstrate the impact of changes in priorities on the part of government, mission bodies, and charitable organisations in the period under analysis. In 1949, the £5,600 under the heading of income included a grant of £1,000 from BELRA, which had quasi-official status at this time with regard to colonial government funding and organisation of leprosy control, £300 from the Native Administrations, £100 for a child adoption scheme, nearly £750 in donations, almost £1400 from medical fees in clinics and maternity wards attached to the leprosy settlement and serving the general public, and £1,450 from St Patrick's, Kiltegan and the MMMs in Drogheda, the parent organisations of the mission. A number of building grants were administered from time to time; these were counted as capital expenditure and not included in the general accounts. Money was spent on transport, charity to patients, catechists, repairs, schools and administration.

By 1963, when a government grant of £2,000 towards electrification brought light and subsequent demands for air-conditioning in the operating theatre, and an x-ray machine,[61] the total income of £34,000 included fees and donations, the sale of embroidery, money from Propaganda Fide in the USA, a recurrent grant from government of £16,050, almost £5,000 from BELRA, £2,000 from the German bishops, and about £1,600 from both the education department and Ogoja County Council. As well as salaries and charity, money was spent on occupational therapy, a nutrition programme and electrical fittings. Money from the Oxford Committee for Famine Relief (OXFAM), the British bishops' fund, and the German Leprosy Relief Association aided the electrification of the settlement, the development of a patient-staffed orthopaedic shoe facility, and physiotherapy.

With regard to incidence of leprosy, statistics in the early years tended to be gross, taking into account the distinction between the majority inpatients and a small number of outpatients. From time to time a note is appended on what treatment is being administered,[62] or where the grants are coming from, but the impression is of a form of document which expands and contracts in direct response to particular local and contemporary conditions, rather than in response to any broader epidemiological imperative.

The UNICEF returns, filled in and returned from the mid-1950s onward, separate patients into classes, whether new or old patients, whether defaulters reinstated, relapses or transfers, whether children, women between sixteen and forty, women over forty, or men. These statistics were useful in tracking the success of various outpatient and inpatient strategies and in generating an overall view of the work conditioned less by the imperatives of a local situation or the agendas of a particular doctor. The multiplication of categories amid the target population also assisted in the development of therapies according to perceived need – the small number of inpatients could be dealt with on a more personal level, and patients referred for surgery and rehabilitation could be assured that attempts were being made to address their needs as a group.

The expansion of the late-1950s, and the focus on developing treatment centres rather than segregation villages, brought Ogoja into line with the trends towards outpatient care seen somewhat earlier in the Government-run schemes. One result of this was that the engagement with patients, sustained and intense in the early years of the Ogoja scheme, typically became less intense and more of a piece with everyday life. In a description of the work at Ogoja in 1964, we are told that:

> A leprosy attendant and a dresser attends [*sic*] the Segregation village and treatment centre. Ulcers are cared for only at the villages, only able bodied patients attend treatment centres and they do so with minimum disturbance of their life two visits a week and patients do not have to travel further than 3 miles to a centre.[63]

This observation is very much at odds with the portrait of evangelical opportunity suggested in the film *Visitation*, a mere seventeen years earlier.

In the years from 1959 to 1962, the number of segregated patients attached to Ogoja Leprosy Settlement dropped from 2,144 to 761, while the total number of patients treated also began to show a fall, from 7,482 in 1959 to 5,294 in 1962, with discharges as cured running at between one and two thousand a year in the early-1960s.[64] An interesting effect of the trends towards outpatient treatment is that the manpower previously provided by the able-bodied segregated patients was now lost to the remaining settlements.[65] This had typically been the case for some time in the Government-run leprosy control areas where numbers had already fallen off sharply by Independence. Chambers presents the ramifications of this change to the Leprosy Advisor in a letter which links the changes in the leprosy problem in Ogoja to that which had already been observed in the Igbo areas of the east. The expenses of comprehensive rehabilitation schemes, orthopaedic care and convalescence services had added to the financial burden of the central settlement.

Particular industries such as weaving and farming, carried out with a rehabilitative aim in mind, attracted government grants and money from the increasing number of Catholic charitable organisations in Europe and North America, and an orthopaedic surgeon was hired and paid for from 1962 to 1964 by the Catholic Medical Mission Board in the USA. The development of these industries highlighted shortcomings in the provision at Ogoja, with an operating theatre and x-ray facilities high on the list of requirements.

Though it was finally clear by the early-1960s that coverage in Ogoja and Abakaliki was adequate, the need in Ogoja to administer leprosy control on an outpatient basis meant that the engagement with the community at large afforded by prior models of leprosy control – where endemic populations were segregated on community land granted for the purpose, and interacted with markets and farmers – had greatly diminished by the early 1960s. In the years prior to Independence, emphasis had been placed on the leprosy settlement village, which had proved very fertile for propaganda purposes, generating tales of suffering and redemption, education and baptism documented through the late-1940s and 1950s in film and in missionary magazines. Articles such as those by lay missionary teacher Lily Murphy in *The Medical Missionary of Mary*, providing vignettes of settlement life,[66] no longer reflected either the work being carried out in the Ogoja Leprosy Scheme, or the way in which its missionary staff wished to be portrayed. The emphasis now shifted to the hospitals at Ogoja and Abakaliki Leprosy Settlements, which were presented as being at the centre of a variety of new surgical and rehabilitative techniques, practised by women of science.[67] This reflected a desire to consolidate and preserve Catholic institutions, and the services these provided to a growing Catholic community, rather than persisting with the groundwork of evangelisation, and marked a step in the increasing politicisation of the Catholic Church in Eastern Nigeria.[68]

While the Ogoja Leprosy Scheme expanded in scale and scope, moves were made across Eastern Nigeria to increase and formalise both the level and the impact of local consultation with regard to leprosy control. This went hand-in=hand with constitutional change across Nigeria through the 1950s which saw provision for elected councils in the Eastern Region from 1950, the abolition of the post of Resident in 1956 and 1957, and the instigation of a federal system for regional self-government in 1956. The effect of this change was to dismantle the unpopular Native Authorities, which were seen as deriving their authority from British colonial power rather than from any basis in local politics.[69] Thus, a 1956 proposal to the Eastern Region Leprosy Advisory Board that a member from each Province be chosen to sit on a board hitherto almost entirely consisting of European administrators, medical experts, and missionary representatives betokened a process of Africanisation proceeding at a rapid pace throughout government services. That the Board in question was consultative and advisory, and that the Nigerians representing the Provinces would be nominated by interested parties[70] was also very much along the lines evolving under the late colonial regime.

At the same time, it was envisaged that these representatives would be at the parapet of a broader effort at consultation, reaching down to Province, and further to Division or County level: the same meeting recommended that local advisory boards would be set up to bring together local representatives, government medical officers and advisors, leprosy superintendents, and mission representatives, in order to discuss issues of local importance regarding the development and use of hospitals and dispensaries. The Leprosy Inspectors Training School at Oji River had become a Rural Health Training School,[71] and it was envisaged that Leprosy Attendants would be absorbed into the newly transformed Rural Health Service which was evolving out of the dispensary system.

The appointment of a representative on the Eastern Region Board from Ogoja Province was not straightforward. The Leprosy Adviser, K.S. Seal, at the Rural Health Headquarters in Oji River, wrote to Sr Visitation Chambers, the Medical Superintendent of the RCM Leprosy Settlement in Ogoja, asking for a recommendation from Ogoja, Ikom and Abakaliki. Chambers referred the matter to McGettrick, who wrote in reply:

> It is hard even to think of anyone who is literate but who is not directly associated with the mission and at the same time has an interest in public affairs.[72]

All the same, it was agreed that Peter Abue, a district councillor from Mbube, near Ogoja, would be recommended. The Ogoja nomination was noted as awaiting approval at the February 1958 meeting of the Eastern Region Board, and was not in evidence at the July 1959 meeting. It was not until the 1960 meeting that confirmation was received of a representative from Ogoja Province, one E.M.A. Ogar, noted as the Ikom representative.

The attitude of the RCM towards county and divisional leprosy advisory boards was similarly cautious, if not downright dubious. Chambers was reported as saying in 1959 that 'from her experience [the boards] were not very helpful. She preferred dealing direct with the District Councils at their general meetings which brought personal contacts with important personalities.'[73] Though the early meetings of these boards were inconclusive, consisting mostly of reports on the work in hand at Ogoja, Ikom, and Obudu given by the medical superintendent, and complaints about withholding or diverting of funding thought to be properly the due of leprosy control work, Ogoja divisional and local leprosy boards continued to meet into the 1960s, with increasingly elevated local representation in the guise of heads of councils sitting alongside the various medical personages.

Given that many of the crucial changes impacting on the organisation and development of leprosy control happened either before or after October 1960, we must ask to what extent Independence was a watershed for Catholic missionaries working in Eastern Nigeria? It was certainly a marker of anxiety, brought about in part by the experience of increased Nigerian involvement in welfare and development politics. Okpara's speech demonstrated what the significance of Nigerian ownership of services might be: that the missionary contract to run educational and health services, informal in spirit if not in letter under the British administration, might become both circumscribed and revocable. The suspicions and fears are clearly expressed in a diocesan circular issued by McGettrick in Ogoja in January 1959, with the purpose of outlining a programme for Catholic action in the Diocese:

> The Communists say: 'tomorrow the world will be ours'. They seem to be on their way to make good their boast. In a single generation a small highly organised group have [gained] control of one third of the world's population.... What the Communists have done in the world we must strive to do in Ogoja – bring the light of the Gospel to the majority of the people through an organised system of teaching Catechism; the few will instruct and save the many.
>
> Hitherto we have relied almost completely on the Schools for contacts and conversions. The system while it brought good results has inherent weaknesses and disadvantages... it is as plain as a pike staff that the Councils and State will secularise the schools if and as soon as they can pay the costs

> of the schools without the assistance of the Managers. We should prepare for that contingency and have a subsidiary organisation established to meet that emergency; otherwise our whole conversion system may be stymied.[74]

Indeed, Communism was not the only perceived threat emerging from the rush towards independence. Even the strategic second string of Catholic healthcare provision was experiencing the pincer pressures of Cold War politics. McGettrick writes:

> The country is changing overnight. One thing is clear that if we are to get any more Medical Institutions going we have to get them inaugurated now. Tomorrow will be too late. American Protestant Missionaries have begun to arrive here in greater and greater numbers. The USA has a Consul General in Lagos and a Representitive [*sic*] in each Region.... They intend to play a stronger hand in the development of Nigeria. All kinds of family planning and use of contraceptives will be advocated on a wider and wider scale... To save our Christian Homes we need Catholic Hospitals and Catholic Doctors. We should have one in every Division.[75]

The difficulties encountered in providing Catholic services to the population of Ogoja are most clearly indicated by the overwhelmingly European profile of senior Catholic clergy in Ogoja. In 1957–8, one report has it that Ogoja had forty-eight European Catholic priests and forty-two European nuns, with no Africans in either category,[76] though the maternity hospital in Kakwagom, between Ogoja and Ikom, had been handed over to a Nigerian order of nuns in 1956.[77] The first priest from Ogoja, the present Bishop Joseph Ukpo, was not ordained until 1965.[78] The recruitment of women for the Sisterhood continued to be *ad hoc* right into the 1960s, with those applicants who presented themselves being sent to a novitiate. In 1963, McGettrick decided to institute a new system of recruitment on a similar model to that of a seminary, with the aim of getting:

> [S]ufficient Native Sisters to staff our Hospitals, Girls' Schools and Colleges – and the Nigerianisation of our staffs is not only desirable but can almost be said to be necessary for the prestige of the Catholic Mission in the Country.[79]

This resolution, made in advance of McGettrick's departure for the first session of the Second Vatican Council, is indicative of the Catholic Church's general re-orientation towards Independent Nigerian politics, as reflected in the joint pastoral letter of the Nigerian hierarchy to the new nation's Catholics on 1 October 1960. In this letter, the Catholic bishops claimed pride 'that [the Church's] contribution to education and her work of drawing together into one social body people from all parts of the country' had assisted in achieving national independence.[80] The concerns of the Church for the continuation and stability of its influence in Africa, given local and international secularising pressures, add a certain piquancy to our vision of the pressures and changes undergone by missionary services in the period of decolonisation.

From the archival material available, it is clear that the Government saw the Ogoja Leprosy Scheme as increasingly conforming to a type. Its peculiarity in earlier years was predicated on its late start, its extremely rapid expansion while leprosy was being successfully tackled elsewhere in Eastern Nigeria, and the seemingly unique difficulties posed by the infrastructural and linguistic terrain of Ogoja. The imposition of co-ordinated policy on Nigerian leprosy control, the material and technical contribution of UNICEF and WHO, and the increasing role of Nigerians in the consultation and administration of all levels of social services brought the Ogoja Leprosy Scheme into parallel with other such schemes. The expanding notions of self-help flagged by politicians such as Michael Okpara, and the growing local and national political sphere open to Africans, further limited the sphere for independent action on behalf of missionaries.

However, the Roman Catholic Mission perceived its own work in a fashion starkly divergent from the notions held by government bodies. This much is obvious from the animated statements issuing from the Bishop's residence in Ogoja in the late-1950s regarding Communism and Protestantism. The ability of the Roman Catholic Mission to mobilise large amounts of international aid for its individual projects gave it strategic leverage in its work, a leverage which contributed to its profile locally as it attempted to integrate education, religious vocations, staff training, general medical work, and leprosy control in a coherent missionary strategy for the nurturing of a Catholic ethos in a political and social situation where this was felt ever more under threat with each passing day. Concerned with preserving its spiritual thrust and influence, and challenged with the negotiation of pitfalls surrounding the provision of a leprosy service, amid changing contours of disease, epidemiology, and treatment, in a rapidly transforming society with rising expectations regarding expatriates contracted to its service, the Roman Catholic Mission managed the evolution from religious agency and colonial servant to development agency and government contractor. In doing so, it offered a template for European engagement in late-colonial and independent Africa entirely at odds with the predominant rhetoric of retreat, significantly prefiguring post-colonial welfare and development relations between Africa and donor nations to the North.

Notes

1. Michael Okpara was a prominent Nigerian nationalist politician, later Premier of the Eastern Region under the federal system in independent Nigeria.
2. 'Minister Opens New Hospital: Team Work Praised', in *Catholic Life*, 11, 3, (March 1956), 1, 8.
3. *Catholic Life*, 11, 3, (March 1956), 2.
4. *Ibid.*
5. *Ibid.* No surname given for Benedict.
6. M.I. Brightmer, 'The Spatial Pattern of Leprosy on the Cross River Region of Nigeria', (PhD, Liverpool, 1994), 65.
7. *The Catholic Encyclopedia*, Vol. IX, (New York: Robert Appleton, 1910) defines canon law as follows: 'Canon law is the body of laws and regulations made by or adopted by ecclesiastical authority, for the government of the Christian organisation and its members.' It should be pointed out that prior to the Second Vatican Council and the subsequent ecumenical mandate, the word 'Christian' in Catholic parlance commonly related to Catholic issues alone.
8. P.A. Talbot, *The Peoples of Southern Nigeria: A Sketch of their History, Ethnology and Languages, with an Abstract of the 1921 Census*, Vol. 1 (Oxford: OUP, 1926), 226–7.
9. T. McGettrick, *Memoirs of Bishop T. McGettrick* (Sligo: Passprint, 1988), 126.
10. H. Willink, *et al.*, *Nigeria: Report into the Commission Appointed to Enquire into the fears of Minorities and the Means of Allaying Them* (London: HMSO, 1958), 36–7.
11. R.L. Sklar, *Nigerian Political Parties: Power in an Emergent African Nation* (Princeton: Princeton University Press, 1963), 13.
12. J.C. Anene, quoted in S.O. Onor, *The Ejagham Nation in the Cross River Region of Nigeria* (Ibadan: Kraft, 1994), 7.
13. Onor, *op. cit.* (note 12), chs. 5 and 6, 118–53, and R. Harris, 'The History of Trade at Ikom, Eastern Nigeria', *Africa*, 42, 2 (1972), 122–39, detail the economic linkages crossing the Cross River hinterland, extending to Mamfe and Bamenda in Cameroon to the east and to the Benue/Plateau area to the north, as well as outlining similarities between dispersed languages and shared customs and rituals among communities throughout the Cross River area.
14. E.O. Erim, 'The Old Ogoja Province under Colonial Rule', in M.B. Abasiattai, *Akwa Ibom and Cross River States: The Land, the People and their Culture* (Calabar: Wusen, 1987), 118–22, and Talbot, *op. cit.* (note 8), outline the process of pacification and military conquest experienced in old

Ogoja Province, north of the Cross River.

15. Quoted in Erim, *ibid.,* 119.
16. K.D. Patterson, *Health in Colonial Ghana: Disease, Medicine, and Socio–Economic Change, 1900–1955* (Waltham, MA: Crossroads, 1981), 73.
17. Clifford, Governor of Ghana in 1913, was also Governor of Nigeria at a later stage, and was crucial in elaborating a new template for the future governance of Nigeria in the wake of Lord Lugard's impact on indirect means of administration, reflected in a famous address to the Nigerian Council in 1920.
18. National Archives, Enugu (NAE), CALPROF 14/5/40. Note dated 12 May 1910 from W. Stewart Snell, Medical Officer, Ogoja, to the District Commissioner, Ogoja.
19. NAE, CALPROF 14/5/40. Note dated 21 July 1911 from A.W.H. Grant, Medical Officer, Ogoja, to the District Commissioner, Ogoja.
20. Brightmer, *op. cit.* (note 6), 65. The listed diseases are referred to by Brightmer as the 'big-five', combinations of which represented a source of grave health concern to Europeans both within and beyond their own borders.
21. *Ibid.*
22. NAE, OGPROF 2/1/1789, 341. Copy of letter dated 13 December 1943, from Dr Harry Hastings to unknown correspondent. Also 2/1/1789, 349. Letter dated 31 January 1944, from the Resident, Ogoja Province to the Secretary, Eastern Provinces, Enugu. These letters date the beginning of leprosy work based at the already extant mission hospital at Uburu to 1927.
23. NAE, OGPROF 2/1/1789, 341 – see above. Hastings notes that treatment at Osu Edda began 'within three months of our first obtaining a lorry'. Also see Muir (1936), 163. Muir writes '[a] native land-owner of the Edda Clan, himself a leper, established a leper village to which other lepers of this clan were gathered. There are now five such villages within a radius of some three to four miles from a central treatment centre at Usu, which is on the main road some ten miles west of Afikpo.'
24. E. Muir, 'Leprosy in Nigeria: A Report on Anti-Leprosy Work in Nigeria with Suggestions for its Development', *Leprosy Review,* 7, 4 (1936), 155–71.
25. NAE, OGPROF 2/1/1789, 338–40. Letter dated 17 December 1943, from Mr R.B. Cardale, District Officer, Afikpo Division, to the Resident, Ogoja Province. Cardale writes 'Dr Hastings' Treatment Centre at Osu proved to be a prototype. Owerri and Onitsha followed his example'.
26. NAE, OGPROF 2/1/1788, 1–5, Letter dated 24 April 1934, from the Resident, Ogoja to the Secretary, Southern Provinces, Enugu. On page 1, the author reports that '1,008 lepers have been counted in a population of 135,930'.
27. Muir, *op. cit.* (note 24), 152. Muir writes 'there are economic, educational,

sociological and other factors which have an important bearing on the leprosy problem. All of these have to be studied if this difficult disease is to be understood and in the end effectively controlled. And it is not sufficient to study them in one country or among one race alone, for they vary in every land and in every province, among every tribe and people.'

28. R.G. Cochrane, *Leprosy in Europe the Middle East and Africa* (London: World Dominion Press, 1928), 62.
29. Cited in Ogoja Convent Files: 'Leprosy in Ogoja Province', by Joseph Barnes. The version of this document in the Ogoja Convent Files consists of ten typed pages and seems to be the most complete copy of the original proposals for leprosy control in Ogoja, presented in 1945.
30. McGettrick, *op. cit.* (note 9), 127.
31. Two important discussions on the history of Irish Catholic missions, one being perhaps the most important general monograph on this history, refer in their titles to the missionary 'movement'. See 'The Modern Missionary Movement' in D. Fennell (ed.), *The Changing Face of Catholic Ireland* (London: Chapman, 1968), and E.M. Hogan, *The Irish Missionary Movement: A Historical Survey, 1830–1980* (Dublin: Gill and Macmillan, 1990).
32. The term 'religious' refers to professed members of the Catholic Church, be they priests, nuns or brothers; thus, the term 'women religious' distinguishes nuns and religious sisters from lay women.
33. The thesis that Irish Catholicism witnessed a devotional revolution in the nineteenth century was first advanced in E. Larkin, 'The Devotional Revolution in Ireland, 1850–1875', *American Historical Review*, 77 (1972), 625–52. The degree to which the transformation in religious expression involved contending cultures of Catholicism or was led and wrought by a small group of clergy has been a matter for study and debate since. However, there is general acceptance that a transformation occurred, resulting in new and powerful institutional and devotional forms.
34. M.P. Magray, *The Transforming Power of the Nuns* (New York: OUP, 1998), 80.
35. See J.J. Ó Ríordáin, *Irish Catholics: Tradition and Transition* (Dublin: Veritas, 1980) for an attempt to situate persistent and superseded forms and traditions of pre-Famine Irish Catholic spirituality amid the growing social and political engagement of Catholic religious during and since the nineteenth century.
36. Magray, *op. cit.* (note 34), 4–5.
37. Hogan, *op. cit.* (note 31), 106–7, attributes this to 'a fear that the practice of certain medical and nursing skills could constitute a threat to chastity and consequently to vocation'.
38. *Ibid.*, 110.

39. *Ibid.*, 107–8.
40. The St Patrick's Missionary Society, founded in Ireland in 1932, had been entrusted with Catholic evangelisation in the districts of Calabar and Ogoja in Eastern Nigeria. The society is based in Kiltegan, Co. Wicklow, giving rise to the common appellation by which they are known.
41. Perhaps tellingly, between 1945 and 1950, when it was decided by the MMM that such work was incompatible with the aims of the order, three MMM sisters were in charge of the house-keeping in Kiltegan. See T. Kiggins, *Maynooth Mission to Africa: The Story of St. Patrick's, Kiltegan* (Dublin: Gill and Macmillan, 1991), 184–5 for more on this episode.
42. Ogoja Convent Files. 'Leprosy in Ogoja Province', by Joseph Barnes.
43. *Ibid.*, 2.
44. *Ibid.*, 4.
45. *Ibid.*, 5–6.
46. A. Buchanan, *Visitation: The Film Story of the Medical Missionaries of Mary* (Drogheda: Medical Missionaries of Mary, 1948) documents the production and scenario of the film, part of which was filmed in Ogoja.
47. J. McGlade, *The Missions: Africa and the Orient* (Dublin: Gill, 1967), 48.
48. Medical Missionaries of Mary, *Medical Missionaries of Mary: Covering the First Twenty Five Years of the Medical Missionaries of Mary, 1937–1962* (Dublin: Three Candles, 1962), 67.
49. From author's interview with Drs Joe and Betty Barnes, 27 March 2000.
50. 'Medical work in Ogoja Prefecture', *The Medical Missionary of Mary*, Vol. 16, 3 (March 1955), 4.
51. Z. Gussow, *Leprosy, Racism and Public Health* (Boulder: Westview, 1989), 224–5.
52. Ogoja Convent Files. Proceedings of the second meeting of the Central Leprosy Board, Enugu, 8th May, 1951, para. 5. This division of funding reflected the recommendations of the 1946 Phillipson report, *Financial Relations Between the Government of Nigeria and the Native Administrations.*
53. R. Schram, *A History of the Nigerian Health Services* (Ibadan: Ibadan University Press, 1971), 356–62.
54. S.G. Browne, *Leprosy* (Basle: Geigy, 1970), 69
55. Ogoja Convent Files. Minutes of the third meeting of the Central Leprosy Board, Lagos, 20th May, 1952. Paragraph 3 paraphrases the remarks to this effect of the new Leprosy Adviser, T.F. Davey.
56. Ogoja Convent Files. Report on Leprosy Control – Eastern Nigeria 1960. Section 1 introduces the history of leprosy control in the Eastern Region of Nigeria to 1960, and states: 'On 30/4/1954 the Government entered into an Agreement with the World Health Organisation and UNICEF for assistance in the expansion of the Programme and this most fruitful arrangement has enabled the work to proceed more effectively and in a much more extensive

way than would have otherwise been possible.'

57. Ogoja Convent Files. Proceedings of the fourth meeting of the Central Leprosy Board, Enugu, 9 November 1954, para. 3.
58. 'Report of Second International Conference on Control of Yaws: Nigeria, 1955', *The Journal of Tropical Medicine and Hygiene,* 60, 2 (February 1957), 27–38, and 3 (March 1957), 62–73.
59. Ogoja Convent Files. Proceedings of the eighth meeting of the Central Leprosy Board, Oji River, 3rd July, 1959. para. 2.4.1–2.4.3.
60. Ogoja Convent Files. Report on Leprosy Control – Eastern Nigeria 1960. Section 3.
61. Ogoja Convent Files. Letter dated 25 March 1964, from Bishop Thomas McGettrick to Bishop G. Olivotti, Auxiliary Bishop of Venice. Olivotti had sent a donation of £1,140 to Ogoja in the hope that a leprosarium could be built and named in honour of Venice. McGettrick suggested an orthopaedic Unit and appended the wish-list of the medical superintendent.
62. Ogoja Convent Files. Annual Report 1948. The Roman Catholic Leper Settlement, Ogoja. This report notes that chaulmoogral [*sic*] oil was the main from of treatment, with some experimental work taking place on Promin. Chaulmoogra oil, injected intradermally, was the treatment of choice in Nigeria between 1936 and the late-1940s in the absence of a better option, though its effectiveness was always in doubt.
63. Ogoja Convent Files. Copy of letter dated 19 February 1964, describing Ogoja leprosy work, from the Medical Superintendent.
64. *Ibid.*
65. Ogoja Convent Files. Letter dated 20th August 1962 from Medical Superintendent, Ogoja L.S. to K.S. Seal, Leprosy Adviser, Oji River.
66. See, for instance, L. Murphy, 'Where Lepers Walk: A Visit to Ogoja Leper Village', *The Medical Missionary of Mary,* 14, 2 (1953), 11–15, and L. Murphy, 'Umaji – A Leper from Ogoja Village', *The Medical Missionary of Mary,* 15, 1 (1954), 11–13.
67. Medical Missionaries of Mary, *op. cit.* (note 48), 81–93, comprising a picture essay, and a statement on missionary method which focuses on development and hopes for Africanisation almost to the exclusion of evangelical aims, demonstrates the growing centrality of medical practice in MMM consciousness of mission at this time.
68. See E.C. Amucheazi, *Church and Politics in Eastern Nigeria, 1945–1966: A Study in Pressure Group Politics* (Lagos: Macmillan, 1986), and D.B. Abernethy, *Church and State in Nigerian Education* (Ibadan: NISER, 1966) for a description of this process, arising largely from the concerns of lay educated Nigerian Catholics.
69. Royal Institute of International Affairs, *Nigeria: The Political and Economic Background* (London: Oxford University Press, 1960), 67.

70. Ogoja Convent Files. Minutes of the [fifth?] meeting of the Eastern Region Leprosy Advisory Committee [*sic*], February [1956], para. 5. 'It was agreed that the membership of the committee be extended to include one member from each Province, to be appointed by the Hon. Minister of Health on the recommendation of the Medical Officer in charge of Leprosy Control in the Province.'
71. *Ibid.*, para. 6.
72. Ogoja Convent Files. Letter from McGettrick to Sr Visitation Chambers, dated 4 October 1957.
73. Ogoja Convent Files. Minutes of the eighth meeting of the Eastern Region Leprosy Advisory Board, 3 July 1959, para. 3–3(d).
74. Ogoja Convent Files. [Ogoja Diocesan] Circular No. 136, Thomas McGettrick, Bishop of Ogoja, January 1959. A copy was issued to each Catholic priest and nun in the Diocese.
75. MMM archives – 1/Dio/8/159 – Letter from Bishop T. McGettrick to Mother Mary Martin, dated 29 January 1959.
76. Amucheazi, *op. cit.* (note 68), 36
77. Ogoja Convent Files. Typescript entitled 'A Brief History of the Medical Missionaries of Mary in Ogoja' (n.d. [1986?]), 10. Kakwagom maternity clinic was handed to the Handmaids of the Holy Child Jesus in 1956, and they built a novitiate there.
78. McGettrick, *op. cit.* (note 9), 138–9.
79. Ogoja Convent Files. Letter dated 19 March 1963, from Bishop Thomas McGettrick to Mother Mary Martin, MMM Drogheda. This letter summarises the content of Diocesan Circular no. 150.
80. *The Catholic Church in an Independent Nigeria: Joint Pastoral Letter of the Nigerian Hierarchy*, 1 October 1960, 3.

Notes on Contributors

Uoldelul Chelati Dirar is from Eritrea and now Associate Professor of African History at the University of Macerata (Italy). He gained his Doctorate in African History from the University of Bologna (Italy). He works on the history of Eritrea during the colonial period. After having studied the role of European missions in colonial Eritrea, his research interests are now shifting to the study of colonial troops (*ascari*) and their impact on social and political identities.

David Hardiman is Professor of History at the University of Warwick. He carried out his doctoral research on modern Indian history at the University of Sussex, the thesis being published as *Peasant Nationalists of Gujarat: Kheda District 1917–1934* (New Delhi: Oxford University Press, 1981). He worked for many years in India at the Centre for Social Studies, Surat, and is the author of *The Coming of the Devi: Adivasi Assertion in Western India* (New Delhi: Oxford University Press, 1987), *Feeding the Baniya: Peasants and Usurers in Western India* (New Delhi: Oxford University Press, 1996), *Gandhi in His Time and Ours* (New Delhi: Permanent Black, 2003), and *Histories for the Subordinated* (New Delhi: Permanent Black, 2006). He is a founder member of the Subaltern Studies group, and has published several articles in *Subaltern Studies*, and edited one of the volumes.

Michael Jennings is a Lecturer in African History and International Development at the Centre for Development Studies, Swansea University. His research focuses on the history of social development (including health and medicine) in East Africa. He has written on popular participation and development in early post-colonial Tanzania, the history of non-governmental organisations in East Africa, as well as on the history of development in the twentieth century more widely. He has also written on Chinese medicine in contemporary Dar es Salaam, and regularly writes briefing documents on a range of current health issues in sub-Saharan Africa.

Linda Beer Kumwenda works at the National Archives, Kew, dealing mainly with the records of the Ministry of Defence. She qualified as a Registered General Nurse in 1988. After working as a ward manager at a medical mission in the North Western Province of Zambia, she gained both a BA and PhD from the School of Oriental and African Studies. Her doctoral thesis, titled 'Healing, Conflict and Conversion: Medical Missions in Northern Rhodesia, 1880s–1954' (2005), examined three missions widely spaced along the spectrum of Protestantism.

Michael C. Lazich is an Associate Professor of History at Buffalo State College. He gained his PhD in the field of Chinese history from the State University of New York. His research and publications have focused primarily on nineteenth-century Sino–American cultural and political relations. In his book, *E.C. Bridgman (1801–1861): America's First Missionary to China* (Lewiston, NY: Edwin Mellen Press, 2000), he examines the role of E.C. Bridgman as a pioneering scholar and cultural intermediary.

John Manton is a post-doctoral research fellow at the Wellcome Unit for the History of Medicine at the University of Oxford, UK. He gained his D.Phil at Nuffield College, Oxford, on a history of medical missions in mid-twentieth-century Nigeria. His current research is in missionary-run leprosy control schemes in relation to the broader context of development, resource control, and decolonisation in Nigeria.

James H. Mills is Director of the Centre for the Social History of Health and Healthcare Glasgow, a research collaboration between the University of Strathclyde and Glasgow Caledonian University. His publications include *Madness, Cannabis and Colonialism: The 'Native Only' Lunatic Asylums of British India, 1857 to 1900* (Basingstoke: Palgrave, 2000), and *Cannabis Britannica: A Social and Political History of Cannabis and British Government, 1800-1928* (Oxford: Oxford University Press, 2003). He is currently Reviews Editor of the *Social History of Medicine.*

Shobana Shankar is Assistant Professor of African History at Lafayette College. Her research focuses on Hausa-speaking communities of Northern Nigeria, and she is currently completing a book-length study of the material and moral dimensions of childhood in Muslim experiences of British colonialism. Her article about leprosy missions and the transformation of Muslim native authority will appear in *Journal of African History.* She has also published on women and health in Islamic

Africa, religious politics in pre-colonial Hausa narrative, and the creation of religious boundaries in British Northern Nigeria.

John R. Stanley teaches at the Kutztown University of Pennsylvania. He gained his PhD in history from the School of Oriental and African Studies in 2003 for a thesis titled 'New Perspectives on the Early China Mission Enterprise: A Study of the Weixian Station's Educational and Medical Enterprise, 1883–1920.'

Timothy Man-kong Wong is an Associate Professor of History at Hong Kong Baptist University. He gained his PhD from the Chinese University of Hong Kong, and is a specialist in the history of Christianity in China, and the history of Hong Kong. He is the author of *James Legge: A Pioneer at Crossroads of East and West* (Hong Kong: Hong Kong Educational Publishing Company, 1996), co-editor of *Wang Tao and the Modern World* [in Chinese] (Hong Kong: Hong Kong Educational Publishing Company, 2000), and co-author of *Centenary History of the Chinese General Chamber of Commerce, Hong Kong* [in Chinese] (Hong Kong: Commercial Press (HK) Ltd., 2002) and *Cross-cultural Perspectives on the History of Christianity in Modern China* [in Chinese] (Taipei: Cosmic Light, 2006).

Index

L

M

T

U

V

W

www.ingramcontent.com/pod-product-compliance
Lightning Source LLC
Chambersburg PA
CBHW071409230926
51613CB00015B/23
9789042021068